PSYCHIATRY – THEORY, APPLICATIONS AND TREATMENTS

ANTIPSYCHOTIC DRUGS

PHARMACOLOGY, SIDE EFFECTS AND ABUSE PREVENTION

PSYCHIATRY – THEORY, APPLICATIONS AND TREATMENTS

Additional books in this series can be found on Nova's website under the Series tab.

Additional E-books in this series can be found on Nova's website under the E-book tab.

PSYCHIATRY – THEORY, APPLICATIONS AND TREATMENTS

ANTIPSYCHOTIC DRUGS

PHARMACOLOGY, SIDE EFFECTS AND ABUSE PREVENTION

THOMAS L. SCHWARTZ
JAMES MEGNA
AND
MICHAEL E. TOPEL
EDITORS

NOVA BIOMEDICAL

New York

For permission to use material from this book please contact us:
Telephone 631-231-7269; Fax 631-231-8175
Web Site: http://www.novapublishers.com

Library of Congress Cataloging-in-Publication Data

ISBN 978-1-62100-071-6

Library of Congress Control Number: 2012941953

Published by Nova Science Publishers, Inc. † New York

CONTENTS

ACKNOWLEDGMENT

Drs. Schwartz and Megna would like to acknowledge the hard work, long hours and indomitable spirit of supervisor, mentor, elite chairman, and gentleman, Dr. Mantosh Dewan. In addition, Ms. Diane Deluca and Dr. Umar Siddiqui should be commended for their help in preparing this book for publication.

Mr. Topel would like to acknowledge the steadfast support and careful guidance provided by his mentors, Drs. John Zajecka and Corey Goldstein, who model intelligent, compassionate care for patients; and his lovely wife, Lauren, whose gently taking all those extra hours of his household duties made his participation possible.

Thomas L. Schwartz, M.D.
Associate Professor, Department of Psychiatry,
SUNY Upstate Medical University, Syracuse, NY, US

James L. Megna, M.D.
Associate Professor, Department of Psychiatry,
SUNY Upstate Medical University, Syracuse, NY, US

Michael E. Topel, M.A.,
Research Coordinator, Department of Psychiatry,
Rush University, Chicago, IL, US

PART I: HISTORY

In: Antipsychotic Drugs
Editors: T.L. Schwartz, J. Megna and M.E. Topel
ISBN: 978-1-62100-071-6

Chapter 1

ANTIPSYCHOTICS: WHERE HAVE WE BEEN? WHERE ARE WE NOW? WHERE ARE WE GOING?

Lewis A. Opler[1*] and Mark G. Opler[2]
[1]Professor of Clinical Psychiatry, Columbia University Medical Center, Adjunct Professor of Psychiatry, NYU School of Medicine, Mount Vernon, NY, US
[2]Assistant Professor, Psychiatry and Environmental Medicine, New York University School of Medicine, New York, NY, US

WHERE HAVE WE BEEN?

Prior to 1952, psychiatrists used medication to control dangerous behavior. Among the agents used were morphine, potassium bromide, chloral hydrate, and barbiturates [1, 2]. The use of barbiturates peaked in the 1930s and 1940s but declined throughout the 1950s after neuroleptics, starting with chlorpromazine, were found not only to have sedative properties but also to treat hallucinations and delusions [3].

The landmark discovery that chlorpromazine was an antipsychotic was serendipitous. A French surgeon, Henri Laborit, was combining medications given before anaesthesia with the goal of decreasing post surgical shock; theorizing that inclusion of an antihistamine would be beneficial, Laborit first included the sedating antihistamine promethazine and subsequently chlorpromazine in what was referred to as a "lytic cocktail." Laborit et al. [4] reported that the inclusion of chlorpromazine was important in stabilizing the autonomic nervous system. But Laborit was particularly impressed by the calmness induced by chlorpromazine. Laborit convinced three psychiatrists at Val de Grace military hospital in Paris to try chlorpromazine in one of their patients, and Hamon et al. [5] reported that, in addition to rapid calming, after 20 days of treatment, the patient was able to "resume normal life."

Pierre Deniker and Jean Delay, psychiatrists at Saint-Anne's Hospital in Paris, subsequently conducted a clinical trial in the hopes that chlorpromazine would be an effective and safe sedative. Like Hamon and colleagues, they reported beneficial effects beyond

* Corresponding author: Lewis A. Opler. Professor of Clinical Psychiatry, Columbia University Medical Center Adjunct Professor of Psychiatry, NYU School of Medicine 765 Gramatan Avenue, Mount Vernon, NY 10552. E-mail: laop1@juno.com.

sedation and published their findings in 1952, reporting that chlorpromazine was an antipsychotic. Psychiatrists world-wide began using chlorpromazine. In psychoanalytically dominated North America, an article by Lehmann and Hanrahan [6] gave credibility to the novel idea that a medication could not just sedate but actually improve psychosis.

As described elsewhere [7,3] both applied chemistry and the new science of behavioral pharmacology lead to a number of standard neuroleptics being developed and marketed from the late 1950s through 1975. First, by making alterations in the side chains, other phenothiazines were synthesized. Chlorpromazine is an aliphatic phenothiazine; thioridazine is a piperidine phenothiazine; and trifluperazine, fluphenazine, and perphenazine are piperazine phenothiazines. By making a minor modification in the phenothiazine ring structure itself, a new class of neuroleptics, the thioxanthenes, was synthesized, and thiothixene became widely used. Behavioral preclinical tests predicting antipsychotic efficacy had emerged, including induction of catalepsy and reversal of conditioned avoidance. Paul Janssen was not looking for a new antipsychotic when he synthesized the butyrophenone haloperidol, but when he found that it caused both catalepsy and reversal of conditioned avoidance, he quickly moved haloperidol into clinical trials, and for many years haloperidol was the most widely used neuroleptic.

Janssen also synthesized the diphenylbutylpiperidine pimozide, approved as an antipsychotic in many European and South American countries. In the United States, pimozide is approved only for Tourette's Disorder but not for psychosis, which Opler and Feinberg [8] have argued is unfortunate given some unique features such as the treatment of delusional disorder and negative symptoms.

The dibenzoxazepine loxapine was also found to be a neuroleptic antipsychotic. Another dibenzoxazepine, clozapine, was the the first atypical antipsychotic, treating psychotic symptoms while causing little or no motor side effects. Neuroleptics by definition cause motor side effects, including early extrapyramidal side effects (EPS) as well as the later choreoathetoid movement disorder tardive dyskinesia (TD), and until the 1970s some assumed that motor side effects and antipsychotic efficacy were inseparable.

Serendipitously, clozapine was derived from the tricyclic antidepressant imipramine, but when it was found to reverse conditioned avoidance in rats, although it did not induce catalepsy, it was entered into clinical trials as an antipsychotic rather than as an antidepressant. Clozapine caused little or no EPS. Clozapine did not cause TD and in some cases where TD was present clozapine actually ameliorated preexisting TD. Additionally, as reported anecdotally and later demonstrated in a randomized double-blind trial [9], clozapine treated psychosis as measured by improvement in the Brief Psychiatric Rating Scale (BPRS) in patients who had failed to respond to several neuroleptic antipsychotics. Clozapine was called an atypical antipsychotic to distinguish it from the neuroleptics. Unfortunately and unexpectedly, it was found that clozapine causes agranulocytosis in approximately 1% of patients, which slowed down its approval in several countries, including the US. Therefore, the clinical trials reported in the landmark study by Kane et al. were important in leading to clozapine's approval in the United States and several other countries as a second line treatment.

Clozapine demonstrated that psychosis could be treated without causing motor side effects, and several pharmaceutical companies started developing compounds in the hopes that they would find other clozapine-like atypical antipsychotics with a better side effect profile.

Where Are We Now

As new atypical antipsychotics were introduced, beginning with risperidone in 1994, olanzapine in 1996, and quetiapine in 1997, they started replacing standard neuroleptics as first line treatment for psychosis. The atypical antipsychotics are still viewed as first line treatment, although two large, non-commercial clinical trials unexpectedly had findings questioning the superiority of all of the atypical antipsychotics, with the noteworthy exception of clozapine, over the older standard neuroleptics [10]. The following comprise the presently available atypical antipsychotics, with more in the pipeline: clozapine, risperidone, olanzapine, quetiapine, aripiprazole, asenapine, iloperidone, and lurasidone.

Clozapine remains the gold standard but is underutilized for several reasons, the main one being concern that it can cause agranulocytosis in approximately 1% of patients. While this is a serious side effect, it can be treated effectively when it occurs. Another rare but serious side effect, myocarditis, is not well understood and there is at present no antidote or treatment.

Given the limitations of the atypical antipsychotics, gaining a better understanding of what it is about clozapine that makes it the gold standard remains a high priority. Unlike the neuroleptics, clozapine blocks 5-HT2 or S2 receptors as well as D2 dopamine receptors.. This additional pharmacologic activity was the basis for development and marketing of most of the atypical antipsychotics –a noteworthy exception is aripiprazole which is unique in being a partial dopamine agonist. But since none of these other atypical antipsychotics is as good as clozapine, the search goes on to determine exactly what makes clozapine different. One compelling idea is that clozapine facilitates glutamate transmission in a subset of channels gated by NMDA-glutamate receptors, as will be discussed below.

Where Are We Going

Several plausible hypotheses exist regarding the etiology of schizophrenia and other psychotic disorders. For example, ten years ago we [11] presented evidence of abnormal phospholipid metabolism in schizophrenia and still believe this is a promising avenue for treatment and research. However, rather than provide a comprehensive inventory of all of the possible findings that may lead to the next generation of antipsychotics, we will instead focus on what we see as the most promising approach: correcting glutamate hypofunction.

The clinical observations that would later lead to the glutamate hypofunction hypothesis of schizophrenia were made 50 years ago by Luby and colleagues [12, 13] who proposed that phencyclidine (PCP) caused a transient psychosis in normal volunteers more like schizophrenia than that caused by lysergic acid diethylamide. At the time, the mechanism of action of PCP was not known. Work by Javitt and colleagues [14, 15] demonstrated that PCP binding blocked the influx of calcium through excitatory channels gated by NMDA-glutamate receptors (NMDARs). Subsequently, Javitt and Zukin [16] proposed that phencylidine psychosis, by creating hypoglutamatergia, caused a psychosis more like schizophrenia than that caused by amphetamine. Specifically, in addition to positive symptoms, PCP psychosis is characterized by negative and cognitive symptoms as well.

If PCP psychosis is a more schizophrenia-like "model psychosis" than both LSD and amphetamine psychosis, then perhaps decreased transmission through NMDARs , in addition to being the mechanism of action of PCP, explains at least in part the neurobiological basis of schizophrenia. There are two allosteric sites in the NMDAR. One, the redox site, binds glutathione, while the other binds glycine and D-serine, both released into the synapse by adjacent astrocytes. Exciting work has shown that adding glycine [17,18], the glycine transport inhibitor sarcosine [19], and D-serine [20] to antipsychotic medications results in decreased symptom severity. The search for medications that facilitate NMDAR function is evidenced by Eli Lilly and Company's clinical trials of LY-2140023 in patients with schizophrenia. LY-2140023 is a prodrug that becomes a glutamate receptor agonist and preliminary reports suggest efficacy without motor and metabolic side effects [21].

Adding N-acetylcysteine, a precursor of glutathione, to maintenance antipsychotic regimens has been shown to decrease symptom severity [22] and auditory sensory processing abnormalities [23] in patients with schizophrenia.

Using what appears to be a different strategy, Pfizer has launched phase 2 clinical trials of phosphodiesterase 10A inhibitors [24].

We hypothesize that PDE10A inhibitors act on astrocytes to promote NMDAR transmission for several reasons. First, PDE10A is potently blocked by papaverine, and one of us (LAO) showed forty years ago that papaverine had robust effects on cyclic AMP levels in cultured astrocytoma cells [25]. Astrocytes were originally named neuroglia by Virchow [26], which literally means neural "glue," reflecting the view that they were inert elements present only to hold neurons in place. In the subsequent years, it has become clear that astrocytes are more than "neural cement" [27]. Solomon's group has made it clear that astrocytes are playing a key role in the functioning of NMDA-glutamate neurotransmission [28]: the astrocytes contain the enzyme serine racemase, which converts L-serine into D-serine, and D-serine occupies the "glycine" allosteric site. Astrocytes also contain D-amino acid oxidase (D-AAO), an enzyme originally identified by Krebs who was appropriately puzzled because a role for D-amino acids in humans who ingest L-amino acids had not been described, which is involved in the degradation of D-serine. The astrocytes are also the source of glycine, as well as the place where glycine is delivered by glycine transport inhibitors where it too is degraded by oxidation. Too few or dysfunctional astrocytes would disrupt NMDA-glutamate transmission because not enough D-serine or glycine would be available. We hypothesize that PDE10A inhibitors, by increasing cycling AMP levels and resulting glycogenolysis in astrocytes, "turn on" astrocytes improving their efficiency, thereby partially ameliorating compromised NMDA-glutamate neurotransmission.

We believe the glutamate hypofunction hypothesis will lead to the next generation of antipsychotics, agents that have better efficacy and fewer side effects than existing neuroleptics and atypical antipsychotics.

However, despite their drawbacks, antipsychotics have transformed our thinking and our treatment of schizophrenia and other psychotic disorders, helping to move persons with psychotic disorders out of long-term care facilities while allowing remission and recovery for many. The brain is complex and yields its secrets slowly: we stand on the shoulders of Laborit, Delay, Deniker, Janssen, and others as we anticipate the next generation of antipsychotics.

REFERENCES

[1] Ban, T. A. Pharmacotherapy of mental illness—a historical analysis. *Prog. Neuropsychopharmacol. Biol. Psychiatry* 2001;25:709-727.

[2] López-Muñoz, F., Ucha-Udabe, R., Alamo, C. The history of barbiturates a century after their clinical introduction. *Neuropsychiatr. Dis. Treat.* 2005;1:329-343.

[3] Healy, D. *The Creation of Psychopharmacology*, Harvard University Press:Cambridge, MA, 2002.

[4] Laborit, H., Huguenard, P., Alluaume, R. Un noveau stabilisater vegetatif (le 4560 RP). *La Presse Medicale.* 1952;60:206-208.

[5] Hamon, J., Paraire, J., Velluz, J. Remarques sure l'action due 4560 RP sure l'agitation maniaque. *Annales Medico-psychologiques* (Paris) 1952:110:331-335.

[6] Lehmann, H. E., Hanrahan, G. E. Chlorpromazine, new inhibiting agent for psychomotor excitement and manic states. *Archives of Neurology and Psychiatry* 1954;71:227-237.

[7] Opler, L. A. Schizophrenia and other psychotic disorders. In: Feinstein, R. E., Brewer, A. A. (eds.) Primary Care Psychiatry and Behavioral Medicine: Brief Office Treatment and Management Pathways. New York, NY, Springer-Verlag, 1999

[8] Opler, L. A., Feinberg, S. S. The role of pimozide in clinical psychiatry: a review. *J. Clin. Psychiatry* 1991;52:221-233.

[9] Kane, J., Honigfeld, F., Singer, J., Meltzer, H. Clozapine for the treatment-resistant schizophrenia. A double-blind comparison with chlorpromazine. *Archives of General Psychiatry* 1988;45:789-796.

[10] Lewis, S., Lieberman, J. CATIE and CUtLASS:can we handle the truth? *Br. J. Psychiatry.* 2008;192:161-163.

[11] Opler, M. G., Opler, L. A. Abnormal phospholipid metabolism in schizophrenia: evidence from epidemiological findings, clinical observations, and preliminary clinical trials. *Front Biosci.* 2001;6:E61-65.

[12] Luby, E. D., Gottlieb, J. S., Cohen, B. D., Rosenbaum, G., Domino, E. F. Model pychoses and schizophrenia. *Am. J. Psychiatry* 1962;119:61-67

[13] Domino, E. F., Luby, E. D. Phencyclidine/schizophrenia: one view toward the past, the other to the future. *Schizophrenia Bulletin* 2012.In press.

[14] Javitt, D. C., Jotkowitz, A., Sircar, R., Zukin, S. R. Non-competetive regulation of phencyclidine/sigma-receptors by the N-methyl-D-aspartate receptor antagonist D-(-)-2-amino-5-phosphonovaleric acid. *Neurosci. Lett.* 1987;78:193-198.

[15] Javitt, D. C., Zukin, S. R. Interaction of [3H]MK-801 with multiple states of the N-methyl-D-aspartate receptor complex of rat brain. *PNASdg US* 1989;86:740-744.

[16] Javitt, D. C., Zukin, S. R. Recent advances in the phencyclidine model of schizophrenia. *Am. J. Psychiatry* 1991; 148:1301-1308.

[17] Heresco-Levy, U., Javitt, D. C., Ermilov, M., Mordel, C., Silipo, G., Lichtenstein, M. Efficacy of high-dose glycine in the treatment of enduring negative symptoms of schizophrenia. *Arch. Gen. Psychiatry* 1999;56:29-36.

[18] Heresco-Levy, U., Ermilov, M., Lichtenberg, P., Bar, G., Javitt, D. C. High-dose glycine added to olanzapine and risperidone for the treatment of schizophrenia. *Biological Psychiatry* 2004;55:165-171.

[19] Tsai, G., Lane, H. Y., Yang, P., Chong, M. Y., Lange, N. Glycine transporter I inhibitor, n-methylglycine (sarcosine), added to antipsychotics for the treatment of schizophrenia. *Biological Psychiatry* 2004; 55:452-456.

[20] Heresco-Levy, U., Javitt, D. C., Ebstein, R., Vass, A., Lichtenberg, P., Bar, G., et.al. D-Serine efficacy as add-on pharmacotherapy to risperidone and olanzapine for treatment refractory schizophrenia. *Biological Psychiatry* 2005;57:577-585.

[21] Mezler, M., Geneste, H., Gault, L., Marek, G. J. LY-2140023, a prodrug of the group II metabotropic glutamate receptor agonist LY-404039 for the potential treatment of schizophrenia. *Curr. Opin. Investig. Drugs* 2010;11:833-845.

[22] Berk, M., Copolov, D., Dean, O., Lu, K., Jeavons, S., Schapkaitz, I., et.al. N-acetyl cysteine as a glutathione precursor for schizophrenia-a double-blind, randomized, placebo-controlled trial. *Biol. Psychiatry* 2008;64:361-8.

[23] Lavoie, S., Murray, M. M., Deppen, P.,_Knyazeva, M. G., Berk, M., Boulat, O., et al. Glutathione precursor, n-acetyl-cysteine, improves mismatch negativity in schizophrenia patients. *Neuropsychopharmacology* 2008;33:2187–2199.

[24] Kehler, J., Nielsen, J. PDE10A inhibitors: novel therapeutic drugs for schizophrenia. *Curr. Pharm. Des.* 2011;17:137-150.

[25] Opler, L. A., Makman, M. H. Mediation by cyclic AMP of hormone-stimulated glycogenolysis in cultured rat astrocytoma cells. *Biochemical and Biophysical Research Communications* 1972, 46:1140-1152.

[26] Virchow, R. *Cellularpathologie*. Hirschwald, Berlin, 1859.

[27] Fields, R. D., Stevens-Graham, B. New insights into neuron-glia communication. *Science* 2002;298:556-562.

[28] Wolosker, H., Blackshaw, S., Snyder, S. H. Serine racemase: a glial enzyme synthesizing D-serine to regulate glutame-N-methyl-D-aspartate neurotransmission. *PNAS* 1999;96:13409-13414.

In: Antipsychotic Drugs
Editors: T.L. Schwartz, J. Megna and M.E. Topel
ISBN: 978-1-62100-071-6

Chapter 2

SECOND GENERATION ANTIPSYCHOTIC MEDICATIONS IN THE TREATMENT OF AFFECTIVE DISORDERS

***Corey N. Goldstein*[1], *Michael E. Topel*[2*] *and John M. Zajecka*[3]**
[1]Medical Director, Women's Board Treatment Research Center, Rush University Medical Center, Chicago, IL, US
[2] Research Coordinator, Department of Psychiatry, Rush University Medical Center, Chicago, IL, US
[3] Director, Women's Board Treatment Research Unit, Associate Professor of Psychiatry, Rush University Medical Center, Chicago, IL, US

ABSTRACT

Introduction: A body of evidence supporting the use of second generation antipsychotics (SGAs) in treatment resistant affective disorders has been accrued in recent years [1] and these medications are now widely prescribed for psychiatric disorders outside of the schizophrenia spectrum. SGAs are thought to affect monoamine transmitters among other neurobiological systems that are hypothesized to play a role in the pathophysiology and treatment of affective disorders [2,3,4].

Conclusion: In the search conducted for this chapter aripiprazole, olanzapine, quetiapine produced a number of positive randomized, controlled trial (RCT) findings. For risperidone, outcomes in located trials were mixed. Medline searches for clozapine, asenapine, paliperidone and ziprasidone did not produce reported RCTs. Aripiprazole, olanzapine and quetiapine have FDA-approval for adjunctive use in MDD. Most SGAs have been approved for acute mania, some for mixed mania; Seroquel XR, and the combination of olanzapine and fluoxetine for bipolar depression. No SGA currently has the indication for mood disorder monotherapy. The articles for this review were located via Medline search of dates up through November of 2011; search terms included "second generation antipsychotic," "atypical antipsychotic," "major depressive disorder," "treatment resistant depression," "dysthymia" and "bipolar disorder."

* Corresponding author E-mail: michael_e_topel@rush.edu.

Introduction

Affective disorders, including bipolar disorder and unipolar depression, remain among the most prevalent illnesses responsible for significant worldwide disability. Despite availability of a growing number of effective treatments, both bipolar disorder and major depressive disorder continue to have significant morbidity and mortality, especially if not adequately treated.

Similarly to other chronic medical illnesses, the evidence supports the importance of achieving and sustaining full symptomatic remission during all phases of the illness. Failure to achieve or sustain remission remains among the most common reasons for the lack of successful treatment outcome, and may contribute to developing greater resistance to treatment with each level of intervention that fails to achieve a full remission.

In recent years there has been more emphasis on early introduction of pharmaceutical agents that provide broad pharmacological action (either as mono- or combination therapy) to achieve remission and increase the chances for full recovery. Development of the second generation antipsychotics provided an option over conventional antipsychotic medications for the management of schizophrenia and psychotic symptoms associated with other illnesses, including affective disorders. Utilization of the various SGAs continued to be studied as options for the management of acute mania and mixed states (as mono- and combination therapies, and in combination with lithium and divalproex), bipolar maintenance treatment, bipolar depression and eventually as adjunctive treatment in various levels of treatment resistance in unipolar depression.

As a class of medications, the SGAs have provided an alternative to conventional antipsychotics for schizophrenia. However, each SGA a unique pharmacological profile that contributes to differences in safety/tolerability profiles and possibly to particular efficacy in the management of the different phases of affective disorders. Further, specific SGAs as well as specific SGA doses have been shown to have greater or lesser efficacy in different diagnostic types and subtypes, and illness phases.

SGAs offer a valuable addition to treatment option arrays in the management of affective disorders. Clinicians are advised to be informed of empirical evidence of dose, safety and tolerability of SGAs for the management of affective disorders at various levels of treatment, initial through more treatment resistant.

Treatment-Resistant Depression

While there may be a lack of consensus in defining precisely the criteria for an "incomplete response" to antidepressant therapy (ADT) (e.g., "treatment refractory," "treatment-resistant," "non-responders," "difficult to treat," or "incomplete responders"), it is widely recognized that many patients do not achieve a complete response (remission), and up to 10% of all depressed patients receiving treatment fail treatment completely [5]. "Treatment resistance," for our purpose, is defined as the failure of at least one adequate trial of an antidepressant medication [6].

We note that the associated public health burden referenced above is derived from all patients with continued symptoms, and this includes those conventionally termed "responders" yet who have not achieved a true remission. Importantly, residual symptoms are associated with an increased risk of relapse [7; 8] impaired social and occupational functioning [9, 10, 11], and, obviously, chronicity [12]. Based on these findings, achieving sustained remission is the commonly accepted "gold-standard" of therapeutic goals [13, 14].

Again, in spite of the continuing swell in both the number and diversity of pharmaceutical medications with antidepressant mechanisms [15] accumulating data indicates that many patients suffering from major depression have persistent symptoms in spite of treatment efforts. To wit, Corey-Lisle et al (2004) reported that "approximately 22% of patients receiving treatment for depression by their primary-care physicians remitted following six months of treatment" [16].

Similarly, Rush et al. (2004) reported only an "11% remission rate among depressed outpatients" following 12 months of ADT in "one of several public-sector community clinics" [17]. In the course of the Sequenced Treatment Alternatives to Relieve Depression(STAR*D) study, Trivedi et al. (2006) followed nearly 3,000 outpatients with MDD who had been prescribed open-label citalopram [18]. The authors reported remission rates of 28-33%. Petersen et al (2005) studied outpatients with MDD enrolled in "one of two hospital-based, academically-affiliated depression specialty clinics" and reported a 20.5-30.7% remission rate among patients receiving a single treatment [19].

Even among patients achieving remission residual symptoms are common [20]. Lingering symptoms are associated with reduced adaptive psychosocial functioning [21], and increased risk of [10] or accelerated [9, 12] relapse rates. The side-effect burden of many ADs is high. Common AD and atypical antipsychotic medication side effects include weight gain, metabolic syndrome, extra-pyramidal symptoms, sexual dysfunction and somnolence (ibid), and it is an obvious consequence that high side-effect burden results in low medication compliance.

Similar to any other medical illness, depression should be treated to full remission, which describes a symptom-free recovery. Remission has now become the standard of care for treating individuals with major depressive disorder (MDD), and should be the goal of treatment. This includes both the patient who responds partially in the first episode, and the patient who may have failed to respond to multiple treatments.

Unfortunately, up to 50% of patients who "respond" to their antidepressant treatment fail to fully "remit" [20]. Data from long-term clinical trials of antidepressant response have estimated that approximately two thirds of patients fail to achieve a full remission [22]. More recent findings from the National Institute of Mental Health's Sequenced Treatment Alternatives to Relieve Depression (STAR*D), suggest that in a community sample of patients with depression, approximately 40% of patients failed to "respond" to an adequate trial of a selective serotonin reuptake inhibitor (SSRI) and over 65% failed to achieve remission [18]. This study went on to show that, even when patients were given a chance to switch antidepressants or augment their treatment to a set sequence of treatment alternatives, they achieved only modest improvement of response or remission and, further, showed high rates of residual symptoms [23; 18]. Furthermore, acute and long-term studies show that high rates of "residual symptoms" remain, or persist, even after treatment of a depressive episode [20; 24]; these residual emotional or physical symptoms of depression significantly increase the risk of relapse and recurrence [10].

In addition to increased risk of relapse and recurrence, there are several other possible consequences of failing to achieve remission, including continued psychosocial impairments, increased use of medical services, potentially worsened prognosis of any comorbid medical/psychiatric illnesses, ongoing risk of suicide and at least the theoretical possibility of the patient becoming "treatment resistant" [25; 26].

FUNDAMENTALS

Major depressive disorder (MDD) as an example of a psychiatric disorder which has a wealth of treatment options available with varying amounts of evidence base to support their use. Broadly, the FDA considers all antidepressants to be equally efficacious as regulatory studies generally show similar effect sizes but differing levels of tolerability. Practicing clinicians know that each antidepressant possesses certain clinical attributes which may help one patient better than the next.

Ideally, psychopharmacologic treatment for MDD uses a broad-spectrum approach. It is key to optimize effect on all potential biological systems early in treatment. This includes consideration of trimonoamine modulation (5HT, NE, DA); selective serotonin increase and the compensatory decrease of NE and DA resulting in fatigue, amotivation, blunted affect, cognitive impairment, sexual side effects, or “tachyphylaxis.” We suggest the early use broad-spectrum AD, and, if response is inadequate, augmentation over switching. Consider possible role of folate-related dysfunction on 5HT, NE, DA (from genetic polymorphism, illness, medication). Consider other neurotransmitter/modulator dysfunction (glutamate, GABA, HPA axis). Finally, consider psychotherapeutic interventions [27].

In order to achieve/maximize remission and prevent TRD, it is essential to confirm diagnoses (new medical/psychiatric, iatrogenic, SUDs?). We place a strong emphasis on education and adherence; the patient should expect remission. The course of the illness may change over time. We ask about and document new or residual “target symptoms,” and consider augmentation or combination pharmacotherapy, potentially combined with psychotherapy.

We also utilize second opinions or consultations. If the response continues to be inadequate, we may switch to another AD treatment with a different mechanism of action (consider “bridging” treatments). We suggest relying on the evidence base, and extant data for informing treatment decision, and tailoring the treatment to the individual over time [28].

It is important to know and follow the evidence-based literature outside of regulatory studies and approvals especially when using off-label or more esoteric combination therapies. When these two rules have sparse support, a clinician should fall back on theoretical applications of known psychotropics based on the particular drug's mechanism of action [29]. For example, understanding that MDD may evolve from a deficiency in available monoamine neurotransmitters, an excess of their receptors, or poor communication from one neuroanatomical area and another, clinicians may elect drugs intended to alter these abnormalities to raise neurotransmitter levels, downregulate receptors, etc. This means that psychopharmacologists must know FDA approvals, be generally aware of the current literature, and understand how each antidepressant works in the brain and how manipulating certain transmitters and receptors may improve target psychiatric symptoms. This approach should provide a high standard of care, which is medico-legally safe, and advanced level of psychopharmacological practice.

AUGMENTATION AND COMBINATION

Augmentation or combination treatment as a treatment strategy, suggested by some authors as preferable to monotherapy as an initial treatment plan is increasingly supported in the literature and in clinical practice. These treatment strategies may increase symptom relief, treatment compliance, and ease side-effect burden [30]. Potential alternative medication strategies in difficult cases include the use of lithium, tricyclic medications, buspirone, combining medications and switching [31]. STAR*D has shown that augmenting early, rather than waiting for treatment failure, increases the likelihood of remission and decreases the chances of relapse (ibid).

Prompt treatment, especially in the index episode predicts a more robust response. Conversely, delaying augmentation in patients showing resistance to monotherapy has been shown to correlate negatively with complete remission and positively with increased chance of relapse, even if complete remission is achieved [32]. There is, however, a lack of consensus among psychiatrists as to what comprises proper, evidence-based treatment for patients with incomplete response, and this is due largely to insufficient data from rigorous studies. Due to the challenge MDD poses to both clinicians and the patients they treat, and, due to the cost to society itself, creating new, effective treatment strategies for MDD is needed urgently to further elevate the standard of care for depression [33].

Switching medications has been shown to be effective treatment strategy in refractory depression, as is augmentation, although, obviously, the quality of patient response to the selected initial medication tends to predict which of the two second-line treatment approaches will be more effective. That said, generally, patients who initially show an incomplete response have shown better improvement with augmentation than that seen with switching [32].

DOCUMENTATION DURING THE MANAGEMENT OF COMBINATION STRATEGIES

For those willing to delve into and provide complex polypharmacy, more energy must go into documenting this decision process in the medical record. It is important for clinicians to keep written records of past and current treatment trials (including doses, duration of each dose, tolerability and efficacy) available at all times. Our group finds it helpful for patients to use some form of life charting technique to ascertain the level of subjective and objective improvement that the patient experiences, as well as to serve as an additional tool to show patterns of response, adherence and other potential factors that may impact outcome (e.g., menstrual cycle, substance use and other factors). It is important to obtain verbal informed consent before all interventions, especially when using combination strategies that are not Food and Drug Administration (FDA) approved (i.e., "off-label"). This informed consent should describe the risk and benefit to the patient, explaining in detail the non-approved status of these combinations and their side -effects. It is important to invite the patient to ask questions, and to involve the patient's significant others whenever possible.

When there is an absence of findings in the literature, clinicians may rely on theoretical ideas of pharmacodynamics, central nervous system physiology, and clinical utility, which suggest that certain deficiencies in specific neurotransmitter systems or receptors may be the underlying, cause of specific depressive symptoms. For example, a MDD patient who remains fatigued and unable to concentrate may preferentially benefit from the use of a drug that enhances noradrenergic activity. Medical records should note a lack of data from the literature and also note the scientific thinking behind the choice of medication(s) used.

We now conclude this brief overview of some principles of complex polypharmacy; the authors will next provide a review regarding the evidence-base for polpypharmacological medication management of MDD. The concept again suggests that clinicians will likely not find a cure-all monotherapy for all of depression (or any other primary psychiatric disorder) and that clinicians' effective practice will likely benefit from an embrace of the use of polypharmacy strategies to gain the targeted "full remission" goal for a majority of their patients.

Atypical Antipsychotic Medications As Augmentation

Use of antipsychotic medications for the treatment of mood symptoms was initially discouraged by the presence of extrapyramidal side effects, but the appearance of second generation atypicals, with reduced side effect profiles, re-opened consideration of the use of antipsychotic agents for mood symptoms. The first reported use of an atypical was by Ostroff and Nelson [34] wherein the authors augmented SSRIs with risperidone in eight non-responsive depressed patients.

The FDA has approved only 2 medications and 1 medicinal food for adjunctive use with ADs inpatients failing to show adequate response to AD monotherapy: quetiapine, aripiprazole and L-methylfolate (ibid). (Note: Symbyax, a combination of fluoxetine and olanzapine, has very recently received approval for treatment resistant depression). This governmental approval is consistent with the findings of the STAR*D study. Significantly, STAR*D references for augmentation, however, did not include antipsychotics, supplements, or stimulant medications. Primarily, data that does exist for stimulant use in treatment of depression supports it as an augmentation rather than as monotherapy [35]. Of these additional approved medications, aripiprazole has been found to be effective in increasing interest and motivation as well as enthusiasm. Aripiprazole does, however, carry a side-effect burden. In a recent acute study of aripiprazole, 18% of subjects experienced akathisia; other common side-effects included headache, somnolence, dizziness, restlessness, insomnia, constipation, diarrhea, nausea, fatigue, blurred vision and upper respiratory infection [36].

The alternative FDA-approved, pharmaceutical, AD-augmenting agent, quetiapine, has beenshown to improve depressive symptoms, especially insomnia and anxiety. It does, however, also carry a side-effect burden. Garakani, et al. (2009) found weight change, symptoms of dizziness, and GI symptoms, the last-mentioned being the only side effect to achieve differentiation from placebo [37]. In extended release quetiapine, McIntyre et al. (2009) found sedation, somnolence, EPS, weight gain, and an increase in fasting glucose [38].

The last few years have added a more bona fide evidence base by way of the growing literature of controlled trials and FDA approvals on the use of the atypical antipsychotics as adjunctive treatment to an antidepressant medication. Atypical antipsychotics act primarily by blocking the D2 and 5HT2A receptors providing antipsychotic, anti-manic, and anti-

neuromuscular side effects. 5HT2A and 2C receptor antagonism may also promote dopamine and norepinephrine activity in the frontal cortex as well. They may also modulate, in varying degrees, several additional serotonin sub-receptors (such as 5HT3, 5HT1b, 5HT2b) and inhibit the reuptake of norepinephrine and serotonin similar to SSRI and SNRI antidepressants.

Uniquely, aripiprazole partially agonizes the DA2 and DA3 receptors promoting increased dopaminergic tone. These have theoretical antidepressant effects. Some agents block H1 histamine receptors and this action is utilized by FDA approved hypnotic agents and anxiolytics.

Further, in subjects with treatment-resistant depression, statistically significant increases in brain-derived neurotropic factor (BNDF) plasma levels of have been observed upon adjunctive use of atypical antipsychotics with various classes and AD medications [39].

Each drug in this class possesses a unique receptor profile which can help the physician pick the appropriate therapy for the individual patient. Some of the above mechanisms at serotonin sub-receptors also apply to certain FDA-approved antidepressants (e.g., mirtazapine, nefazodone, trazodone), increasing the possibility that the atypical antipsychotics may be effective treatments for anxiety and depression.

The atypicals also possess many pharmacodynamic properties that a modern day psychopharmacologist must be aware of to pick the best drug for each patient. Some have more antidepressant effect, more antipsychotic effect, more sedation, more activation- all based upon receptor affinity profiles. Many of these agents have antipsychotic or manic effects at high doses and antidepressant effects at lower doses. The future or advanced psychopharmacologist should be aware of these minor properties which may lend nuance while treating each individual patient [40].

Addressing the atypicals in depression, Barbee et al. conducted a retrospective chart review to determine the effectiveness of olanzapine, risperidone, quetiapine and ziprasidone as adjunctive treatment agents in patients with treatment-resistant depression [41]. The overall response rate was 65%. As to side effects, it was found that weight gain was associated with olanzapine; nausea, anxiety, depression were associated with risperidone; and sedation was associated with quetiapine and ziprasidone (ibid). Nelson and Papakostas (2010) conducted an extensive meta-analysis of RCTs investigating atypical antipsychotic augmentation in major depressive disorder resistant to previous treatment [42].

Results indicated that atypical antipsychotics are significantly effective augmentation agents in treating MDD but do involve a notable side-effect burden. The authors noted that efficacy did not significantly vary between the atypical antipsychotic medications tested (i.e., olanzapine, risperidone, quetiapine, aripiprazole) (ibid).

Increasing data suggest that the use of some atypical antipsychotics appears to cause a higher incidence of metabolic disorders. With increased data and approvals, more of these agents are being used and outside of monitoring for extrapyramidal and tardive dyskinesia side effect, it is uniformly recommended to monitor metabolic parameters as well at baseline and regular intervals with all atypical antipsychotics set forth in guidelines by the American Psychiatric Association and American Diabetes Association [43].

With regard to the above-stated suggestion, the clinician must use careful judgment in the administration of these drugs in combination with antidepressant medications, coupled with patient education and regular monitoring. Moreover, because these are dopamine-blocking drugs, the typical warnings exist for the monitoring of all extrapyramidal syndromes.

Amisulpiride

Cassano and Jori (2002) conducted an acute, randomized, double-blind, parallel group, multicenter trial of amisulpride (50 mg o.d.) and paroxetine (20 mg o.d.) in 272 patients with MDD. The results between groups was not statistically significant [44]. Lecrubier and others (1997) conducted a 6 month, multicenter, controlled trial comparing amisulpride (50 mg/d) to imipramine (100 mg/d) in 219 patients meeting DSM-III-R criteria for primary dysthymia, dysthymia with major depression or major depression in partial remission as measured by the CGI, MADRS, ERD, and SANS. The authors reported significant differences between groups' scores on all measures [45].

Aripiprazole

Aripiprazole was the first pharmacological agent to receive formal FDA prescription approval (2007) as an adjunctive treatment for inadequate response to a monotherapy antidepressant. This was based on the outcome of two six-week studies conducted by Berman [46] and by Marcus [47]. The study conducted by Berman et al. [46] found remission and response rates to be higher in the aripiprazole augmentation group versus placebo (15.7% versus 26.0%) and (23.8% versus 33.7%), respectively. The mean dose of aripiprazole in this trial was approximately 11 mg/day with akathisia being a leading side effect. The later replication by Berman et al. in 2008 confirmed the previous findings [48]. The standards for this prescription approval are considered higher than the medical food standards applied to methylfolate.

In addition to the 5-HT modulating effects via the 5HT2A blockade and 5HT1A stimulation of these receptors, aripiprazole has a unique pharmacological property as a "partial" dopamine receptor agonist as well (as noted above). Our group reported on the augmenting effects of aripiprazole to poor responders to SSRI or venlafaxine XR monotherapy for unipolar depression [49] with resultant mean HDRS score reduction at endpoint of 10.8. Open-label prospective trials replicated this result [50].

Successful pilot studies then led to fully controlled regulatory trials. These trials have shown definitive efficacy of aripiprazole as an adjunctive treatment agent and with less stringency as a monotherapy in patients with treatment-resistant depression [15, 50, 51 52, 53, 54, 55]. These studies have shown the onset of aripiprazole activity as early as week one of treatment, at doses lower than those used in schizophrenia or mania.

Our group has found success in starting patients on low doses (occasionally only 1 mg/day) and gradually increasing the dose to minimize akathisia.

Other aripiprazole controlled trials have also suggested its augmentation efficacy, and still other studies suggest efficacy in bipolar disorder [56, 57] as monotherapy or adjunctively to antidepressant medication. In a 3-week, double-blind study, Keck et al. found aripiprazole monotherapy to be superior to placebo in a group (n=262) with an acute manic or mixed episode [58]. Vieta et al. found adjunctive aripiprazole to be more effective than lithium or valproate alone in reducing bipolar mania [99]. Reviews and meta-analyses [42, 59, 60] of the data have also supported the efficacy of aripiprazole in this population.

In a study of aripiprazole with bipolar depression, Thase et al. [61] measured MADRS scores in depressed without psychotic features bipolar patients during two, identical RCTs last eight weeks each. Patients were randomized to aripiprazole monotherapy or placebo, and while statistically significant differences were seen in weeks 1-6, at endpoint, aripiprazole did not achieve statistical significance.

Asenapine

This sublingual atypical antipsychotic is approved (in the both US and EU) as monotherapy and adjuctively for the treatment of mania and bipolar I disorder. Asenapine is active via combined antagonism at the 5HT2A and D2 receptors, although its exact mechanism of action has not been fully uncovered. There have been three RCTs studying the efficacy of asenapine in acute mania or mixed states bipolar I disorder; 2 monotherapy studies conducted by McIntyre et al. [62, 63] and one adjuctive study by Calabrese et al [64]. Although all three were low-powered studies, each showed efficacy compared with placebo in treating manic symptoms.

Clozapine

The efficacy of clozapine for treatment-resistant mania was examined in a 13-week prospective study of 25 subjects diagnosed with acute mania in bipolar disorder or schizoaffective disorder-bipolar subtype with inadequate response and/or reported adverse events to lithium, anticonvulsants, or neuroleptics. All subjects were treated with clozapine monotherapy. Eighteen subjects (72%) exhibited marked improvement on the Young Mania Rating Scale, and eight (32%) exhibited marked improvement on the BPRS. The bipolar patients as compared to schizo-affective patients, and the non-rapid as compared to rapid cyclers, had significantly greater improvement in total BPRS score.

Olanzapine

Olanzapine is a relatively simple atypical and does not possess SSRI, NRI, 5HT1a agonism, and is not an accepted monotherapy for depression, but with the added SSRI potential of fluoxetine, it has well-controlled trials and regulatory data supporting its use in depression. Overall, the evidence in support of the olanzapine-fluoxetine combination earned FDA approvals for bipolar depression and for treatment resistant MDD. A small sample (n=20) controlled trial suggested that prospective treatment with an antidepressant may be necessary to achieve the rapid trajectory sometimes associated with olanzapine augmentation in MDD [66].

Tohen et al. initially reported that olanzapine as monotherapy, or in combination with fluoxetine, produced a greater reduction of core depressive symptoms compared to placebo in Bipolar I depressed patients (2003), resulting in FDA approval for the treatment of depression associated with bipolar I disorder [67]. Shelton et al. conducted a double-blind trial of olanzapine with fluoxetine versus either agent alone with treatment-resistant unipolar depression [68]. Olanzapine plus fluoxetine produced significantly greater improvement than either monotherapy from baseline. Increased appetite and weight gain occurred among patients treated with olanzapine. There were no significant differences between treatment groups with regard to extrapyramidal symptoms (EPS) or adverse drug interactions. Thase et al. replicated Shelton's 2001 findings in a group of unipolar depressed patients [69], yet subsequent trials failed to replicate the findings [70; 71]. Rothschild et al. [72] compared olanzapine and fluoxetine to olanzapine and placebo in patients with psychotic depression (n=124). Outcomes showed that the olanzapine + fluoxetine decreased mean HRSD scores by -20.9 (p=0.001); olanzapine monotherapy = -14.9; placebo = -10.4). The authors' simultaneously published replicated trial produced similar results. Meyers et al. [73] also studied psychotic depression; one group was given olanzapine + sertraline (OS) and the control, olanzapine + placebo (OP). The OS group showed greater rates of remission over the placebo group, with final remission rates resting at 41.9% for OS and 23.9% for OP.

Quetiapine

Quetiapine is now likely the next most extensively studied atypical antipsychotic in the treatment of bipolar and unipolar depression and a leader in the evidence base along with lithium controlled data. Early trials assessed quetiapine immediate release, while more recent trials have used the extended release version (XR.) A unique combination of direct and indirect pharmacological actions mediated with quetiapine and its active metabolite, norquetiapine, may underpin its clinical antidepressant properties. The high affinity and inhibitory actions on the norepinephrine transporter and potent 5HT2A,C receptor antagonism, 5HT1a receptor agonism and histamine-1 receptor antagonism give it the theoretical potential to ameliorate not only psychosis, and mania, but also depression, anxiety, and insomnia [74].

Early open-label trials supported the efficacy of a range of doses (50mg and above) of quetiapine to improve antidepressant efficacy in partial responders. At lower doses (less than 150 mg/day), the augmenting antidepressant effects of quetiapine to partial responders to monotherapy antidepressants may have been partly due to rapid improvement of sleep, anxiety or improving sexual function.

However, higher doses (>150 mg/day) may provide a broader pharmacological profile on the serotonin, dopamine and noradrenergic system that may provide a more direct antidepressant effect of quetiapine and have been demonstrated in both bipolar depression monotherapy and in MDD augmentation studies [74]. Quetiapine was the first pharmacological treatment to receive FDA-approval as a monotherapy for the depressed phase in bipolar I and II. Two consecutive controlled trials supported this efficacy [75, 76] and two additional large, placebo-controlled trials also support the use of quetiapine XR as an adjunctive treatment for inadequate response to various antidepressants in MDD [77, 78]. Side effects suggested higher rates of sedation, somnolence, dizziness, weight gain and metabolic issues increasing when doses exceed 150mg/d.

In another study of patients with MDD comorbid with anxiety, McIntyre and Gendron [79] found remission rate (MADRS ≤8) rates to be statistically insignificant compared with placebo. Earley, McIntyre, Wang et al. [80] studied QTP XR compared with escitalopram and with placebo, finding no significant differences between the groups' scores measuring response or remission. Katila, Meezhebovsky, Mulroy, et al. [81] studied 338 geriatric (≥66 y.o.) patients with MDD randomized to monotherapy QTP XR or placebo. The active medication group achieved greater rates of both response and remission ($p<0.001$ in each case) with a mean dose of 160mg/d.

Chaput, et al. [82] studied quetiapine adjunctive to cognitive behavior therapy in 22 treatment-resistant depressed patients, with a significant finding for the active treatment group on both the HDRS and the MADRS. Bauer, Pretorius, Constant and colleagues [83] conducted a large-scale RCT of quetiapine XR adjunctive to venlafaxine, citalopram, setraline, escitalopram, fluoxetine, paroxetine or duloxetine in MDD. Both 150mg and 300mg daily showed significant reductions (P=<0.01) in mean MADRS scores compared with placebo. Weisler, Joyce, McGill and others (2009) found MADRS scores significantly decreased as compared with placebo at monotherapy quetiapine doses of 50mg (P=0.01), 150mg (P=0.001) and 300mg (P=0.001) [84].

In the same year, Cutler, Montgomery, Feifel, et al. conducted a 6-week randomized trial of quetiapine (150 or 300mg/d), duloxetine 60 mg/d or placebo [85]. Response was found in both doses of QTP; remission only in the higher dose. In an 8-week trial of quetiapine XR v. placebo in 310 patients with major depressive disorder, patients treated with QTP XR showed significantly greater rates of response compared with placebo [86]. A 52-week maintenance RCT of QTP XR in MDD was conducted by Liebowitz, Lam, Lepola and colleagues (2010); 776 remitted patients were randomized to QTP XR or placebo [87]. The QTP XR group had a significantly reduced risk of experiencing a (predefined) depressive episode ($p < 0.001$). The sole trial of quetiapine in psychotic depression studied QTP in combination with venlafaxine with the HDRS as primary outcome. Response to the combination was greater than to venlafaxine alone, but comparable imipramine monotherapy. Remission rates separated the combination from imipramine monotherapy but not from venlafaxine monotherapy [88].

Our group may start quetiapine at the lower dose range, but increases doses toward 300 mg/day as either a monotherapy or adjunctive treatment. Use of quetiapine XR allows for once-per-day dosing in the evenings.

Modern psychopharmacologists must be aware of the evidence base and the drug's mechanism of action in order to choose medications appropriately, but also must be aware of the technology that goes into making pills. Instant release drugs have a higher initial side effect burden i.e. sedation within 30 minutes where slow release products allow for lower plasma levels, less severe side effects that may linger into the day.

Immediate release quetiapine is given at bed time and the high drug plasma levels allow greater initial sedation that may promote sleep (a side effect if sleepiness occurs during the day, but a positive clinical effect if insomnia is treated at night). The slow release product is given 4 hours before bed time as peak plasma levels and sedation occurs later. Some patients require the hypnotic effect and prefer the immediate release and others who prefer to avoid daytime sedation may choose the slow release.

Risperidone

Hirose and Ashby completed an open-pilot study of fluvoxamine plus risperidone as an initial antidepressant therapy [89] where 76% achieved remission, 17% achieved response, and two were not responsive. Adverse effects were mild, without cases of EPS, nausea or vomiting. Rapaport, Gharabowi and Caruso studied 241 treatment-resistant depressed patients prospectively treated with and failed citalopram, but responding to citalopram + risperidone

[90]. In the 24-week maintenance phase, patients on active medication relapsed more slowly than did the placebo group patients; relapse rates, ultimately, were the same between groups. A similar study was conducted [91] in which 63 treatment-resistant, depressed, older adults unresponsive to escitalopram yet responsive to the AD + risperidone were compared to placebo for 6 months. Results reflected those of the first study: relapse, albeit more slowly, in the active medication group compared with placebo. Mahmoud, Tandina, Turkoz and others [92] conducted the first short-term trial of risperidone augmentation of AD monotherapy in treatment-refractory depressed patients. The combination was superior to AD + placebo in producing response (46% v. 29.5%) and remission (24.5% v. 11%). Reeves, Batra, May, et al. [93] compared risperidone adjunctive to AD to placebo adjunctive to AD in patients with a depressed episode and suicidal ideation. The active combination was superior to placebo, more notably in depressive symptom reduction overall than in suicidal ideation reduction specifically.

Also in 2006, Keither, Garlow, Ryan and others reported an open-label study which showed monotherapy risperidone's efficacy in depressed patients who failed to respond to monotherapy SSRI [94]. Keitner et al. [95] reported on a controlled study in which MDD patients who were not responsive to antidepressant monotherapy were randomized to risperidone or placebo where subjects in both groups improved significantly, however, the odds of remitting were significantly better for patients in the risperidone arm than for those in the placebo arm.

Sulpiride

Ruther, Degner, Munzel, et al. [96] conducted a parallel-group RCT comparing sulpiride (150-300 mg) to placebo in 177 patients with mild to moderate depressive symptoms as measured by the HAMD. Change in HAMD score from baseline to last visit favored the active medication group by 2.5 points. This change was statistically significant ($p = 0.0007$). CGI score outcomes were similar. The mean dose for the active group was 181 mg/d.

Ziprazidone

In an open label trial conducted by Papakostas et al., patients with MDD who had failed to respond to an adequate trial of an SSRI were treated with ziprasidone [97] and at the end of the trial, 61.5% were classified as responders with 38.5% remittance. The use of ziprasidone appeared safe with no severe adverse events and no clinically significant QTc prolongation. Dunner et al. reported on a group of MDD subjects who were randomized to single-blind continuation of monotherapy sertraline or received ziprasidone adjunctive treatment [98]. There was a numerically significant greater improvement in the adjunctive treatment group compared to the monotherapy sertraline.

Of note, the remission rate in the sertraline/ziprasidone 160 mg/day group was 21% and 5% for the other two group.

Conclusion

This chapter serves as a review of how to manage patients with treatment resistant depression where monotherapy has failed to treat patients to remission. Polypharmacy may be the rule rather than the exception [99] when a clinician attempts to help a patient reach full remission of MDD symptoms, and is gaining popularity when side-effects need to be alleviated in order for the patient to remain adherent to otherwise successful long-term medication management. It further illuminates for the reader where limited approvals regarding augmentation/combination exist, and further, how the astute psychopharmacologist must command knowledge of the off-label literature. Finally, readers must note that there are more open-label and anecdotal reports than controlled studies. There is often a dearth of stringent evidence base for certain medication combinations as the clinician strives to obtain the ideal remission of symptoms. When needed stringent data is unavailable, clinicians are advised to rely on knowledge of the drug's mechanism of action, and select rational polypharmacy approaches where non-overlapping pharmacodynamic properties may successfully address and ameliorate residual symptoms. All of the above must be carefully weighed against risk-benefit and cost-benefit analyses.

Appendix 1. Second Generation Antipsychotics

Second Generation Antipsychotics

Amisulpride (Solian)
Aripiprazole (Abilify)
Asenapine (Saphris)
Blonanserin (Lonasen)
Clotiapine (Entumine)
Clozapine (Clozaril)
Iloperidone (Fanapt)
Lurasidone (Latuda)
Mosapramine (Cremin)
Olanzapine (Zyprexa)
Paliperidone (Invega)
Perospirone (Lullan)
Quetiapine (Seroquel)
Remoxipride (Roxiam)
Risperidone (Risperdal)
Sertindole (Serdolect)
Sulpiride (Sulpirid, Eglonyl)
Ziprasidone (Geodon, Zeldox)
Zotepine (Nipolept)

Appendix 2. Acute Mania

Acute Mania: FDA-Approved Monotherapy (2011)

		Acute Mania	Mixed Mania	Pediatric	
	lithium*	√			
	valproate*	√	√		
	carbamazepine*	√	√**		
	Aripiprazole	√		√	
	Asenapine	√	√		
	chlorpromazine	√			
	Olanzapine	√	√**		
	quetiapine*	√	√		
	risperidone	√	√		
	Ziprasidone	√	√		

* Includes extended-, delayed-, sustained-release formulations

** Only extended-release

Acute Mania: FDA-Approved Combination Treatments with Lithium or Valproate*

aripiprazole	√
olanzapine	√
quetiapine*	√
risperidone	√

Evidence-Based Acute Mania Studies

		Category A	Only Category C, D	Category A
		Positive		Negative or Failed Trials
	Carbamazepine	√		
	Lithium	√		
	Valproate	√		
	Aripiprazole	√		
	Asenapine	√		
	Chlorpromazine		√	
	Haloperidol	√		
	Olanzapine	√		
	Paliperidone	√		
	Quetiapine	√		
	Risperidone	√		
	Ziprasidone	√		

Evidence-Based Acute Mania Studies (Continued)

		Category A	Only Category C, D	Category A
		Positive		Negative or Failed Trials
TREATMENT RESISTANT				
	Clozapine	√		
	ECT	√		
	Lamotrigine		√	
	Gabapentin		√	
	Oxcarbazepine		√	
	Topiramate		√	
	Licarbazepine			
** *FDA-approved*				

*Adapted from Sachs, G. S., et al. NCDEU, 2011.

Appendix 3. Bipolar Depression

Acute Bipolar Depression: FDA-Approved Treatments

olanzapine/fluoxetine combination	√
quetiapine*, **	√

*includes extended-release formulation

**includes bipolar II

Acute Bipolar Depression Studies: Evidence-Based*

	Category A			Category B, C
	Positive	Failed or Negative	Negative	
aripiprazole		X		
bupropion + MS		X		
imipramine		X		
imipramine + lithium		X		
lamotrigine	X	X		
lithium		X	X **	X
olanzapine	X			
olanzapine + fluoxetine	X			
paroxetine		X	X **	
paroxetine + MS		X		
paroxetine + lithium		X		
quetiapine***	X			
ECT				X
VNS				X

* Adapted from Sachs GS, et al. NCDEU, 2011

** lithium < placebo, quetiapine > placebo

*** bipolar I and II

MS = mood stabilizer

Maintenance Therapy for Bipolar I FDA-Approved (2011)

	Monotherapy	Combination with Lithium or Valproate
carbamazepine	X	
lamotrigine	X	
lithium	X	
apripiprazole	X	X
olanzapine	X	
quetiapine		X
risperidone	X	X
ziprasidon		X
VNS		X

*Includes extended-release formulation
**Long-acting

Bipolar Maintenance Studies-Evidence-Based*

	Category A - Positive	Category A - Neg or Failed	Category A - Negative	Category C
aripiprazole	X			
imipramine		X	X	
lamotrigine	X			
lithium	X		X	
olanzapine	X			
risperidone	X**, X***			
quetiapine	X**, X***			
valproate	X			
ziprasidone	X**			
VNS				X
ECT				X

*Adapted from Sachs, G. S., et al. NCDEU, 2011.
**as adjunctive therapy
***extended-release/long-acting formulations

APPENDIX 4. SGAS IN MDD

SGAs in Major Depressive Disorder

Adjuctive Indications
seroquel XR Aripiprazole Monotherapy (evidence suggests)
Seroquel XR

REFERENCES

[1] Shelton, R. C., Osuntokun, O., Heinloth, A. N., Corya, S. A. Therapeutic options for treatment resistant depression. *CNS Drugs* 2010; 24:131-61.

[2] Delgado, P. L. "Depression: the case for a monoamine deficiency. *J. Clin. Psychiatry* 2000; 61: 7-11.

[3] Blier, P., Szabo, S. T. "Potential mechanisms of action of atypical antipsycotic mdications in treatment-resistant depression and anxiety. *J. Clin. Psychiatry* 2005; 66: 30-40.

[4] Lee, S., Jeong, J., Kwak, Y., Park, S. K. "Depression research: where are we now?" *Mol. Brain* 2010; 3: 8.

[5] Goren, J. L., Strategies for treatment refractory depression. *Journal of Pharmacy Practice* 2001;14:478-486

[6] Carvahlo, A. F., Machado, J. R., Cavalcante, J. L. Augmentation strategies for treatment-resistant depression. *Current Opinion in Psychiatry* 2008; 22:7–12.

[7] Van Londen, L., Molenaar, R. P., Goekoop, J. G., et al.Three- to 5-year prospective follow-up of outcome in major depression. *Psychol. Med.* 1998;28:731-5.

[8] Thase, M. E., Simons, A. D., McGeary, J., et al. Relapse after cognitive behavior therapy of depression: potential implications for longer courses of treatment. *Am. J. Psychiatry* 1992;149:1046-52.

[9] Judd, L. L., Akiskal, H. S., Maser, J. D., et al. Major depressive disorder: a prospective study of residual subthreshold depressive symptoms as predictor of rapid relapse. *J. Affect. Disord.* 1998;50:97-108.

[10] Paykel, E. S., Ramana, R., Cooper, Z., et al. Residual symptoms after partial remission: an important outcome in depression. *Psychol. Med.* 1995;25:1171-80.

[11] Miller, I. W., Keitner, G. I., Schatzberg, A. F., et al. The treatment of chronic depression, part 3: psychosocial functioning before and after treatment with sertraline or imipramine. *J. Clin. Psychiatry* 1998;59:608-19.

[12] Judd, L. L., Paulus, M. J., Schettler, P. J., et al. Does incomplete recovery from first lifetime major depressive episode herald a chronic course of illness? *Am. J. Psychiatry* 2000;157:1501-4.

[13] Zajecka, J. M. Treating depression to remission. *J. Clin. Psychiatry* 2003;64:7-12.

[14] Thase, M. E. Evaluating antidepressant therapies: remission as the optimal outcome. *J. Clin. Psychiatry* 2003;64:18-25.

[15] Papakostas, G. I., Fava, M. Monoamine-based Pharmacotherapy. In: Licinio, J., Wong, M. L. editors. *Biology of Depression: From Novel Insights to Therapeutic Strategies*, First Edition. Weinheim: Wiley-VCH Verlag, 2005: 87-140.

[16] Corey-Lisle, P. K., Nash, R., Stang, P., et al. Response, partial response, and nonresponse in primary care treatment of depression. *Arch. Intern. Med.* 2004;164:1197-204.

[17] Rush, A. J., Trivedi, M., Carmody, T. J., et al. One-year clinical outcomes of depressed public sector outpatients: a benchmark for subsequent studies. *Biol. Psychiatry* 2004;56:46-53.

[18] Trivedi, M. H., Rush, A. J., Wisniewski, S. R., et al. Evaluation of outcomes with citalopram for depression using measurement-based care in STAR*D: implications for clinical practice. *Am. J. Psychiatry* 2006;163:28-40.

[19] Petersen, T., Papakostas, G. I., Posternak, M. A., et al. Empirical Testing of Two Models for Staging Antidepressant Treatment Resistance. *J. Clin. Psychopharmacol.* 2005, 25: 336-341.

[20] Nierenberg, A. A., Keefe, B. R., Leslie, V. C., et al. Residual symptoms in depressed patients who respond acutely to fluoxetine. *J. Clin. Psychiatry* 1999;60:221-5.

[21] Papakostas, G. I., Petersen, T., Denninger, J. W., et al. Psychosocial functioning during the treatment of major depressive disorder with fluoxetine. *J. Clin. Psychopharmacol.* 2004a;24:507-11

[22] Kupfer, D. J., Spiker, D. G. Refractory depression: prediction of non-response by clinical indicators. *J. Clin. Psychiatry* 1981;42:307-312.

[23] Rush, A. J., Kraemer, H. C., Sackheim, H. A., et al. Report by the ACNP Task Force on response and remission in major depressive disorder. *Neuropsychopharmacoly* 2006;31:1841-1853.

[24] Weissman, M. M., Prusoff, B. A., Klerman, G. L. Personality and prediction of long-term outcome of depression. *Am. J. Psychiatry* 1978;135:797-800.

[25] Thase, M. E. Introduction: Defining remission in patients treated with antidepressants. *J. Clin. Psychiatry* 1999;60:3-6.

[26] Hirschfeld, R. M., Keller, M. B., Panico, et al. The National Depressive and Manic Depressive Association consensus statement on the undertreatment of depression. *JAMA* 1997;277:333-340.

[27] Zajecka, J. M. Augmentation strategies to increase antidepressant tolerability. *J. Clin. Psychiatry*. 2007;68: 10:23-7.

[28] Blier, P., Keller, M. B., Pollack, M. H., et al. Preventing recurrent depression: long-term treatment for major depressive disorder. *J. Clin. Psychiatry* 2007;68:e06.

[29] Stahl, S. M. Stahl's essential psychopharmacology: Neuroscientific Basis and Practical Applications. Cambridge: Cambridge University Press 2008.

[30] Fava, M., Rush, A. J. Current status of augmentation and combination treatments for major depressive disorder: a literature review and a proposal for a novel approach to improve practice. *Psychother. Psychosom.* 2006;75:139-53.

[31] Fleurence, R., Williamson, R., Jing, Y., et al. A Systematic Review of Augmentation Strategies for Patients with Major Depressive Disorder. *Psychopharmacol. Bull.* 2009;42:57-90.

[32] Rush, A. J. STAR*D: What Have We Learned? *Am. J. Psychiatry* 2007,164:2, 201-4.

[33] Montgomery, S. A. Why do we need new and better antidepressants? *International Clinical Psychopharmacology* 2006;21: S1-S10.

[34] Ostroff, R. B., Nelson, J. C. Risperidone augmentation of selective serotonin reuptake inhibitors in major depression. *J. Clin. Psychiatry* 1999;60:256-9.

[35] Chiarello, R. J., Cole, J. O. The use of psychostimulants in general psychiatry. A reconsideration. *Arch. Gen. Psychiatry* 1987 ;44:286-95.

[36] Berman, R., Fava, M., Thase, M., et al. Aripiprazole augmentation in major depressive disorder: a double-blind, placebo-contolled study in patients with inadequate response to antidepressants. *CNS Spectrums* 2009;14: 197-206

[37] Garakani, A., Martinez, J. M., Marcus, S., et al. A randomized, double-blind, and placebo-controlled trial of quetiapine augmentation of fluoxetine in major depressive disorder. *Int. Clin. Psychopharmacol.* 2008;23:269-75.

[38] McIntyre, R. S., Muzina, D. J., Adams, A., et al. Quetiapine XR efficacy and tolerability as monotherapy and as adjunctive treatment to conventional antidepressants in the acute and maintenance treatment of major depressive disorder: a review of registration trials. *Expert Opin. Pharmacother.* 2009;10:3061-75. Review.

[39] Yoshimura, R., Ikenouchi-Sugita, A., Hori, H., et al. Adding a low dose atypical antipsychotic drug to an antidepressant induced a rapid increase of plasma brain-derived neurotrophic factor levels in patients with treatment-resistant depression. *Progress in Neuro-Psychopharmacology and Biological Psychiatry* 2010, 34, 308–312

[40] Schwartz, T. L., Stahl, S. M. Treatment strategies for dosing the second generation antipsychotics. *CNS Neurosci. Ther.* 2011;17:110-7.

[41] Barbee, J. G., Conrad, E. J., Jamhour, N. J. The effectiveness of olanzapine, risperidone, quetiapine and ziprasidone as adjunctive treatment agents in treatment-resistant major depressive disorder. *J. Clin. Psychiatry* 2004;65:975-981.

[42] Nelson, J. C. and Papakostas, G. I. Atypical antipsychotic augmentation in major depressive disorder: A meta-analysis of placebo-controlled randomized trials. *American Journal of Psychiatry* 2010;166:980–991.

[43] American Diabetes Association, American Psychiatric Association. Consensus development conference on antipsychotic drugs and obesity and diabetes. *J. Clin. Psychiatry* 2004;65:267-272.

[44] Cassano, G. B., Jori, M. C.; AMIMAJOR Group. Efficacy and safety of amisulpride 50 mg versus paroxetine 20 mg in major depression: a randomized, double-blind, parallel group study. *Int. Clin. Psychopharmacol.* 2002;17:27-32.

[45] Lecrubier, Y., Boyer, P., Turjanski, S., et al. Amisulpride versus imipramine and placebo in dysthymia and major depression. *Journal of Affective Disorders* 1997;43: 95-103.

[46] Berman, R. M., Marcus, R. N., Swanink, R., et al. The efficacy and safety of aripiprazole as adjunctive therapy in major depressive disorder: a multicenter, randomized, double-blind, placebo-controlled study. *J. Clin. Psychiatry* 2007;68:843-53.

[47] Marcus, R. N., McQuade, R. D., Carson, W. H., et al. The efficacy and safety of aripiprazole as adjunctive therapy in major depressive disorder: a second multicenter, randomized, double-blind, placebo-controlled study. *J. Clin. Psychopharmacol.* 2008;28:156-65.

[48] Berman, B. M., Fava, M., Thase, M. E., et al. Aripiprazole adjunctive treatment of major depressive disorder: a double-blind, placebo-controlled study in patients with inadequate response to antidepressants. *CNS Spectrums* 2009;14:197-206.

[49] Zajecka, J., Gutierrez, S., Mackey, I. Adjunctive treatment with aripiprazole to partial responders on SSRIs or SNRIs for depression. *Poster presented at the 45th Annual Meeting of the New Clinical Drug Evaluation Unit*, June 6-9, 2005, Boca Raton, Florida.

[50] Schwartz, T. L., Nasra, G. S., Chilton, M. S. Aripiprazole adjunctive treatment of selective and serotonin norepinephrine reuptake inhibitors in treatment of major depressive disorder. *Primary Psychiatry* 2007;14:67-69.

[51] Simon, J. S., Nemeroff, C. B. Aripiprazole adjunctive treatment of antidepressants for the treatment of partially responding and nonresponding patients with major depressive disorder. *J. Clin. Psychiatry* 2005;66:1216-1220.

[52] Worthington, III J. J., Kierys, G., Wygant, L. E., et al. Aripiprazole as an augmentor of selective serotonin reuptake inhibitors in depression and anxiety disorder patients. *Int. Clin. Psychopharmacol.* 2005;20:9-11.

[53] Patkar, A. A., Masand, P. S., Pae, C., et al. A randomized, double-blind, placebo-controlled trial of augmentation with an extended release formulation of methylphenidate in outpatients with treatment-resistant depression. *J. Clin. Psychopharmacol.* 2006;26:653–656

[54] Adson, D. E., Kushner, M. G., Fahnhorse, T. A. Treatment of residual anxiety symptoms with adjunctive aripiprazole in depressed patients taking selective serotonin reuptake inhibitors. *J. Affect. Disord.* 2005;86:99-104.

[55] Pae, C. U., Patkar, A. A., Jun, T. Y., et al. Aripiprazole adjunctive treatment for treatment of patients with inadequate antidepressant response. *Depression and Anxiety* 2007;24:522-526.

[56] McIntyre, R. S., Cohen, M., Zhou, J., et al. Asenapine in the treatment of acute mania in bipolar I disorder; a randomized, double-blind, placebo-controlled trial. *J. Affect. Disord.* 2010;122: 27-38.

[57] Thase, M. E., Jonas, A., Khan, A., Bowden, C. L., et al. Aripiprazole Monotherapy in Nonpsychotic Bipolar I Depression: Results of 2 Randomized, Placebo-Controlled Studies. *Journal of Clinical Psychopharmacology* 2008; 28:13-20

[58] Keck, P. E. Jr, Marcus, R., Tourkodimitris, S., et al. A placebo-controlled, double-blind study of the efficacy and safety of aripiprazole in patients with acute bipolar mania. *Am. J. Psychiatry* 2003;160:1651-8.

[59] Papakostas, G. I. Managing partial response or nonresponse: switching, augmentation, and combination strategies for major depressive disorder. *J. Clin. Psychiatry* 2009;70:16-25.

[60] Arbaizar, B., Dierssen-Sotos, T., Gómez-Acebo, I., et al. Aripiprazole in major depression and mania: meta-analyses of randomized placebo-controlled trials. *General Hospital Psychiatry* 2009;31: 478-483.

[61] Thase, M. E., Jonas, A., Khan, A., Bowden, C. L., Wu, X., McQuade, R. D., Carson, W. H., Marcus, R. N., Owen, R. Aripiprazole monotherapy in nonpsychotic bipolar i depression: results of 2 randomized, placebo-controlled studies. *Journal of Clinical Psychopharmacology*: 2008, 28, 1, 13-20.

[62] McIntyre, R. S., Cohen, M., Zhao, J., et al. A 3-week, randomized, placebo-controlled trial of asenapine in the treatment of acute mania in bipolar mania and mixed states. *Bipolar Disord.* 2009;11:673-86.

[63] McIntyre, R. S. Pharmacology and efficacy of asenapine for manic and mixed states in adults with bipolar disorder. *Expert Rev. Neurother.* 2010;10:645-9.

[64] Calabrese, J., Stet, L., Kotari, H., et al. Asenapine as adjunctive treatment for bipolar mania; results of a placebo-controlled, 12-week study and a 40-week extension. *Eur. Psychiatry* 2010;25 : 1447.

[65] Calabrese, J. R., Kimmel, S. E., Woyshville, M. J., et al. Clozapine for treatment-refractory mania. *Am. J. Psychiatry* 1996;153:759-64.

[66] Parker, G., Brotchie, H., Parker, K. "Is combination olanzapine and antidepressant medication associated a more repid response trajectory than antidepressant alone?" *Am. J. Psyciatry* 2005;162: 796-8.

[67] Tohen, M., Ketter, T. A., Zarate, C. A., et al. Olanzapine versus divalproex sodium for the treatment of acute mania and maintenance of remission: a 47-week study. *Am. J. Psychiatry* 2003;160:1263-1271.

[68] Shelton, R. C., Tollefson, G. D., Tohen, M., et al . A novel augmentation strategy for treating resistant major depression. *Am. J. Psychiatry* 2001;158:131-4.

[69] Thase, M. E., Corya, S. A., Osuntokun, O., et al. A randomized, double-blind comparison of olanzapine/fluoxetine combination, olanzapine, and fluoxetine in treatment-resistant major depressive disorder. *J. Clin. Psychiatry* 2007;68:224-36.

[70] Corya, S. A., Williamson, D., Sanger, T. M., et al. A randomized, double-blind comparison of olanzapine/fluoxetine combination, olanzapine, fluoxetine, and venlafaxine in treatment-resistant depression. *Depress Anxiety.* 2006;23:364-72.

[71] Shelton, R. C., Williamson, D. J., Corya, S. A., et al. Olanzapine/fluoxetine combination for treatment-resistant depression: a controlled study of SSRI and nortriptyline resistance. *J. Clin. Psychiatry* 2005;66:1289-97.

[72] Rothschild, A. J., Williamson, D. J., Tohen, M. F., et al. A double-blind, randomized study of olanzapine and olanzapine/fluoxetine combination for major depression with psychotic features. *J. Clin. Psychopharmacol.* 2004;24:365-73.

[73] Meyers, B. S., Flint, A. J., Rothschild, A. J., et al. A double-blind randomized controlled trial of olanzapine plus sertraline vs olanzapine plus placebo for psychotic depression: the study of pharmacotherapy of psychotic depression (STOP-PD). *Arch. Gen. Psychiatry.* 2009;66:838-47.

[74] Goldstein, J. M., Christoph, G., Grimm, S., et al. Unique Mechanism of Action for the Antidepressant Properties of the Atypical Antipsychotic Quetiapine. Presented at the 160th Meeting of the American Psychiatric Association, May 19-24, 2007, San Diego, California.

[75] Calabrese, J. R., Keck, P. E., Macfadden, W., et al. A randomized, double-blind, placebo-controlled trial of quetiapine in the treatment of bipolar I or II depression. *Am. J. Psychiatry* 2005;162:1351-1360.

[76] Thase, M. E., Mcfadden, W., Weisler, R. H., et al. Efficacy of quetiapine monotherapy in bipolar I and II depression: a double-blind, placebo-controlled study (the BOLDER II study). *J. Clin. Psychopharmacol.* 2006;26:600-9.

[77] El-Khalili, N., Joyce, M., Atkinson, S., et al. Adjunctive extended-release quetiapine fumarate (quetiapine XR) in patients with major depressive disorder and inadequate antidepressant response. *Poster presented at the 161st Annual Meeting of the American Psychiatric Association,* May 3-8, 2008, Washington, DC.

[78] Earley, W., McIntyre, A., Bauer, M., et al. Efficacy and tolerability of extended release quetiapine fumarate (quetiapine XR) as add-on to antidepressants in patients with major depressive disorder (MDD): results from a double-blind, randomized, phase III study. *Poster presented at the 46th Annual Meeting of the American College of Neuropsychopharmacology*, December 9-13, 2007, Boca Raton, FL

[79] McIntyre, A., Gendron, A., McIntyre, A. Quetiapine adjunct to selective serotonin reuptake inhibitors or venlafaxine in patients with major depression, comorbid anxiety, and residual depressive symptoms: a randomized, placebo-controlled pilot study. *Depress Anxiety* 2007;24:487-94.

[80] Earley, W., McIntyre, A., Wang, G., et al. Double-blind study of the efficacy and tolerability of extended release quetiapine fumarate (quetiapine XR) monotherapy in patients with major depressive disorder (MDD). *8th International Forum on Mood and Anxiety Disorders.* Vienna, Austria; 2008. p. P10.

[81] Katila, H., Mezhebovsky, I., Mulroy, A., et al. Efficacy and tolerability of once-daily extended release quetiapine fumarate (quetiapine XR) monotherapy in elderly patients with major depressive disorder (MDD). *8th International Forum on Mood and Anxiety Disorders.* Vienna, Austria; 2008. p. P23.

[82] Chaput, Y., Magnan, A., Gendron, A. The co-administration of quetiapine or placebo to cognitive-behavior therapy in treatment refractory depression: a preliminary trial. *BMC Psychiatry* 2008; 28:8:73.

[83] Bauer, M., Pretorius, H. W., Constant, E. L., et al. Extended-release quetiapine as adjunct to an antidepressant in patients with major depressive disorder: results of a randomized, placebo-controlled, double-blind study. *J. Clin. Psychiatry* 2009; 70:540–549.

[84] Weisler, R., Joyce, M., McGill, L., et al. Extended release quetiapine fumarate monotherapy for major depressive disorder: results of a double-blind, randomized, placebo-controlled study. *CNS Spectr.* 2009, 14, 299-313.

[85] Cutler, A. J., Montgomery, S. A., Feifel, D., et al. Extended release quetiapine XR monotherapy in major depressive disorder: a placebo-and duloxetine-controlled study. *Journal of Clinical Psychiatry* 2009, 70, 526-39.

[86] Bortnick, B., El-Khalili, N., Banov, M., et al. Efficacy and tolerability of extended release quetiapine fumarate (quetiapine XR) monotherapy in major depressive disorder: a placebo-controlled, randomized study. *J. Affect. Disord.* 2011;28:83- 94.

[87] Liebowitz, M., Lam, R. W., Lepola, U., et al. Efficacy and tolerability of extended release quetiapine fumarate monotherapy as maintenance treatment of major depressive disorder: a randomized, placebo-controlled trial. *Depress Anxiety* 2010;27: 964-76.

[88] Wijkstra, J., Burger, H., van den Broek, W. W., et al. Long-term response to successful acute pharmacological treatment of psychotic depression. *J. Affect. Disord.* 2010;123:238-42.

[89] Hirose, S., Ashby, C. R. Jr. An open pilot study combining Risperidone and a selective serotonin reuptake inhibitor as initial antidepressant therapy. *J. Clin. Psychiatry* 2002;63:733-736.

[90] Rapaport, M. H., Gharabawi, G. M., Canusco, C., et al. Effects of risperidone augmentation in patients with treatment-resistant depression: results of open-label treatment followed by double-blind continuation. *Neuropsychopharmacology* 2006, 31, 2505-13.

[91] Alexopoulos, G. S., Canuso, C. M., Gharabawi, G. M., et al. Pseudo-controlled study of relapse prevention with risperidone augmentation in older patients with resistant depression. *American Journal of Geriatric Psychiatry* 2008;16: 21-33.

[92] Mahmoud, R. A., Pandina, G. J., Turkoz, I., et al. Risperidone for treatment-refractory major depressive disorder: a randomized trial. *Ann. Intern. Med.* 2007;147:593-602

[93] Reeves, H., Batra, S., May, R. S., et al. Efficacy of risperidone augmentation to antidepressants in the management of suicidality in major depressive disorder: a randomized, double-blind, placebo-control pilot study. *Journal of Clinical Psychiatry* 2008; 69: 1228-336.

[94] Keither, G. I., Garlow, S. J., Ryan, C. E., et al. Risperidone adjunctive treatment for patients with difficult-to-treat major depression. *Poster presented at the 159th Annual Meeting of the American Psychiatric Association*, May 20-25, 2006, Toronto, Canada.

[95] Keitner, G. I., Garlow, S. J., Ryan, C. E., et al. A randomized, placebo-controlled trial of risperidone augmentation for patients with difficult-to-treat unipolar, non-psychotic major depression. *Journal of Psychiatric Research.* 43:205-14.

[96] Rüther, E., Degner, D., Munzel, U., Brunner, E., et al. Antidepressant action of sulpiride. Results of a placebo-controlled double-blind trial. *Pharmacopsychiatry* 1999;32:127-35.

[97] Papakostas, G., et al. Ziprasidone adjunctive treatment of selective serotonin reuptake inhibitors (SSRIs) for SSRI-resistant major depressive disorder. *J. Clin. Psychiatry* 2004;65:217-21.

[98] Dunner, D. L., Amsterdam, J. D., Shelton, R. C., et al. Efficacy and tolerability of adjunctive ziprasidone in treatment-resistant depression: a randomized pilot study. *J. Clin. Psychiatry* 2007;68:1071-1077.

[99] Vieta, E., T'joen, C., McQuade, R. D., et al. Efficacy of adjunctive aripiprazole to either valproate or lithium in bipolar mania patients partially nonresponsive to valproate/lithium monotherapy: a placebo-controlled study. *Am. J. Psychiatry*, 2008 165, 10, 1316-25.

In: Antipsychotic Drugs
Editors: T.L. Schwartz, J. Megna and M.E. Topel
ISBN: 978-1-62100-071-6

Chapter 3

ANTIPSYCHOTIC DRUGS AND CHILDREN: THE GOOD, THE BAD, AND WHAT TO DO ABOUT IT

Cliff McKinney
Mississippi State University, MS, US

ABSTRACT

Despite the fact that the Food and Drug Administration has approved the use of antipsychotic drugs for children in very few situations (i.e., the use of risperidone for the management of irritability associated with Autism and Schizophrenia, and the use of risperidone or aripiprazole for manic and mixed episodes experienced in the context of Bipolar I Disorder), the use of antipsychotic drugs to treat children has become increasingly prevalent for a wide range of disruptive behavior including children experiencing symptoms of Oppositional Defiant Disorder and Conduct Disorder. Although research on antipsychotic drugs in children has increased, mechanisms of action and long-term outcomes continue to be understood inadequately. Even though these medications may alleviate some problems in some cases, a plethora of side effects which range from mild to lethal exist. In fact, one of the side effects (i.e., somnolence/sedation) may be the reason why these medications reduce disruptive behavior in children. Research on the use of particular antipsychotic drugs (i.e., risperidone, aripiprazole, olanzapine) to treat children is reviewed and both positive and negative effects of these drugs when used to treat children are summarized. Following a discussion of the positive and negative effects, safety guidelines and other recommendations are made to encourage proper treatment of children when antipsychotic drugs are being considered.

INTRODUCTION

Although antipsychotic medications were developed originally to assist with the treatment of psychotic disorders in adults, these medications also are being used to treat both psychotic and non-psychotic disorders in children (Sivaprasad, Hassan, & Handy, 2006). Traditional antipsychotic medications were used in the past despite ongoing concerns about negative effects associated with these medications, but the introduction of atypical antipsychotic medications, which have less severe and frequent side effects compared to traditional antipsychotic medications, has led to more frequent use (Croarkin, Emslie, & Mayes, 2008; Erdogan et al., 2008; Sivaprasad et al., 2006; Zito, Safer et al., 2008). In fact, several recent studies (e.g., Farrell, Fisher, & McCabe, 2010; Olfson, Blanco, Liu, Moreno, & Laje, 2006; Sivaprasad et al., 2006; Staller, Wade, & Baker, 2005; Zito, Safer, et al., 2008) conducted in various places of the world (i.e., United Kingdom, Netherlands, Germany, and the United States) indicate an increasing trend in the use of atypical antipsychotic medications. Specifically, those studies found that 74 to 95% of psychiatrists have prescribed atypical antipsychotic medication to children, that 65 to 86% of psychiatrists prescribed those medications for a non-psychotic condition (i.e., Disruptive Behavior Disorder, Mood Disorder, Anxiety Disorder, Pervasive Developmental Disorder, Intellectual Disability, Eating Disorder), that office visits including treatment with antipsychotic medications increased by over 500% from 1993 to 2002, that 18.3% of visits to psychiatrists and 9.2% of all mental health visits involve treatment with atypical antipsychotics, and that 92.3% of those visits involve treatment with atypical antipsychotic medications.

The increase in the use of atypical antipsychotic medications to treat children has occurred despite the fact that the use of these medications is largely unapproved by the Food and Drug Administration (FDA). Specifically, The FDA has approved the use of risperidone in the treatment of irritability associated with Autism in children aged 5 to 16 years and the use of both risperidone and aripiprazole in the treatment of manic and mixed episodes associated with Bipolar I Disorder in children aged 10 to 17 years and Schizophrenia in children aged 13 to 17 years (Croarkin et al., 2008; Greenaway & Norris, 2009; Scott & Dhillon, 2008; Stigler & McDougle, 2008). Although these are the only FDA approved uses of atypical antipsychotic medications in children, these medications also are used to treat children with other disorders (Findling, 2003; Greenaway & Elbe, 2009; Mehler-Wex, Romanos, Kirchheiner, & Schulze, 2009; Ritchie & Norris, 2009; Stigler & McDougle, 2008). In fact, approximately 50 to 75% of children are prescribed medication off label (Findling, 2003; Zito, Derivan et al., 2008).

Clearly, the above research demonstrates the dramatic increase in the use of atypical antipsychotic medications to treat a wide range of disorders in children. Both positive and negative effects of the use of atypical antipsychotic medications have been observed (McKinney & Renk, 2011).

THE GOOD

Many studies have examined the effects of atypical antipsychotic medications for treating children. In particular, risperidone has been examined most followed by aripiprazole, olanzapine, and other atypical antipsychotic medications. In some cases, research provides support for the short-term efficacy of these medications.

For example, Troost et al. (2005) examined the use of risperidone over a 6 month period in children (age 5 to 17 years) who exhibited severe disruptive behavior (e.g., tantrums, aggression, or self-injurious behavior) in the context of an Autism Spectrum Disorder. Of the 36 children, 26 of them experienced a decrease in disruptive behavior. Further, children who continued use of the medication relapsed less than children who had their use discontinued. The Research Units on Pediatric Psychopharmacology Autism Network (2005) replicated the study by Troost et al. (2005) and found similar results (i.e., participants experienced a decrease in disruptive behavior and less relapse if continued on risperidone compared to those whose use was discontinued). Scott and Dhillon (2008) also examined the use of risperidone in 156 children (age 5 to 17 years) diagnosed with Autism during two 8-week randomized, double-blind trials and found that disruptive and stereotypic behavior decreased with the use of risperidone.

Croonenberghs et al. (2005) conducted a multisite (i.e., 32 sites across 12 counties) study to examine the use of risperidone in children (age 5 to 14 years) who exhibited below average intelligence (i.e., IQs ranging from 36 to 84). They found that the use of risperidone in children with below average intelligence was generally safe and effective (i.e., low percent of adverse events and reduction in disruptive behavior). Reyes, Olah, Csaba, Augustyns, and Eerdekens (2006) examined the use of risperidone over a 3-year period in children (age 6 to 16 years) diagnosed with a Disruptive Behavior Disorder and below average intelligence (i.e., IQs ranging from 35 to 84). Positive effects noted within the first year of treatment were maintained over the 2-year extension period. Findling, Aman, Eerdekens, Derivan, and Lyons (2004) examined the use of risperidone over a 48 week period in 107 children (age 5 to 12 years) who exhibited severe disruptive behavior and below average intelligence (i.e., IQs ranging from 36 to 84). In this study, risperidone was associated with significant reductions of disruptive behavior and long-term improvement. Reyes, Buitelaar, Toren, Augustyns, and Eerdekens (2006) conducted a multisite study across eight countries that examined the effects of risperidone over 6 months on 527 children (age 5 to 17 years) diagnosed with a Disruptive Behavior Disorder and who varied in intelligence (i.e., 190 children with IQs between 55 and 84 and 145 children with IQs over 84). Children who received risperidone experienced a significantly longer delay in relapse compared to children who did not receive risperidone, suggesting that risperidone has long-term efficacy. Haas, Karcher, and Pandina (2008) conducted a 1-year extension study on 232 children (age 5 to 17 years) diagnosed with a Disruptive Behavior Disorder and found a decrease in disruptive behavior symptoms in children receiving risperidone.

Caldwell, Malterer, Umstead, and McCormick (2008) compared the effects of cognitive-behavioral therapy and risperidone to the effects of cognitive behavioral therapy only in 129 children (age 13 to 18 years) diagnosed with childhood onset Conduct Disorder. It was found that children receiving risperidone in addition to cognitive behavioral therapy experienced significant decreases in disruptive behavior compared to both baseline and children receiving cognitive behavioral therapy only. De Deyn and Buitelaar (2006) reviewed 19 open-label, double-blind studies investigating the effects of risperidone on disruptive behavior across the age span, including some of the studies discussed above. Results indicated that the safety and tolerability of low-dose risperidone was good overall.

Although risperidone is the most well studied atypical antipsychotic medication used in children, olanzapine and aripiprazole also have been studied more recently as a treatment for children. Masi et al. (2006) examined the use of olanzapine in children (aged 11 to 17 years) diagnosed with Conduct Disorder and in psychosocial treatments. They found that the type of aggression displayed by children predicted treatment response. Specifically, children who displayed impulse affective aggression responded better to treatment than children who displayed controlled-predatory aggression. Handen and Hardan (2006) also examined the use of olanzapine over 8 weeks in 16 children (age 13 to 17 years) diagnosed with a Disruptive Behavior Disorder and below average intelligence (i.e., IQs ranging from 36 to 79). Results of the study indicated significant reductions in disruptive behavior. With regard to aripiprazole, Greenaway and Elbe (2009) completed a research review and suggested findings similar to research examining risperidone and olanzapine but cautioned that less research has been completed on aripiprazole as compared to risperidone.

THE BAD

Although antipsychotic medications may have efficacy in treating children as suggested by the research summarized above, this usage is problematic for several reasons. First, a plethora of side effects related to atypical antipsychotic medications exist. Second, children appear to be at a higher risk for side effects, such as sedation, weight gain, Movement Disorders, and so forth, compared to adults (Findling, 2003; Zito, Derivan et al., 2008). Third, although recent research has begun examining the effects of risperidone in children in great detail, less research has examined the effects of other atypical antipsychotic medications. Specifically, olanzapine and aripiprazole have received little attention, and quetiapine, ziprasidone, and other medications in this class have received even less attention. Finally, although short-term effects are better known, long-term effects are less studied or unknown. Thus, the efficacy of atypical antipsychotic medications must be weighed against their potential costs.

As noted in the introduction of this chapter, a possible explanation for the increase of antipsychotic medication in the treatment of children may be related to the introduction of atypical antipsychotic medications, which have a less severe side effect profile compared to traditional antipsychotic medications. Although atypical antipsychotic medications indeed have less severe side effects than traditional antipsychotic medications, it still must be emphasized that negative side effects, or adverse events, exist.

One particularly concerning adverse event is Neuroleptic Malignant Syndrome (NMS), a rare iatrogenic reaction to antipsychotic medications that is potentially fatal (Croarkin et al., 2008; Greenaway & Elbe, 2009; Neuhut, Lindenmayer, & Silva, 2009). Although this disorder is not well understood, symptoms may include "rigidity, fever, increased serum creatine phosphokinase levels, leukocytosis, autonomic instability, tachypnea, delirium, and diaphoresis" (Croarkin et al., 2008, p. 1158) in addition to altered mental status and tachycardia (Neuhut et al., 2009). Croarkin et al. (2008) and Neuhut et al. (2009) report a low incidence rate of NMS in adults but state that there is a lack of information regarding NMS in children. In addition to NMS, severe movement problems including extrapyramidal symptoms, dystonia, tremor, akathisia, and tardive dyskinesia are associated with atypical antipsychotic medications (Correll & Kane, 2007; Farrell et al., 2010; Greenaway & Elbe, 2009; Haas et al., 2008; Reyes, Olah et al., 2006; Scott & Dhillon, 2008; Zito, Derivan et al., 2008). Another serious adverse event is cardiac problems including tachycardia, QTc interval prolongation, and cardiac arrest (Greenaway & Elbe, 2009; Ray, Chung, Murray, Hall, & Stein, 2009; Ritchie & Norris, 2009). Although the adverse events described above all have a low incidence, the effects are of great severity and lethal in some cases (e.g., NMS, cardiac arrest).

The most common adverse event associated with atypical antipsychotic medications is weight gain beyond normal maturation (Varley & McClellan, 2009). Nearly every study examining the use of atypical antipsychotic medications in children reports this side effect (Caldwell et al., 2008; Croonenberghs et al., 2005; Findling et al., 2004; Fraguas et al., 2008; Greenaway & Elbe, 2009; Haas et al., 2008; Handen & Hardan, 2006; Research Units on Pediatric Psychopharmacology Autism Network, 2005; Reyes, Olah et al., 2006; Scott & Dhillon, 2008; Troost et al., 2005; Zito, Derivan et al., 2008). This is a particularly concerning adverse event given how common it is and given increasing concerns regarding childhood obesity (e.g., childhood obesity associated with negative physical and psychological outcomes and targeted by several programs in the United States; Fraguas et al., 2008). Other metabolic and hormonal adverse events include increased appetite, nausea, vomiting, constipation, increased saliva, dry mouth, gastrointestinal bleeding, hyperglycemia, dyslipidemia, liver function changes, hyperprolactinemia, and hyperthyroidism (Coskun & Mukaddes, 2008; Erdogan et al., 2008; Fraguas et al., 2008; Greenaway & Elbe, 2009; Scott & Dhillon, 2008; Zito, Derivan et al., 2008).

Somnolence, fatigue, and lethargy appear to be the most frequent adverse events following weight gain (Caldwell et al., 2008; De Deyn & Buitelaar, 2006; Greenaway & Elbe, 2009; Scott & Dhillon, 2008; Troost et al., 2005) and may occur in 26 to 78% of cases (Caldwell et al., 2008; Greenaway & Elbe, 2009). This adverse event is especially important given that somnolence, fatigue, and lethargy are mutually exclusive with the symptoms (i.e., disruptive behaviors) most frequently targeted by atypical antipsychotic medications. A sleepy, tired child by definition is less likely to engage in disruptive behavior. Thus, atypical antipsychotic medications may be effective due to a side effect of the medication rather than being used to target specific symptoms.

Many other adverse events have been reported and include edema (Akdag, Fettahoglu, & Ozatalay, 2009), sexual dysfunction (e.g., frequent penile erections; Wadoo & Chalhoub, 2009), headache (Greenaway & Eble, 2009), upper respiratory tract infection (Scott & Dhillon, 2008), and epistaxis (Coskun & Mukaddes, 2008). Although the adverse events described above are certainly concerning, perhaps of greatest concern is what is not reported. Specifically, adverse events may be underreported by 80 to 95% (Elbe, 2009; Hazell & Shakir, 2006), suggesting that the actual occurrence of adverse events is much, much higher than that demonstrated in the extant literature.

Aside of the negative effects described above, a large proportion of children treated with atypical antipsychotic medications discontinue treatment due to loss of or no efficacy or an increase in severity of symptoms (Croonenberghs et al., 2005; Handen & Hardan, 2006; Research Units on Pediatric Psychopharmacology Autism Network, 2005; Reyes, Buitelaar et al., 2006; Troost et al., 2005). In fact, Troost et al. (2005), Reyes, Buitelaar et al. (2006), and Handen and Hardan (2006) reported that 28% (10 out of 36), 21% (113 out of 527), and 25% (4 out of 16) of their samples, respectively, discontinued treatment due to the lack of initial or continued response to atypical antipsychotic medications or worsening of symptoms. Further, many treatment responders ultimately discontinue use of the medication due to an adverse event.

What to Do About It

The first step in deciding what to do about a child who may benefit from the use of atypical antipsychotic medication is to determine if such medication is necessary. Many psychosocial and behavioral interventions are highly effective for the symptoms targeted by atypical antipsychotic medications.. For example, parent management training, collaborate problem solving, parent-child interaction therapy, empathy and social skills training, promoting prosocial behavior and problem-solving skills, and other treatments are all effective at treating children who are commonly prescribed atypical antipsychotic medications and are validated extensively (Kazdin, 1995, 2007). Some children, such as those experiencing a Pervasive Development Disorder or Intellectual Disability, may be particularly difficult to treat, making the use of atypical antipsychotic medication quite attractive (i.e., improve their behavior simply by taking medicine). Even in these cases, however, psychosocial and behavioral interventions are recommended as the first line of treatment. Specifically, Conduct Disorder and Autism, disorders that are perceived traditionally to be difficult to treat, have psychosocial and behavioral treatments which are validated highly (e.g., early intensive behavioral interventions; Eldevik et al., 2009; Kazdin, 2007; Shaw, Bruce, Ouimet, Sharma, & Glaser, 2009).

Overall, a psychosocial or behavioral treatment should be considered the treatment of choice, and these interventions should be implemented even if atypical antipsychotic medications are used in treatment. De Deyn and Buitelaar (2006), among others (e.g., Farrell et al., 2010; McKinney & Renk, 2011; Shaw et al., 2009), recommend that treatment of children begins with psychosocial and behavioral interventions and not medication. They suggest that if psychosocial interventions are ineffective, medications to treat the primary diagnosis may be used (e.g., a stimulant for Attention-Deficit/Hyperactivity Disorder). If this approach does not improve the situation, non-specific medications may be considered (e.g., the use of atypical antipsychotic medications to treat disruptive behavior) in addition to primary therapy and only as a last resort.

McKinney and Renk (2011) offer additional recommendations when deciding upon the use of atypical antipsychotic medications to treat children. Specifically, atypical antipsychotic medications should be used only when 1) a reasonable etiology for the child's condition is established, 2) at least three psychosocial/behavioral interventions have been attempted, 3) a rationale for the lack of effectiveness of the interventions is provided, 4) the targeted symptoms are determined to be wholly intransigent, and 5) the targeted symptoms would cause more potential harm than the worst reasonably expected side effects (e.g., somnolence and weight gain may be preferred over head trauma resulting from self-injurious behavior).

When atypical antipsychotic medications are used, Zito, Derivan et al. (2008) recommend monitoring the effects of the medications closely and using the lowest dosage necessary to achieve positive effects. Although side effects still occur at lower doses, they occur less frequently and with less severity (Findling et al., 2004).

Finally, in research completed by Sivaprasad et al. (2006), it was found that many medical doctors share concerns about best practices regarding atypical antipsychotic medications. Specifically, doctors expressed their concerns about 1) the occurrence of adverse events, 2) a lack of clear monitoring guidelines and difficulties monitoring outpatients, 3) differences between adults and children, 4) off-label use of atypical antipsychotic medications, 5) increases in parental concerns and media attention (e.g., cases of children on atypical antipsychotic medications dying), 6) a lack of consensus on the use of atypical antipsychotic medications with children, 7) a difficulty gaining expertise in the use of atypical antipsychotic medications, and 8) pressure to provide a quick cure and appease pharmaceutical companies. Consistent with the above recommendations, these doctors further stated that the use of atypical antipsychotic medications is recommended only when absolutely necessary, in the smallest possible dose for the shortest possible duration, and in conjunction with other psychological treatments. Also, these doctors suggested obtaining a second opinion, conducting a risk-benefit analysis, and openly discussing possible issues with parents before making a decision to prescribe atypical antipsychotic medications to children.

CONCLUSION

The use of atypical antipsychotic medications in children has increased dramatically worldwide. Overall, many research studies demonstrate at least some efficacy for the use of atypical antipsychotic medications, particularly risperidone, in the treatment of children. Specifically, many children who are treated with atypical antipsychotic medications experience a decrease in disruptive behavior. These benefits must be weighed against the costs associated with atypical antipsychotic medications. A large proportion of children who take these medications do not respond well (e.g., no initial or continued response or worsening of symptoms) and most all experience some sort of adverse event, some of which are debilitating and lethal. In all cases, other methods of treatment should be considered first as suggested in the recommendations described above. Finally, researchers who conduct research on atypical antipsychotic medications and professionals who prescribe atypical antipsychotic medications must proceed with great caution and follow recommendations suggested here and elsewhere. Until more data are available, less risky interventions should be used and children receiving atypical antipsychotic medications should be monitored very closely (Sivaprasad et al., 2006;Varley & McClellan, 2009).

REFERENCES

Akdag, S. T., Fettahoglu, E. C., & Ozatalay, E. (2009). Pedal edema induced by low-dose risperidone monotherapy in a child. *Journal of Child and Adolescent Psychopharmacology, 19*, 481-482.

Caldwell, M. F., Malterer, M., Umstead, D., & McCormick, D. J. (2008). A retrospective evaluation of adjunctive risperidone treatment in severely behaviorally disordered boys receiving psychosocial treatment. *Journal of Child and Adolescent Psychopharmacology, 18*, 34-43.

Correll, C. U., & Kane, J. M. (2007). One-year incidence rates of tardive dyskinesia in children and adolescents treated with second-generation antipsychotics: A systematic review. *Journal of Child and Adolescent Psychopharmacology, 17*, 647-655.

Coskun, M., & Mukaddes, N. M. (2008). Possible risperidone-related gastrointestinal bleeding or epistaxis in two pediatric cases. *Journal of Child and Adolescent Psychopharmacology, 18*, 299-300.

Croarkin, P. E., Emslie, G. J., & Mayes, T. L. (2008). Neuroleptic malignant syndrome associated with atypical antipsychotics in pediatric patients: A review of published cases. *Journal of Clinical Psychiatry, 69*, 1157-1165.

Croonenberghs, J., Fegert, J. M., Findling, R. L., De Smedt, G., Van Dongen, S., & the risperidone Disruptive Behavior Study Group. (2005). Risperidone in children with Disruptive Behavior Disorders and subaverage intelligence: A 1-year, open-label study of 504 patients. *Journal of the American Academy of Child and Adolescent Psychiatry, 44,* 64-72.

De Deyn, P. P., & Buitelaar, J. (2006). Risperidone in the management of agitation and aggression associated with psychiatric disorders. *European Psychiatry, 21,* 21-28.

Elbe, D. (2009). Commentary to QTc prolongation associated with atypical antipsychotic use in the treatment of adolescent-onset Anorexia Nervosa. *Journal of the Canadian Academy of Child and Adolescent Psychiatry, 18,* 64.

Eldevik, S., Hastings, R. P., Hughes, J. C., Jahr, E., Eikeseth, S., & Cross, S. (2009). Meta-analysis of early intensive behavioral intervention for children with autism. *Journal of Clinical Child and Adolescent Psychology, 38*, 439-450.

Erdogan, A., Atasoy, N., Akkurt, H., Ozturk, D., Karaahmet, E., Yalug, I., Yalug, K., Ankarali, H., & Balcioglu, I. (2008). Risperidone and liver function tests in children and adolescents: A short-term prospective study. *Progress in Neuropsychopharmacology and Biological Psychiatry, 32*, 849-857.

Farrell, D., Fischer, J., & McCabe, P. C. (2010). Tardive dyskinesia with typical and atypical antipsychotic medications in children and adolescents. In P. C. McCabe, S. R. Shaw, P. C. McCabe, S. R. Shaw (Eds.), *Psychiatric disorders: Current topics and interventions for educators* (pp. 60-70). Thousand Oaks, CA: Corwin Press.

Findling, R. (2003). Dosing of atypical antipsychotics in children and adolescents. *Primary Care Companion Journal of Clinical Psychiatry, 5,* 10-13.

Findling, R. L., Aman, R. G., Eerdekens, M., Derivan, A., & Lyons, B. (2004). Long-term, open-label study of risperidone in children with severe disruptive behaviors and below-average IQ. *American Journal of Psychiatry, 161,* 677-684.

Fraguas, D., Merchan-Naranjo, J., Laita, P., Parallada, M., Moreno, D., Ruiz-Sancho, A., Cifuentes, A., Giraldez, M., & Arango, C. (2008). Metabolic and hormonal side effects in children and adolescents treated with second-generation antipsychotics. *Journal of Clinical Psychiatry, 69*, 1166-1175.

Greenaway, M., & Elbe, D. (2009). Focus on aripiprazole: A review of its use in child and adolescent psychiatry. *Journal of the Canadian Academy of Child and Adolescent Psychiatry, 18,* 250-260.

Haas, M., Karcher, K., & Pandina, G. J. (2008). Treating Disruptive Behavior Disorders with risperidone: A 1-year, open-label safety study in children and adolescents. *Journal of Child and Adolescent Psychopharmacology, 18*, 337-346.

Handen, B. L., & Hardan, A. Y. (2006). Open-label, prospective trail of olanzapine in adolescents with subaverage intelligence and Disruptive Behavior Disorders. *Journal of the American Academy of Child and Adolescent Psychiatry, 45,* 928-935.

Hazell, L., & Shakir, S. A. (2006). Under-reporting of adverse drug reactions: A systematic review. *Drug Safety, 29*, 385-396.

Kazdin, A. E. (1995). *Conduct Disorder in childhood and adolescence* (2nd ed.). Newbury Park, CA: Sage.

Kazdin, A. E. (2007). Psychosocial treatments for conduct disorder in children and adolescents. In P. E. Nathan & J. M. Gorman (Eds.), *A guide to treatments that work* (3rd ed.; pp. 71-104). New York, NY: Oxford University Press.

Masi, G., Milone, A., Canepa, G., Millepiedi, S., Mucci, M., & Muratori, F. (2006). Olanzapine treatment in adolescents with severe conduct disorder. *European Psychiatry, 21,* 51-57.

Mehler-Wex, C., Romanos, M., Kirchheiner, J., & Schulze, U. M. E. (2008). Atypical antipsychotics in severe Anorexia Nervosa in children and adolescents: Review and case reports. *European Eating Disorders Review, 16*, 100-108.

McKinney, C., & Renk, K. (2011). Atypical antipsychotic medications in the management of disruptive behaviors in children: Safety guidelines and recommendations. *Clinical Psychology Review, 31,* 465-471.

Neuhut, R., Lindenmayer, J. P., & Silva, R. (2009). Neuroleptic malignant syndrome in children and adolescents on atypical antipsychotic medication: A review. *Journal of Child and Adolescent Psychopharmacology, 19*, 415-422.

Olfson, M., Blanco, C., Liu, L., Moreno, C., & Laje, G. (2006). National trends in the outpatient treatment of children and adolescents with antipsychotic drugs. *Archives of General Psychiatry, 63,* 679-685.

Ray, W. A., Chung, C.P., Murray, K. T., Hall, K., & Stein, C. (2009). Atypical antipsychotic drugs and the risk of sudden cardiac death. *New England Journal of Medicine, 360*, 225-235.

Research Units on Pediatric Psychopharmacology Autism Network. (2005). Risperidone treatment of autistic disorder: Longer-term benefits and blinded discontinuation after 6 months. *American Journal of Psychiatry, 162,* 1361-1369.

Reyes, M., Buitelaar, J., Toren, P., Augustyns, I., & Eerdekens, M. (2006). A randomized, double-blind, placebo-controlled study of risperidone maintenance treatment in children and adolescents with Disruptive Behavior Disorders. *American Journal of Psychiatry, 163,* 402-410.

Reyes, M., Olah, R., Csaba, K., Augustyns, I., & Eerdekens, M. (2006). Long-term safety and efficacy of risperidone in children with Disruptive Behavior Disorders. *European Child and Adolescent Psychiatry, 15,* 97-104.

Ritchie, B., & Norris, M. L. (2009). QTc prolongation associated with atypical antipsychotic use the treatment of adolescent-onset Anorexia Nervosa. *Journal of the Canadian Academy of Child and Adolescent Psychiatry, 18,* 60-63.

Scott, L. J., & Dhillon, S. (2008). Spotlight on risperidone in irritability associated with Autistic Disorder in children and adolescents. *CNS Drugs, 22*, 259-262.

Sivaprasad, L., Hassan, T., & Handy, S. (2006). Survey of atypical antipsychotic medication use by child and adolescent psychiatrists. *Child and Adolescent Mental Health, 11,* 164-167.

Shaw, S. R., Bruce, J., Ouimet, T., Sharma, A., & Glaser, S. (2009). Young children with developmental disabilities and atypical antipsychotic medications: Dual diagnosis, direction, and debate. *Journal of Early Childhood and Infant Psychology*, 537-55.

Staller, J. A., Wade, M. J., & Baker, M. (2005). Current prescribing patterns in outpatient child and adolescent psychiatric practice in central New York. *Journal of Child and Adolescent Psychopharmacology, 15,* 57-61.

Stigler, K. A., & McDougle, C. J. (2008). Pharmacotherapy of irritability in Pervasive Developmental Disorders. *Child and Adolescent Psychiatric Clinics of North America, 17,* 739-752.

Troost, P. W., Lahuis, B. E., Steenhuis, M. P., Ketelaars, C. E. J., Buitelaar, J. K., Van Engeland, H., Scahill, L., Minderaa, R. B., & Hoekstra, P. J. (2005). Long-term effects of risperidone in children with autism spectrum disorders: A placebo discontinuation study. *Journal of the American Academy of Child and Adolescent Psychiatry, 44,* 1137-1144.

Varley, C. K., & McClellan, J. (2009). Implications of marked weight gain associated with atypical antipsychotic medications in children and adolescents. *Journal of the American Medical Association*, 302, 1811-1812.

Wadoo, O., & Chalhoub, N. (2009). Risperidone-induced sexual dysfunction in a prepubertal child: A case report. *Journal of Psychopharmacology, 23*, 727-728.

Zito, J. M., Derivan, A. T., Kratochvil, C. J., Safer, D. J., Fegert, J. M., & Greenhill, L. L. (2008). Off-label psychopharmacologic prescribing for children: History supports close clinical monitoring. *Child and Adolescent Psychiatry and Mental Health, 2*, 24.

Zito, J. M., Safer, D. J., Jong-van den Berg, L. T. W., Janhsen, K., Fegert, J. M., Glaeske, G., & Valluri, S. C. (2008). A three-country comparison of psychotropic medication prevalence in youth. *Child and Adolescent Psychiatry and Mental Health, 2*, 26.

PART II: PHARMOCOKINETICS / PHARMACODYNAMICS / APPLICATIONS

In: Antipsychotic Drugs
Editors: T.L. Schwartz, J. Megna and M.E. Topel
ISBN: 978-1-62100-071-6

Chapter 4

PHARMACOKINETIC PROPERTIES OF SECOND GENERATION ANTIPSYCHOTICS

Kristina Bedynerman [*] ***and James Megna***
SUNY Upstate Medical University, Syracuse, NY, US

ABSTRACT

Introduction: Pharmacokinetic properties determine how the body will release, absorb, distribute, metabolize and excrete a particular agent. The purpose of this chapter is to review literature pertaining to the clinical aspects of pharmacokinetic properties. We will discuss the pharmacokinetic properties of each 2nd generation antipsychotic and the associated theoretical and evidence based implications for clinical practice.

Conclusion: Understanding pharmacokinetic properties of 2nd generation antipsychotics may be utilized as an important tool in guiding clinical practice. What the body does with a drug may impact its efficacy, tolerability and toxicity which subsequently may impact clinical outcomes. Considering pharmacokinetic properties of an agent may influence our treatment decisions and, therefore, represents, an important tool in our knowledge and application of psychopharmacology.

INTRODUCTION

Pharmacokinetics may be simply defined as what the body does to the drug, as opposed to pharmacodynamics which may be defined as what the drug does to the body [1]. In other words, pharmacokinetic properties determine how the body will release, absorb, distribute, metabolize and excrete a particular agent. Each antipsychotic has a unique pharmacokinetic profile which may play a role in its efficacy, tolerability and toxicity. We will discuss the pharmacokinetic properties of each 2nd generation antipsychotic and the associated theoretical and evidence based implications for clinical practice. For the purpose of structure we will

* Corresponding author: Kristina Bedynerman; SUNY Upstate Medical University, 750 East Adams Street, Syracuse, NY 13210; Ph (315) 464-3100; Fax (315) 464-3178; E-mail: Bedynerk@upstate.edu

describe each antipsychotic in the decreasing order of their respective half life (t 1/2), which is defined at the amount of time needed to decrease the drug plasma concentration by 50%.

ARIPIPRAZOLE

Aripiprazole is approved for the treatment of schizophrenia (dosed 10-15mg a day), bipolar disorder (dosed 15 mg a day), adjunctive treatment of major depressive disorder (dosed 2-15 mg a day), as well as for agitation associated with schizophrenia and bipolar disorder (dosed 9.75 mg used intramuscularly) [2].

Aripiprazole has the longest half life out of all second generation antipsychotics, 75 hours. It takes approximately 5 t ½'s in order to achieve complete drug clearance, which theoretically means that it may take a little over 15 days to completely clear aripiprazole from the circulation. This long clearance may theoretically contribute to the longer time needed to observe the individual following an overdose as well as the longer time needed to achieve complete resolution of symptoms, especially in vulnerable populations such as children [3]. One retrospective study linked longer acting second generation antipsychotics with lower risk of hospital admissions/ED visits for adults with schizophrenia [4]. A combination of aripiprazole's, long t 1/2 as well as its high affinity for the D2/D3 receptor, may also have implications in cross titration to another antipsychotic agent, as it may take up to two weeks to clear aripiprazole from the system and subsequently observe the effect of the up titrating agent [5]. Aripiprazole is mostly fecally excreted which suggests that no dose adjustment is required for patients with known renal impairment. [2] Aripiprazole is a substrate for the 2D6 and 3A4 isozymes, therefore caution should be advised when it is used in conjunction with a potent 2D6 inhibitors such as fluoxetine and paroxitine. [2] Aripiprazole's dose may thus need to be decreased under such circumstances.

Aripiprazole is available in tablets, oral solution (Diskmelt) and as an injection. Oral tablets reach peak plasma concentration in 3-5 hours and are 86% bioavailable. In comparison, the intramuscular injection is 100% bioavailable and reaches its peak plasma concentration in 1-3 hours [2]. Also, the plasma concentration of the aripiprazole injection is 90% higher 2 hours after administration then that of the aripiprazole tablet.

Furthermore, the systemic exposure of the 2 formulations in a 24 hour period appears to be generally similar. Based on these pharmacokinetic properties, we can theoretically understand why the intramuscular injection would likely be more efficacious in an acute setting at the expense of a greater side effect burden. Similarly, the oral solution appears to be slightly more bioavailable (with increased plasma concentration) compared to the tablet [2], which may theoretically offer more acute efficacy at the cost of potential side effects.

OLANZAPINE

Olanzpaine is approved for the treatment of schizophrenia (dosed 10 mg a day), bipolar disorder, manic mixed (dosed 5-20 mg a day), bipolar disorder, depressive episode (dosed 5-12.5 mg a day), treatment resistant depression (dosed 5-20 mg a day), and also as treatment for agitation associated with schizophrenia and bipolar disorder, dosed 10 mg intramuscularly.

Olanzapine has a t 1/2 of 21-54 hrs, on average 37 hrs. As discussed with aripiprazole, the longer t 1/2 may contribute to more lasting effects in the case of an overdose, which may warrant a longer monitoring period. In addition, the therapeutic effects/side effects may linger long after the drug has been discontinued, which should be considered in guiding clinical treatment and outcome.

Olanzapine is metabolized by the CYP 450 1A2, 2D6 isozymes, and is also a substrate for 2C19. It is excreted primarily by urine (57%) and feces (30%) [6]. Smoking induces the 1A2 enzyme and therefore plasma concentrations of olanzapine may be lowered by smoking, which may have clinical implications. A 2004 case report demonstrated decreased olanzapine plasma levels and subsequent clinical decline in a 30 year old schizophrenic male who re-started smoking once discharged from the inpatient unit [7]. Inversely, abrupt smoking cessation, which may result from hospitalization, may contribute to increased olanzapine plasma concentrations and, therefore, contribute to increased potential for side effects such as extrapyramidal symptoms [8].

Olanzapine is available in tablets, oral disintegrating tablets, as a short acting intramuscular injection, as well as a depot injection under the brand name of Zyprexa Relprevv. According to the manufacturer, olanzapine is eliminated extensively by first pass metabolism, with approximately 40% of the dose metabolized before it reaches systemic circulation [6]. Oral olanzapine reaches its maximum plasma concentration in 6 hours following ingestion. The intramuscular injection, however, reaches its peak concentration within 15-45 minutes and, secondary to avoiding first pass metabolism, achieves a peak plasma concentration 5 times that of the oral tablet [6]. Based on this package insert information maximum, the plasma concentration of 5 mg of injectable Zyprexa may be equivalent to 25 mg of an oral tablet. This may explain the efficacy of utilizing the intramuscular injection vs. an oral tablet formulation in the treatment of acute psychotic agitation at the expense of increased side effect burden. Theoretically, the oral disintegrating tablet also avoids the first pass effect which may result in a more rapidly achieved and higher peak plasma concentration. However, there are no data from head to head studies available at this time in support of this hypothesis. Lastly, there are some data that indicate the olanzapine sublingual tablet improves compliance [9].

Zyprexa Relprevv is a depot injection which allows for slower release of drug and may allow for biweekly to monthly dose administration.

Zyprexa Relprevv is indicated for those who are already taking the oral formulation and require a conversion to a depot administration. A 10 mg a day dose is equivalent to 210 mg intramuscularly every 2 weeks, or 405 mg intramuscularly every 4 weeks for a period of 8 weeks, then 150 mg intramuscularly every 2 weeks or 300 mg intramuscularly every 4 weeks. Conversion schedules are also available for 15 mg and 20 mg equivalent regimens [10]. The t 1/2 of Zyprexa Relprevv is 30 days [10].

Therefore, as discussed earlier, it could take up to 5 half lives, or in this case up to 5 months, to fully clear the drug. According to the manufacturer, 3 months may be required to reach plasma steady state. Zyprexa Relprevv is only available as a depot injection, in a registered and approved healthcare facility that can observe patients for at least 3 hours following administration for a potential delirium/sedation syndrome [10].

LOPERIDONE

Iloperidone is FDA approved for the treatment of schizophrenia and it is one of the newer antipsychotics available. It has a complicated titration schedule starting with 1mg twice daily for 1 day, then 2mg twice daily and then increased by 4mg/day daily until the efficacious dose of 12-24 mg/day is reached.

It has a t 1/2 of 18-36 hours, is extensively metabolized through the liver, and is a substrate for the 2D6 and 3A4 isozymes. Subsequently, those who are poor 2D6 and 3A4 metabolizers will have longer t 1/2's, e.g. 36 hours instead of 18. In addition, the iloperidone dose should be halved when co-administered with a strong 2D6 inhibitor such as fluoxetine or paroxetine [11]. It is primarily excreted by the urine (45-58%) and feces (20%). No renal or hepatic dose adjustment is required per the manufacturer [11].

ASENAPINE

Asenapine is one of the newest antipsychotics on the market. It has FDA approval for the treatment of schizophrenia and bipolar mania at doses of 10-20 mg/day, starting with 5mg twice a day and increasing up to 10 mg twice a day.

It has a half life of 24 hours and it is a substrate for the 1A2 isozyme. Therefore, levels of asenapine may increase with administration of a 1A2 inhibitor such as fluvoxamine. However, based on crossover studies, smoking, which induces the CYP 1A2 isozyme does not appear to have an effect on the pharmacokinetics of asenapine. Asenapine's metabolism does depend significantly on hepatic function therefore it is contraindicated for those with hepatic impairment.

The unique feature of asenapine is that it is only available for sublingual administration.12 Following sublingual administration, asenapine is rapidly absorbed with peak plasma concentrations occurring within 0.5 to 1.5 hours. The sublingual administration may avoid first pass metabolism, thereby contributing to increased plasma concentration of the drug. However, even by avoiding the first pass effect asenapine's absolute bioavailability is only 35% in contrast to the <2% bioavailability with an oral tablet formulation, which may explain why the oral formulation is not currently available. 12 Water and food should be avoided for 10 minutes following administration due to their contribution to decreasing asenapine's absorption. In a crossover study, food consumption immediately prior to sublingual administration decreased asenapine's uptake by 20% while consumption of food 4 hours after the administration decreased it by 10% [12]. Asenapine's absorption may decrease by as much as 19% when water is administered 2 minutes afterwords, compared to a 10% decrease after water consumption 5 minutes following asenapine's administration [12].The opposite is true of ziprasidone and lurasidone which need to be taken with food [21, 22]. Asenapine is excreted 50% by urine and 40% by feces. Therefore, no dose adjustment is required for patients with renal impairment [12].

Paliperidone

Paliperidone is FDA approved for the treatment of schizophrenia and schizoaffective disorder, dosed once daily at 6-12 mg. It is the active metabolite of risperidone and has a t 1/2 of 23 hours and is excreted 80% renally. As a result, a dose adjustment is required for those with renal impairment [13].

Since paliperidone is the active metabolite of risperidone, it requires little work by the liver's P450 enzyme system which may eliminate concerns for drug to drug interactions or individual metabolism intervariability. In addition, no dose adjustment is required for patients with impaired hepatic function. Paliperidone is dosed once a day through the osmotic-controlled release oral delivery system (OROS), which may reduce dose frequency, contribute to more stable drug concentrations, and may improve tolerability [14, 15].

Paliperidone is also available as a long acting injectable under the brand name invega sustenna (paliperidone palmitate). It is unique in that it is administered monthly with no oral supplementation needed for the first 3 weeks of treatment as it is with risperdal consta [16, 17]. However, tolerability to either oral risperidone or paliperidone is required prior to initiation of treatment [16]. Invega sustenna is administered in the deltoid muscle with a dose of 234 mg on treatment day one and then with 156 mg one week later. The recommended monthly maintenance is 117mg, with a range of 39 mg to 234 mg based on individual efficacy and tolerability [16].

The t 1/2 of invega sustenna (paliperidone palmitate) ranges from 25-49 days and the release of the drug starts as early as day 1 and lasts for as long as 126 days, reaching maximum plasma concentration at a median Tmax of 13 days [16]. Paliperidone palmitate is poorly soluble in water and therefore dissolves slowly after intramuscular injection before being hydrolyzed to paliperidone and absorbed into the circulation. This slow release mechanism may explain why such a high initial dose is needed in order to achieve therapeutic plasma concentration. The initial plasma levels of invega sustenna following a 234 mg dose of are within the exposure range observed with 6-12 mg of extended release oral paliperidone [16].

Similar to paliperidone extended release tablets, invega sustenna is 80% renally excreted, therefore a dose adjustment is recommended for mild renal impairment. The recommended dose of invega sustenna for mild renal impairment is 156 mg on day 1 and 117 mg on treatment day 8. Thereafter, monthly injections of 78 mg follow. The use of invega sustenna is not recommended in those with moderate and severe renal impairment. No dose adjustment is required for patients with mild or moderate hepatic impairment and it has not been studies in those with severe hepatic impairment.

Risperidone

Risperidone is one of the oldest atypical antipsychotics next to clozapine. It has a t 1/2 of 20 hours and it is a substrate for 2D6. Excretion is 70% renal, therefore, dose adjustment is required for those with renal impairment.

It is FDA approved for the treatment of schizophrenia, bipolar disorder, manic or mixed episode with an average dose of 3-4mg/day. It is also approved for the treatment of irritability in autism at lower doses of 1-3mg/day [17].

Risperidone is available as an oral solution, a tablet and an oral disintegrating tablet under the brand name risperdal M-Tab, and as a depot injectable under the brand name Risperdal Consta.

According to the manufacturer the absolute oral availability of risperidone is 70%. Following oral administration of solution or tablet, mean peak plasma concentrations occur at about 1 hour. 17 Pharmacokinetic studies show that Risperdal M-tab and Risperidone oral solution are bioequivalent to risperidone tablets [17].

Risperdal consta is available as a depot injection in 25 mg, 37.5mg or 50 mg dosage aliquots that can be initiated following an established tolerability to risperidone tablets or solution [18]. Risperdal consta utilizes a microsphere technology in which less than 1% of the medication is available upon initial injection while the remainder is slowly released, reaching therapeutic plasma concentration 3 weeks following initial injection. Therefore, it is imperative to continue oral supplementation for a period of 3 weeks. The therapeutic dose is then gradually decreased from weeks 4-6 and then dropped by week 7 [18].

A few studies have compared long acting injectable second generation antipsychotics with oral antipsychotics in terms of efficacy, rates of relapse and extrapyramidal symptoms. Some studies suggest that long acting injectables are advantageous in terms of efficacy with fewer extrapyramidal symptoms in early episode psychosis [19]. However, a recent study comparing injectable risperidone to a physician choice oral antipsychotic treatment demonstrated no significant advantage in efficacy or rates of rehospitalization in those patients treated with long acting injectable risperidone. Furthermore, according to this study, patients who received long acting injectable risperidone reported more adverse events at the injection site and more extrapyramidal symptoms [20]. One of the limitations of this study is that long acting injectable risperidone was compared to a "physician choice" oral antipsychotic which may have confounded the results.

LURASIDONE

Lurasidone was FDA approved for the treatment of schizophrenia in October of 2010. It comes in a 40mg and 80 mg tablet and should be consumed with food (at least 350 cal) to allow for therapeutic plasma concentrations to be reached. It is a pregnancy category B drug which has shown no known teratogenic effects in mice or rabbits. The only other antipsychotic that is category B in pregnancy is clozapine. Lurasidone is metabolized by the CYP 3A4 isozyme and, therefore, should not be used with a strong 3A4 inhibitor such as ketocanozole, or strong inducers such as rifampin and phenytoin. Lurasidone has a t 1/2 of 18 hours [21].

ZIPRASIDONE

Ziprasidone is FDA approved for the treatment of schizophrenia at doses of 20-80 mg twice a day, bipolar disorder, manic or mixed episode, dosed at 40-80 mg twice a day, as well as for acute psychotic agitation at a dose of 10 mg administered intramuscularly [22].

It has a short half life of 7 hours and has been found efficacious as a twice a day administered medication. The relatively short t 1/2 theoretically may contribute to increased withdrawal symptoms when ziprasidone is discontinued abruptly, however there is no clinical evidence available to support this hypothesis.

Ziprasidone is well absorbed after oral administration, reaching peak plasma concentrations in 6-8 hours with an absolute bioavailability of approximately 60% in the presence of food, which may increase the bioavailability up to two fold. Therefore, if the ziprasidone dose is ineffective at controlling symptoms it would be clinically prudent to assess whether the medication is being taken with food or not. Also, this property may be utilized in a dosing up or down titration of ziprasidone by adding or removing food consumption without changing the actual dose. Bioavailability of ziprasidone administered intramuscularly is 100% and peak plasma concentration occurs within 60 minutes with a slightly shorter t 1/2 of 2-5 hours [22].

Although ziprasidone is greater than 99% protein bound, its in vitro plasma protein binding was not shown to be altered by coumadin or propranolol, both of which are highly protein bound drugs. Ziprasidone also did not alter the binding of coumadin or propranolol in human plasma which likely indicates that the interaction of ziprasidone with other highly protein bound agents via displacement is minimal [22].

Ziprasidone is mostly fecally excreted and highly metabolized by the liver with less than 1% of the drug excreted unchanged. Therefore, no dose adjustment is required for those with renal impairment. However, because it is largely metabolized by the liver, hepatic impairment may increase plasma concentration by 13-34%, yet a dose adjustment for those with hepatic impairment is not advised by the manufacturer. Ziprasidone does not appear to inhibit or induce any of the CYP 450 isozymes, however, it is a substrate for CYP3A4. Therefore, concomitant administration of a CYP 3A4 inducer, such as carbamazepine, or a CYP 3A4 inhibitor, such as ketoconazole, may affect the plasma concentration by as much as 35-40%. Interestingly, less than 1/3 of ziprasidone's metabolism is mediated by the cytochrome P450 system with the majority of the metabolic action mediated via aldehyde oxidase reduction. This may minimize drug-drug interactions since aldehyde oxidase does not appear to be affected by metabolic inhibitors or inducers. [22]

QUETIAPINE

Quetiapine has two formulations: immediate release (IR) and extended release (XR). Quetiapine IR is FDA approved for the treatment of schizophrenia divided doses of 150-750mg/day (2-3 times). It is also approved for the treatment of manic episodes of bipolar disorder at doses of 400-800mg/day for twice a day administration. In addition, it is approved for the treatment of depressed episodes of bipolar illness at a dose of 300mg-600mg at night

[23]. Quetiapine XR has the same FDA approvals with the addition of treatment resistant unipolar depression augmentation at a dose of 150-300mg at night [24].

The difference between the two formulations (XR vs. IR) is that the IR has a slightly shorter t 1/2 of 6hrs compared to 7-12 hrs for the XR. In addition the XR has a slower time to peak concentration, which may improve tolerability, resulting in faster titration time schedules. The XR can be initiated at a 300mg dose, unless the patient is elderly or debilitated, and the IR needs to be titrated slower starting with 50 mg BID. Both drugs are extensively metabolized by the liver into the active metabolite norquetiapine and are substrates for the 3A4 P450 isozyme. Therefore, dose adjustment of quetiapine may be necessary if it is administered with a strong CYP3A4 inducer such as phenytoin or an inhibitor such as ketoconazole [23]. Some dose adjustment may be required for patients with severe hepatic dysfunction however no adjustment is required for patients with renal impairment [23].

Bioavailability of quetiapine XR has been shown to be impacted by a high fat meal in a dose related fashion. As per the manufacturer, bioavailabilty of quetiapine XR increases by as much as 44%-52% following a high fat meal for the 50mg tablet. While bioavailability for a 300mg tablet increased by 20-22% [24]. However, a light meal of approximately 300 calories had no impact on quetiapine's plasma concentration. Therefore, the manufacturer recommends that quetiapine XR be consumed with a light meal or without food [24].

Bioavailability of quetiapine IR was also shown to be marginally affected by administration with food [23].

Conclusion

Understanding pharmacokinetic properties of 2nd generation antipsychotics may be utilized as an important tool in guiding clinical practice. What the body does with a drug may impact its efficacy, tolerability and toxicity which subsequently may impact clinical outcomes. Considering pharmacokinetic properties of an agent may influence our treatment decisions and, therefore, represents, an important tool in our knowledge and application of psychopharmacology.

References

[1] Benet, Z. L. Pharmacokinetics: Basic Principles and Its Use as a Tool in Drug Metabolism. *Drug Metabolism and Drug Toxicity*. J. R. Mitchell and M. G. Horning (eds.), Raven Press: New York 1984, 199-200.

[2] Aripiprazole package insert. http://packageinserts.bms.com/pi/pi_ bilify.pdf.Accessed March 13, 2012.

[3] Melhem, S., Katz, K., Jameson, A., et al. Prolonged toxicity in a 2 year old after accidental ingestion of aripiprazole. *Pediatric Emergency Care* 2009; 25:105-6.

[4] Broder, M. S., Bates, J. A., Jing, Y., et al. Association between second generation antipsychotic medication half life and hospitalization in the community treatment of adult schizophrenia. *J. Med. Econ*. 2011;15:105-11.

[5] Grunder, G., Fellows, C., Januschek, H., et al. Brain and plasma pharmacokinetics of aripiprazole in patients with schizophrenia: an (18) fallypride PET study. *Am. J. Psychiatry* 2008; 165: 988-95.

[6] Olanzapine package insert. http://pi.lilly.com/us/zyprexa-pi.pdf. Accessed Mar. 13, 2012.

[7] Chiu, C., Lu, M., Huang, M., et al. Heavy smoking, reduced olanzapine levels and treatment effects. *The drug monitoring* 2004;26: 579-81.

[8] Zullino, D. F., Delssert, D., Eap, C. B., et al. Tobacco and cannabis smoking cessation can lead to intoxification with clozapine or olanzapine. *Int. Clin. Psychopharmocol.* 2002; 17:141-3.

[9] San, L., Casillas, M., Cuidad, A., et al. Olanzapine orally disintegrating tablet; a review of efficacy and compliance. *CNS Neuropsychi. Ther.* 2008;14: 203-14.

[10] Ralprevv package insert. http://www.accessdata.fda.gov/drugsatfda_ docs/label/ 2009/022173lbl.pdf. Accessed Mar. 13, 2012.

[11] Iloperidone package insert. http://www.pharma.us.novartis.com/ product/pi/pdf/ fanapt.pdf. Accessed Mar. 13, 2012.

[12] Asenapine package insert. http://www.spfiles.com/pisaphrisv1.pdf. Accessed Mar. 13, 2012.

[13] Paliperidone package insert. http://www.accessdata.fda.gov/drugsatfda_ docs/label/ 2009/021999s013s014lbl.pdf. Accessed Mar. 13, 2012.

[14] Conley, R., Gupta, S. K., Sathyan, G. Clinical spectrum of the osmotic-controlled release oral delivery system (OROS), an advanced oral delivery form. *Curr. Med. Res. Opin.* 2006; 22:1879-92.

[15] Pani, L., Marchese, G. Expected clinical benefits of paliperidone extended release formulation when compared with risperidone immediate release. *Expert Opin. Drug Deliv.* 2009; 6:319-31.

[16] Invega sustenna package insert. http://www.janssenmedicalinformation. com/assets/pdf/products/files/Invega%20Sustenna/pi/LIB-INVS-069329-09.pdf. Accessed Mar. 13, 2012

[17] Risperidone package insert. http://www.risperdal.com/sites/default/ files/shared/pi/risperdal_uspi.pdf. Accessed Mar. 13, 2012.

[18] Risperdal consta package insert. http://www.risperdalconsta.com/sites/ default/ files/RisperdalConstaPI.pdf#zoom=100. Accessed Mar. 13, 2012,

[19] Emsley, R., Oosthuizen, P. M., Koen, L. M., et al. Oral versus injectable antipsychotic treatment in early psychosis: Post hoc comparison of two studies. *Clin. Ther.* 2008; 30: 2378-2386.

[20] Rosenheck, R. A., Krystal, J. H., Lew, R., et al. Long Acting Risperidone and Oral Antipsychotics in Unstable Schizophrenia. *N Engl. J. Med.* 2011; 364: 842-851.

[21] Lurasidone package insert. http://www.latuda.com/LatudaPrescribing Information.pdf. Accessed Mar. 13, 2012.

[22] Ziprasidone package insert. http://medicaidprovider.hhs.mt.gov/pdf/ geodonrxinfo.pdf. Accessed Mar. 13, 2012.

[23] Quetiapine package insert. http://www1.astrazeneca-us.com/pi/Seroquel. pdf. Accessed Mar. 13, 2012.

[24] Quietiapine, X. R. package insert. http://www1.astrazeneca-us.com/pi/ seroquelxr.pdf. Accessed Mar. 13, 2012.

In: Antipsychotic Drugs
Editors: T.L. Schwartz, J. Megna and M.E. Topel
ISBN: 978-1-62100-071-6

Chapter 5

TRANSLATING BASIC SCIENCE INTO CLINICAL PRACTICE WHILE DOSING THE SECOND GENERATION ANTIPSYCHOTICS

Thomas L. Schwartz,[1*] Umar Siddiqui[1] and Stephen M. Stahl[2,3]

[1]Department of Psychiatry, State University of New York Upstate Medical University, NY, US
[2]Department of Psychiatry, University of California San Diego, San Diego, CA, US
[3]Department of Psychiatry, Cambridge University, UK

ABSTRACT

Introduction: The second generation antipsychotics are often utilized in the treatment of schizophrenia, bipolar depression, bipolar mania, autism, major depressive disorder, anxiety disorder, sleep disorder, pervasive developmental disorder, conduct disorder and attention deficit hyperactivity disorder. Each agent is unique in its pharmacodynamic profile and knowledge of basic pharmacology science may allow for unique dosing strategies while treating specific disorders. A MEDLINE and recent textbook review was conducted regarding current and investigational second generation antipsychotics and cross-referenced with searches for major mental disorders.

Conclusion: The second generation antipsychotics are clearly approved for the treatment of psychosis and mania at higher doses which highly utilize dopamine-2 receptor antagonism for efficacy and serotonin-2a receptor antagonism for extrapyramidal side effect tolerability. Otherwise, each agent has a unique pharmacodynamic profile where some agents carry more, or less antidepressant, anxiolyic, or hypnotic properties. This review suggests ways clinicians may utilize basic science information and clinical trial results to formulate and optimize second generation antipsychotic treatment plans.

* Corresponding author: Thomas L. Schwartz, M.D., Department of Psychiatry State University of New York Upstate Medical University, 713 Harrison Street Syracuse, NY, US. Tel.: 315464-31 66. Fax: 315 464-3163. E-mail: schwartt@upstate.edu.

INTRODUCTION

The first generation antipsychotics (FGA) were approved in the 1950's and were utilized in a very focused manner. These drugs were approved to treat one psychiatric disorder, schizophrenia. The FGA are clear dopamine-2 (D2) receptor antagonists pharmacodynamically. The higher potency FGA are very clean drugs in regard to promoting antipsychotic effects and the low potency FGA have additional pharmacodynamics that dictate a myriad of additional adverse effects. FGA were not only uni-dimensionally used to treat psychosis but were dosed unidimensionally by systematically increasing dopamine-2 receptor (D2) blockade, to inhibit dopaminergic hyperactivity in the mesolimbic dopamine pathway in order lower psychotic symptoms. The clinical practice goal was to reach a high FGA dose to help ameliorate the patient's symptoms. This simple strategy has become more complicated as newer, second generation antipsychotic agents (SGA) were developed. This article reviews and suggests clinical dosing strategies for clinicians to use while dosing the SGA by blending basic and clinical science knowledge.

SECOND GENERATION ANTIPSYCHOTIC DOSING

With the introduction of the second generation, or atypical, antipsychotics in the mid-1990's it became apparent that these agents were better tolerated by creating less extrapyramidal symptoms (EPS) and tardive dyskinesia (TD), but also were more challenging in regards to establishing dosing regimens that optimally balanced efficacy and tolerability. For example, risperidone, was approved for rapid dose escalation within 3 days to a 6 mg divided dose. The FDA and makers of risperidone advertised low incidence EPS, but prescribers quickly identified remarkable EPS rates with this aggressive dosing strategy thus affecting overall patient compliance and therefore overall effectiveness. Good clinical practice dictated a slower, albeit off-label, titration rate to spare this side effect burden. Olanzapine was approved next, and it was suggested to dose this drug at 10 mg per day initially. Worried after aggressive risperidone dosing experiences, clinicians often would dose olanzapine more slowly and at lower ineffective doses. As a result, this agent had less EPS issues, but did not have initial and readily apparent efficacy compared to the package insert information. Consequently, the dose of olanzapine was often clinically raised to over 10 mg per day as clinical experience showed that this created better antipsychotic efficacy.

The next three approved SGAs, quetiapine, ziprasidone, and aripiprazole, had similar initial subtherapeutic dosing issues but were ideally to be dosed in practice at 600 mg, 160 mg, and 30 mg, respectively. Again, clinicians often would under utilize these in fear of adverse effects but likely at the expense of solid efficacy in some patients [1]. It does seem apparent that clinicians have become more comfortable with the aforementioned agents' full dosing range over the years in regard to treating schizophrenia and perhaps the full dosing range of the newest SGAs (asenapine, iloperidone, lurasidone) will follow suit [2].

Dosing the SGAs also became more difficult as pharmaceutical companies began to investigate treating other psychiatric disorders such as bipolar mania, bipolar depression, and unipolar major depressive disorder. The FDA package insert and suggested dosing strategies appear to be 'loading' strategies in regards to treating acute mania. Clinicians are asked to dose the agents very high initially and very quickly to achieve antimanic efficacy within a few days. Risperidone again here is dosed from 4 to 6 mg, but olanzapine is to be initiated at 15 mg, quetiapine at 600 mg, ziprasidone at 120 mg, aripiprazole at 30 mg, and asenapine at 20mg which may be considered aggressive in some cases as these initial doses for mania compared to initial doses of these same agents when used to treat schizophrenia are higher in nature [3–5]. Clinicians now must make an accurate diagnosis, and per the FDA, dose agents more or less aggressively depending on said diagnosis. The final and most recent complication in regard to clinical dose is the approval and use of aripiprazole and quetiapine XR for the adjunctive treatment of major depressive disorder (MDD) [6,7]. The former agent is initially dosed at 2–5 mg instead of the usual 10–30 mg noted previously for schizophrenia and mania. The latter agent is dosed from 50 mg initially to either 150 mg or 300 mg in MDD. These two dosing strategies have clinicians come full circle and back to lower and slower dosing strategies for use in this new patient population.

Looking back to the schizophrenia population, the dosing strategy for efficacy is still similar to the FGA. Clinicians should start at the low FDA recommended dose but titrate upwards until efficacy or intolerable side effects occur. The problem occurs when patients also have comorbid illnesses. What if a patient has schizoaffective disorder or MDD following the resolution of a psychotic break? What dosing strategy should then be used low, middle, or high dose? Patients also may become resistant clinically to the drug they are taking, or may develop side effects that require a change of antipsychotics. Switching among the original first generation agents was relatively easy as clinicians could use a table of potency values [8] and switch drugs in short order in most cases. The newer, atypical antipsychotics really do not have a potency chart to guide instant cross-titrations and often require a more gradual cross titration approach. Dosing again has become increasingly complicated in these transitional titration windows and there are often conflicts between the evidence base for dosing in these situations versus dosing in clinical practice [9]. This review will now discuss and establish specific dosing issues and strategies regarding each individual SGA includinig the most recently approved lurasidone and offer some considerations for the now experimental cariprazine. Using each SGA's individual pharmacodynamic and pharmacokinetic properties may best guide clinical practice when formal studies do not exist to guide treatment. The authors will begin discussion about those SGAs with more simple pharmacological properties and move towards those with more complexity.

Specific Dosing Strategies

Common Features

All second-generation antipsychotic agents are D2 receptor antagonists [10]. This is similar to first generation antipsychotics that have been available since the 1950's. This allows a lowering of limbic dopaminergic hyperactivity in schizophrenia or mania leading next to clinical effectiveness and ideally a reduction of psychosis and/or mania. Some SGAs have a higher affinity for this action and can loosely be assigned a potency (affinity) level in rank order (high to low D2 affinity) as follows: aripiprazole, risperidone, paliperidone, ziprasidone, olanzapine, iloperidone, asenapine, and quetiapine [11–13]. The exact positioning on this pathway is difficult to assess as some studies are conducted in vitro, some in vivo, and oftentimes different laboratories will use differing assessment protocols.

SGA potency values are also difficult to completely assess as all of the SGAs antagonize serotonin-2a (5HT-2a) receptors as well as D2 receptors [10]. The SGA are sometimes delineated as serotonin-dopamine antagonists (SDA) which better describe their collective mechanism of action. This common pharmacodynamic property (5HT-2a) serves a few important functions. First, this antagonism makes these agents fairly selective for antagonizing the limbic dopamine system while sparing other dopamine pathways. 5HT-2a receptor antagonism allows more dopamine activity and neurotransmission to occur in the nigrostriatal system to avoid EPS, which in the mesocortical system to avoid iatrogenically induced negative symptoms, may allow subtle improvement in negative symptoms [14,15], and finally in the tuberoinfundibular pathway to help avoid prolactinemia and its sequelae. Ultimately, 5HT-2a receptor antagonism allows the SGA to be named "atypical" in that they have a much lower rate of TD and EPS than the first generation typical antipsychotics. This common, dual receptor antagonism pharmacodynamic profile amongst the SGAs actually makes them selective agents in that they dampen dopaminergic activity where it is critical for the treatment of positive schizophrenia symptoms and mania while remarkably lowering potential EPS. As noted above, FDA regulatory trials suggest a clear dosing and titration schedule, which gives clinicians a reproducible set of results for their patients. Each SGA has a very unique pharmacokinetic and pharmacodynamic profile which lends each SGA to a set of unique dosing strategies that may not be found in each drug's official FDA package insert. The following section will take the reader through the similarities and discrepancies between clinical trial results and those sometimes used in the trenches of clinical practice for a myriad of patients with variable diagnoses and comorbidities.

Risperidone

This drug is absorbed consistently after ingestion and has high affinity for D2 receptor antagonism. An average dose in schizophrenia or bipolar mania is 3–4 mg/d [16,17]. Dosing for autism in children or adolescents is 1–3 mg/d [18]. There appears to be state (diagnosis) dependent dosing in that lower doses may better treat younger patients with autism and agitation where slightly higher doses are needed to stop bipolar mania or psychosis in adults. This makes dynamic sense as higher doses will allow for better D2 receptor occupancy and blockade. Once this antagonism reaches 60% or more, antipsychotic effects likely occur. At lower doses, this drug likely has little antipsychotic effect.

Risperidone is not indicated for depression or anxiety, but evidence exists for its efficacy in these areas nonetheless. In resistant depression, lower than 'antipsychotic' doses (0.5–3 mg/d) were found to be effective in a 4 week study by Keitner et al. allowing for faster response, remission and improved quality of life when used as an augmentation strategy [19]. A smaller, open-label study suggested that low dose risperidone also helped Selective Serotonin Reuptake Inhibitor (SSRI) non-responsive depressed patients to improve and promoted elevated brain derived neurotrophic levels (BDNF) [20]. A small, randomized, cross-over study suggested that even lower dosed (0.5–2 mg/d) risperidone was effective in treating depression and suicidality symptoms in particular [21]. This series of risperidone for depression findings brings the authors to a very important point and likely a commentary that will run throughout this article. The SGA are drugs that can function on multiple levels to treat different symptoms and syndromes. Risperidone here makes the case that moderate to high doses, 3 mg/d and above, are needed for antipsychotic and antimanic potential. Three milligrams per day and less seem to help depressive symptoms. It follows that there is a relative lack of D2 receptor blockade at these low doses, so where does the antidepressant effect come from? One study suggests that BDNF increases at low risperidone doses. Perhaps consistent with other literature, this neurotrophic factor allows for healthier neuronal connectivity and neurotransmission to alleviate depression [22]. Outside of the BDNF hypothesis, what does risperidone's pharmacodynamic profile suggest to clinicians? Risperidone has affinity, even at low doses, to antagonize 5-HT2a receptors. This effect tends to maintain or even increase dopaminergic activity in select dopamine pathways [10]. When this occurs in the nigrostriatal system, there is less risk for EPS. If this occurs in cortical pathways, more DA activates the frontal lobe, which may allow for better attention, concentration, and executive functioning. These cognitive symptoms are often noted and are diagnostic for depression and certain anxiety disorders. All SGAs possess this property to some degree. If they can promote selective dopaminergic activity in certain brain areas at these low doses, antidepressant effects may be seen in the absence of antipsychotic effects. Risperidone is a fairly Spartan drug in terms of additional pharmacologic binding properties. It possesses 5HT-2a receptor blockade and may promote BDNF at low doses affording treatment of depressive symptoms. At higher doses, the D2 receptor antagonism becomes stronger and allows, likely for a dose–response curve where antipsychotic and antimanic effects occur.

Paliperidone

This drug is the active metabolite of risperidone noted above. It is approved for treating psychosis from schizophrenia at doses of 6–12 mg/d [23,24]. A recently published case report suggests its effectiveness as an augmentation medication in patients with treatment resistant MDD [25]. Several case reports and an open label study in children suggest paliperidone at a dose of 3-12mg/day is effective in treating irritability associated with autistic disorder [26, 27, 28]. As the active metabolite of risperidone it offers a very similar DA-2/5HT-2a receptor antagonism to the risperidone parent product. Despite a limited evidence base, it could be theorized that palidperidone might have the same ability as risperidone to treat MDD or autistic symptoms but this has not been supported by stringently designed studies as yet. This metabolite seems to have less orthostasis and metabolic risks than the parent drug according to its receptor pharmacology and its available data [24,29].

In consideration of dosing of this atypical antipsychotic, the fact that paliperidone is an active metabolite of a known antipsychotic in a controlled release formulation may lead some clinicians to erroneously believe that there are only minor differences between paliperidone and parent drug, risperidone. Clinicians should be alerted that 1 mg of paliperidone is not equal to 1 mg of risperidone. A common mistake is to start patients on 3 mg of paliperidone, incorrectly assuming that it requires up titration like risperidone and that 3 mg of paliperidone is more or less the same as 3 mg of risperidone. Actually, 6 mg paliperidone is a better starting dose for paliperidone. An increase to 9 mg starting the second week of treatment, or even to 12 mg starting the third week of treatment may result in better efficacy. Like most atypical, starting at a higher dose or escalating the dose more quickly may be beneficial if the patient is in imminent risk of relapse, or if the patient has always needed higher doses of antipsychotics, or if the patient has persistent troublesome symptoms despite relatively high doses of the previous antipsychotic. Tolerability may become more problematic with faster dose escalation. On the other hand, lower doses may be useful if the patient is very sensitive to side effects, at least at the start of dosing.

Olanzapine

Olanzapine is the SGA with the molecular structure most similar to that of clozapine [3,30]. Olanzapine is absorbed consistently after ingestion and has a relatively high affinity (though less than risperidone and paliperidone) for D2 receptor antagonism. An average dose in schizophrenia or bipolar mania is 10–15 mg/d [31,32]. For dosing in the persistently mentally ill, Citrome and Kantrowitz (2009) naturalistic data studies suggest an average dose of 22.5 mg/d with greater than 50% of patients receiving above FDA regulatory dose limits. The authors also comment on anecdotal case reports of patients taking 60 mg/d with good effect [33]. A follow-up prospective study regarding 10, 20, 40 mg/d doses did not reveal statistical improvement at the higher dose, but did reveal a clear side effect, dose–response curve for weight gain and prolactinemia [34]. A larger, 20 versus 40 mg/d study suggested no difference in doses except patients with more significant baseline psychotic symptoms responded preferentially to the higher, 40 mg/d dose [35]. These data reinforce clinical experience in that the more severely ill, or psychotic, a patient is, a higher dose of antipsychotic is needed. This makes theoretical sense. As a clinician increases an SGA's dose, there is an increase D2 receptor occupancy and antagonism. Increasing dopamine blockade at greater doses lowers psychotic symptoms. Sometimes, off-label dosing above regulatory guidelines is needed for ultimate symptom reduction. Similar to other off-label practices, full informed consent and increased drug monitoring should proceed and follow super dosing practices. Escalating doses makes pharmacodynamic sense as higher doses allow for greater DA-2 receptor occupancy. Once this reaches 60% or more, antipsychotic and antimanic effects should occur. Olanzapine is not approved for dosing in autism. Olanzapine monotherapy is not indicated for MDD or anxiety, but some evidence in these areas exists [36,37]. Interestingly, when olanzapine is combined with the unipolar MDD antidepressant, fluoxetine, it is considered as an FDA approved combination medication therapy for either bipolar depression or treatment resistant unipolar depression. Dosing in these two types of depression is as follows for olanzapine to fluoxetine ratios: 3–18 mg/d plus 25–75 mg/d [38,39].

Olanzapine itself, has a slightly more complicated pharmacodynamic profile when compared to risperidone and paliperidone. It binds to D2 receptors. It also has the ability to antagonize 5-HT2a receptors also lowering EPS rates when compared to the FGAs. Olanzapine blocks 5HT-2c receptors as well. This action at 5HT2c receptors is more potent than noted for the previous two SGAs (risperidone and paliperidone) and could contribute to its broader diagnostically-based clinical effectiveness. 5HT2c receptor blockade may allow better norepinephrine and dopamine cortical activity through enhancing the mesocortical pathway's ability to activate hypofunctioning dorsolateral prefrontal cortex (DLPFC) areas

[10]. Enhancing DLPFC activity in this manner might theoretically enhance cognition, attention, concentration, and executive functioning. Olanzapine also has higher affinities to antagonize cholinergic muscarinic receptors (AChm) and histamine-1 (H-1) receptors. Anti-cholinergic dry mouth, constipation, blurred vision, memory problems, sedation, weight gain, and metabolic disorder side effects are likely to occur, as such [40].

The SGA class carries FDA warnings now about increasing the risk of metabolic disorders. Olanzapine, carries one of the highest risks based upon the full evidence base available. Patients with a strong family or personal history of diabetes, hypertension, hypercholesterolemia should be screened prior to use of olanzapine (or any SGA) and throughout its longitudinal use. In fact, this practice should likely be implemented for all psychotropics known to promote weight gain or metabolic abnormalities metabolic [41–47].

Quetiapine

This drug was also initially approved to treat psychosis associated with schizophrenia and for bipolar mania in a manner comparable to risperidone and olanzapine. Higher doses (400–800 mg/d) are required to control symptoms as well [48,49]. D2 receptor antagonism of quetiapine is weak compared to all other SGA and may be considered as a low potency drug. This does not suggest it has low effectiveness, but rather requires greater dosing milligrams to achieve a 60% receptor occupancy to alleviate psychosis or mania. For example, 4mg of risperidone or 15 mg of olanzapine may prove effective where 400–800 mg of quetiapine is needed to diminish psychotic or manic symptoms in the average patient. This low affinity may foster quetiapine's lower EPS side effect profile as a substantial benefit [50].

A slow release, once daily version of quetiapine is also approved which may improve compliance. Absorption of the immediate and slow release products is predictable, though the slow release product achieves peak plasma levels, and likely sedating side effects, 3–4 hours post dose. In regards to super dosing quetiapine higher than the FDA regulatory standards, Citrome et al. (2007) reported that 40% or more of persistently ill patients received greater that 750 mg/d in a naturalistic study setting [51]. Another review also suggested that the use of quetiapine at doses greater than 800 mg/d (up to 2400 mg/d) has been noted in anecdotal reports [52].

It is approved as a monotherapy for bipolar depression and also as an augmentation strategy when it is added to SSRI or SNRI antidepressants, in unipolar MDD. Unlike the off-label use of risperidone in depression, multiple, confirmative, regulatory studies have consistently shown that lower doses of quetiapine are quite effective in treating MDD patients. 300 mg/d (which is not effective in psychosis or mania management) will treat bipolar depression as a monotherapy and 150–300 mg will treat MDD as an augmentation approach [53,54]. Quetiapine also has limited data for treating anxiety at doses of 50–300 mg/d [55–57]. There is a large scale, controlled study in patients suffering from generalized anxiety disorder (GAD) who were partial or nonresponders to SSRI monotherapy. Quetiapine here, used as an augmentation strategy at lower doses (50-150mg/day) was effective compared to placebo [58]. A similar trial that utilized the slow release quetiapine XR preparation at doses of 150 and 300mg/day also revealed its effectiveness in treatment of GAD [59]. Treating depression or anxiety at these lower doses likely does not inhibit dopamine transmission and therefore depression treatment responses are likely not from the drug's antipsychotic property. This might engender a conversation about atypical antipsychotics being misnamed in that the SGA seem to be effective in treating more than just schizophrenia induced psychosis.

Quetiapine is the only SGA approved as a monotherapy for bipolar depression. In observing its unique pharmacodynamic profile the authors can speculate as to its translational ability to be an effective antipsychotic, anti-manic, and antidepressant all at once. Quetiapine has an active metabolite, norquetiapine, and when its properties and the parent drug's are combined, many antidepressant and anxiolytic properties seem to emerge [60]. This drug has increased H-1 (histamine) receptor antagonism and similar to olanzapine may promote sedation and metabolic disorder as such. H-1 receptor antagonism is the theoretical mechanism of anxiolysis utilized by the FDA approved agent, hydroxyzine [50]. H-1 receptor blockade can produce fatigue as a side effect but also somnolence as a bona fide clinical hypnotic effect. Over the counter diphenydramine and doxylamine products are approved for treating insomnia as is the recently FDA approved low dose doxepin hypnotic agent which is a tricyclic antidepressant when dosed at much higher ranges [61].

Outside of providing clinically needed hypnosis or anxiolysis, sometimes these can be perceived as side effects that may cause patients to stop taking this medication. Quetiapine has very low to negligible anticholinergic activity so these side effects are largely avoided. Quetiapine has 5HT-2a and 2c antagonism, which lowers EPS rates and improves cognition theorectically as discussed for other SGAs. The norquetiapine metabolite has two relevant pharmacological properties. First, it potentiates 5HT-1a receptor agonism. The serotonergic, FDA approved anxiolytic buspirone and the antidepressant vilazodone both work through this purported mechanism [50,62]. This metabolite also has a potent norepinephrine reuptake inhibitor (NRI) property which is similar to NRI properties possessed by FDA approved unipolar antidepressants such as venlafaxine, duloxetine, bupropion, nortryptiline, and desipramine [50]. Similar to these FDA approved agents in clinical practice, one might expect improvements in cognition, energy, concentration, depression, and anxiety as a result.

Again, it is likely that at lower doses of quetiapine, the drug is less effective at antagonizing and lowering dopamine activity resulting in an inability to treat psychosis and mania at low doses, but clinically is able to treat depression at these lower doses due to serotonergic and noradrenergic pharmacodynamic properties that are supported by large scale regulatory trials confirming clinical efficacy [63,64].

Quetiapine's side effect rate is well noted for its ability to cause sedation, but to have favorable EPS rates, and a fair risk for metabolic disorder. Until recently, it was unclear if metabolic symptoms emerged in a dose-dependent fashion, where higher atypical doses might subject patients to higher metabolic abnormalities.

Conversely and specifically, might any dose of quetiapine convey metabolic risk (weight gain, hyperlipidemia, or hyperglucosemia). Quetiapine XR in particular has now been studied from 50 to 600 mg/d in a myriad of psychiatric disorders and large scale studies now suggest that doses of 150 mg/d may be safer than those at 300 mg/d.

For example, weight gain and hyperglycemia were found to be comparable to placebo rates, whereas 300 mg/d use nearly doubled these side effects' prevalence in acute studies. This data was obtained when quetiapineXR was being studied for antidepressant augmentation in unipolar depression and it is unclear if this dose-adverse effect curve would hold true in other psychiatric disorders [4].

Ziprasidone

This drug is indicated for schizophrenia and bipolar mania treatment [65-67]. It has a higher affinity for D2 receptor antagonism and treats psychosis and mania with doses of 120–160 mg/d. Using the maximal FDA dose in the schizophrenia and bipolar populations has been found to promote longer, sustained ziprasidone adherence and compliance amongst patients which is contrary to the thought that higher doses always yield higher side effect rates and subsequent discontinuation of the medication.

In theory these ziprasidone dose escalation findings are likely due to clear dose–response effects where at the higher doses, symptoms are likely controlled more effectively by improved D2 receptor blockade. Patients remain on ziprasidone longer due to improved clinical effectiveness in other words [68].

The same author observed that dosing often reached superdose amounts above the regulatory maximum of 160 mg/d. Oftentimes an average of 206 mg/d was used for the treatment of more refractory, state-hospitalized patients [69]. Almost half of patients were treated at doses greater than the approved maximum of 160 mg/d [51]. Ziprasidone appears to have the greatest anecdotal evidence for superdosing above the usual FDA approved limits.

Ziprasidone possesses the common serotonin-dopamine antagonist (SDA) properties well documented previously for other SGA agents. It furthermore antagonizes 5-HT1a receptors and inhibits NRI similar to norquetiapine, the metabolite of quetiapine that was discussed in the previous section. Ziprasidone appears to be unique in its ability to also act as an SSRI and inhibit the serotonin transporter system [70,71].

This SSRI mechanism is commonly used to treat unipolar depression and many anxiety disorders(social anxiety, generalized anxiety, obsessive-compulsive, and post traumatic-stress disorder). Unlike quetiapine and the olanzapine–fluoxetine combination, ziprasidone is not approved for the treatment of depression or anxiety, and has fewer published data regarding its potential antidepressant effects compared to the limited data of risperidone in depression or anxiety [72]. Its supportive evidence for treating MDD is stronger than that for paliperidone, asenapine, iloperidone, or latuda.

Stahl and Cutler et al. [73] suggest that in clinical practice, similar to quetiapine, Ziprasidone may be effective in treating anxiety and depression at low doses where DA-2 receptor antagonism is not needed. Large-scale studies in bipolar depression have failed to show consistent results, but smaller studies and those that focus on dysphoric symptoms of mania have concluded with positive results [72,74,75].

One open-label study for a unipolar depression augmentation approach and another for treatment resistant generalized anxiety, both lower 80 mg/d doses, were effective in reducing symptoms [76,77], but a follow-up study in depression was less conclusive, especially at higher doses [78].

Similar to lower dosed risperidone and quetiapine, lower doses of ziprasidone may be effective in the treatment of anxiety or depression, where higher doses are needed for mania or psychosis.

Pharmacokinetically, ziprasidone is unique in that it requires to be taken with food to allow for adequate absorption and bioavailability. [67] Lurasidone, discussed later, also must be taken with food. It is clearly a drug that should be taken twice a day per regulatory agencies and studies.

In regards to adverse effects, this agent is clinically known to be one of the safest in avoiding remarkable weight gain and metabolic disorders when compared to other SGAs and was the first SGA noted to prolong QTc cardiac intervals [79].

Aripiprazole

Aripiprazole could be named an *atypical* atypical. It is a unique SGA as it is actually a partial D2 receptor agonist. It is the only SGA to utilize an agonist property at the D2 receptor instead of full antagonistic properties [10]. Aripiprazole, therefore may have dopamine balancing properties is it can partially stimulate dopamine receptor activity in areas of low dopamine concentration (partial agonism), and also can block the full agonist endogenous dopamine in areas of high dopamine concentration. A partial agonist is functionally a partial antagonist in the presence of a full agonist ie. endogenous dopamine. Aripiprazole in theory might stimulate DA activity in the hypofrontal mesocortical DA pathway and lower DA hyperactivity in the mesolimbic system which is felt to be the origin of mania and psychotic symptoms.

Aripiprazole is fairly unique in another property where it is also a dopamine-3 (DA-3) receptor partial agonist. This property likely does not add to antipsychotic or antimanic activity but might, in fact, lend to promoting dopamine transmission in fronto-cortical areas. This may have pro-cognitive and antidepressant effects in clinical practice as static dopamine activity may be increased over time [10]. Aripiprazole carries previously mentioned 5HT2a receptor antagonism (similar to all SGA) and 5HT-1a receptor partial agonism properties (similar to quetiapine and ziprasidone), which again diminishes EPS, promotes cognition, and antidepressant potential.

In regard to dosing, aripiprazole shows a difference depending upon which psychiatric disorder is being treated (also similar to other SGAs). Originally approved for treating psychosis due to schizophrenia at doses starting from 15 mg up to 30 mg/d, this drug was secondarily approved to treat mania starting at a full loading dose of 30 mg/d [5,80,81]. This higher dosing strategy uses aripiprazole's high D2 receptor affinity (despite partial D2 receptor agonism) to lower DA neurotransmission. There is very little literature evidence showing super dosing above the approved limit of 30 mg/d. Citrome et al.'s (2007) review suggests a 10% superdosing in a New York State hospital system [51].

A few years back, aripiprazole was approved for the treatment of unipolar depression as an augmentation in those patients who failed to respond to initial antidepressant dosing. Aripiprazole was the first FDA approved drug for use in this manner for MDD, where quetiapineXR was approved second [5,82]. Dosing in MDD is again low and ranges from 2 to 15 mg/d with the average dose approximately 10 mg/d, which is much lower than doses used in schizophrenia or mania [83]. At these doses, a reduction in dopamine transmission is likely not achieved, nor required. Instead, promoting dopamine, norepinephrine and serotonin likely occurs as the principal mechanism of action. More recently, this drug was approved for treating irritability due to autism in children also in lower doses of 2– 15 mg/d [84].

In regard to treating anxiety disorders, this drug should theoretically be effective as it contains robust activity partially agonizing 5HT-1a receptors similar to the mechanism of action for the FDA approved anxiolytic buspirone (mentioned in regards to norquetiapine and ziprasidone previously). Small open-label studies exist for GAD and panic disorder (PD) with effectiveness noted in these patients at doses averaging 13.9 mg/d [85, 86]. Again, similar to previous discussion, SGAs at lower doses (including aripiprazole) seem to be effective in treating depression and anxiety where higher doses are required for mania and schizophrenia.

In regards to tolerability, aripiprazole is known for its higher probability of inducing akathisia (sometimes greater than 20%) [5]. This may be due to its high D2 receptor affinity, but also may be due to its overall monoaminergic activity where restlessness and agitation may be confused with more traditional akathisa clinically. This agent, similar to ziprasidone, is felt to be more metabolically friendly in regards to minimizing weight gain based side effects and metabolic side effects as well. Finally, this drug is known to be a p450 2D6 liver enzyme substrate. Its daily dosing should be halved to a maximum daily dose of only 15 mg/d in patients who are simultaneously taking a strong 2D6 inhibitor such as fluoxetine or paroxetine [5].

Asenapine

Asenapine is approved for treating schizophrenia or bipolar mania [87–90]. Similar to other SGAs, asenapine may treat these symptoms with a lower risk of EPS due to its D2/5HT-2a receptor blockade mechanism of action. This drug's structure is similar to the antidepressant mirtazapine [81] and may promote cortical serotonin and norepinephrine activity in a similar manner, but to date there are no MDD trials to prove effectiveness in this area [91]. PUBMED and MEDLINE searches suggest no evidence for using it in the treatment of depression or anxiety, but preclinical animal models continue to show precortical monoamine activity elevations suggesting promise in these areas. Asenapine partially agonizes 5HT-1a receptors, and antagonizes 5HT-2a, and 5HT-2c receptors. As discussed earlier, these pharmacodynamic properties offer anxiolytic, pro-cognitive and antidepressant potential respectively and theoretically.

Dosing typically is 5 mg twice daily with a maximum daily dose allowed up to 20 mg [87]. Manic patients may be started at 10mg twice daily in a loading dose strategy. Unique to this SGA is that it must be taken sublingually and without food or drink 15 min thereafter to ensure absorption [87]. This is the exact opposite of ziprasidone and lurasidone oral tablets which require food to be adequately absorbed. This drug is a known substrate for the CYP450 1A2 liver enzyme system and asenapine blood levels may increase when administered with CYP450 1A2 inhibitors such as fluvoxamine. Very little experience and no literature exist for use of this agent outside the dose range of 10– 20 mg/day. Given the clear evidence that aripiprazole, quetiapine, and quetiapine XR are used at low doses to treat MDD, if clinicians were to use asenapine off-label for MDD, the authors would suggest use of 5-10mg/d as low doses here, should also be effective for treating depressive and/or anxious states.

Iloperidone

Iloperidone is approved for the treatment of schizophrenia [92,93]. Similar to other SGAs, iloperidone may treat these symptoms with a lower risk of EPS due to its D2/5HT2a receptor blockade properties. This drug also has no substantiative evidence (MEDLINE/PUBMED) yet for using it for treating bipolar mania, bipolar depression, MDD or anxiety. It's pharmacodynamic profile [94] suggests some interesting treatment possibilities in these clinical areas however. Its relative lack of 5HT-1a receptor agonism, 5HT-2c receptor antagonism, and selective serotonin/norepinephrine reuptake inhibitor (SNRI) potential allows for a pharmacodynamic profile more similar to that of risperidone, paliperidone, and olanzapine than that of quetiapine, ziprasidone, or asenapine [92,93].

The recommended starting dose for iloperidone is 1 mg twice daily. It has a complicated titration schedule and requires increases to reach the target dose range of 6–12 mg twice daily. These daily dosage adjustments proceed from 2 mg twice daily, 4 mg twice daily, 6 mg twice daily, 8 mg twice daily, 10 mg twice daily, and 12 mg twice daily on days 2, 3, 4, 5, 6, and 7, respectively. Efficacy was demonstrated at a dose range of 6 to 12 mg twice daily for schizophrenia [95,96].

This drug is a known substrate for the CYP450 2D6 liver enzyme system and iloperidone blood levels may increase when administered with CYP2D6 inhibitors such as paroxetine or fluoxetine (similar to precautions noted for aripiprazole). Iloperidone also has been noted to increase cardiac QTc intervals by 9 msec and carries precautions similar to that of ziprasidone [92].

Lurasidone

Lurasidone is the most recently approved SGA and may have the most recent dose finding studies available. Pharmacodynamically, it is an SDA just like all other SGA previously mentioned. Comparably, it has high affinity for both 5HT7 and 5HT2A receptors, moderate affinity for 5HT1A and alpha 2 receptors, and minimal affinity for H1 histamine and M1 cholinergic receptors. It tends not to be less sedating and comparable to ziprasidone and aripiprazole, may have a less deleterious impact upon metabolic factors. 5HT7 receptor antagonism theoretically may provide improved sleep and wakefulness properties via circadian mechanisms.

In regards to dosing, as there is often little, to no sedation, the starting dose of 40 mg is often used and is an effective antipsychotic dose. This drug requires food for improved absorption and effectiveness, similar to ziprasidone. If a patient develops initial side effects, then the first few days can be taken without food, thus lowering absorption and bioavailability and its over all dose in the patient's system. Clinically, this may improve initial tolerability albeit at an initial sub therapeutic dose now. [26] Initial regulatory studies suggested that for maximum long-term efficacy, doses up to 120 mg per day (divided doses) could be useful in some patients. The recommended FDA dose range is 40-80mg per day with food. [95] Most recently, newer post-regulatory studies have shown that the dose may be escalated as high as 160mg per day. This superdosing strategy, given all at bedtime may actually improve tolerability. [96]

There may be moderate EPS with lurasidone, but this often is reduced if lurasidone is given at night. Large scale clinical trials show robust antidepressant efficacy in bipolar depression and additional trials are ongoing in mixed depression (depression with subsyndromal symptoms of mania). The receptor binding profile of lurasidone at 5HT7, 5HT1A and alpha 2 receptors may theoretically offer its potential antidepressant efficacy. [29]

Cariprazine

Cariprazine is a novel atypical antipsychotic drug that is undergoing regulatory trials currently for the treatment of schizophrenia and bipolar mania. It is felt to exhibit a high selectivity and affinity for dopamine D3 (agonism similar to aripirazole) and D2 receptors (antagonism like all SGA) and moderate affinity for the serotonin 5-HT1A receptor antagonism [97, 98, 99]. Cariprazine is rapidly absorbed, with high oral bioavailability and a long plasma elimination t ½ [98]. Data from a phase II randomized ,double blind, placebo controlled, flexible dose study demonstrated that Cariprazine at a dose of 3- 12 mg/day was well tolerated and effective in the treatment of acute mania associated with bipolar I disorder. Recently preliminary results from a phase III trial of cariprazine in patients with acute mania associated with bipolar disorder were consistent with the results observed in the two previously completed placebo-controlled studies in this patient population. [97, 99]

Brexpipirazole

This antipsychotic is also likely an 'atytpical atypical' in that it is a partial D2 receptor agonist similar to aripiprizole mentioned previously. The same partial agonist property theories and applications may be applied to this agent though it is still experimental and not available as of yet. Dosing data and information is, like cariprazine just above, limited given ongoing regulatory studies and a paucity of published information. It is being investigated for use in schizophrenia comparable to other SGA, but also has apparent studies investigating MDD and ADHD. [100]

Summary

The SGAs share similar mechanisms of action in regards to treating psychosis and mania and for reducing EPS risks and this article sought to discuss this class of psychotropics from the most simplistic SGA, pharmacodynamically speaking, to the most complicated. The authors concluded briefly with the two most recently approved SGAs and a current experimental SGA that is in the midst of regulatory trials in order to bring the reader up to date regarding the basic science data and clinical, real world application of these agents.

In general, all of the SGAs possess the pharmacologic actions needed to ameliorate psychosis, some if not all of the SGAs have properties to ameliorate mania, and more recently some SGAs have shown ability to treat depression and autism. The authors have attempted to describe how these properties lend themselves to treating psychosis, mania, depression, and sometimes anxiety in clinical practice as well. In summary, to stop mania or psychosis, it is a clear principle that each SGA must be used near the peak of its daily dose range. This optimizes D2 receptor blockade. This also increases the risk for EPS (akathisia, parkinsonism, dystonia, etc.). The second principle suggests that some of the SGA are now well-defined multifunctional drugs [101, 97]. They have FDA approvals in areas of adult or child schizophrenia and bipolar disorder, autism, and depressive disorders. Many of the non-dopaminergic properties of these drugs occur at their lower dose ranges and lend themselves to treat depressive disorders in particular. Side effects are likely less at lower doses, which is common amongst most classes of medications. With the advent of studying depressive disorders at lower doses, regulatory data are starting to reveal this fact in a more stringent manner. These agents may be flexibly used as monotherapies and appear to be antidepressant/anxiolytic at one dose and antimanic/antipsychotic at higher doses. As add-on or augmentation therapies, the dose range is also varied depending upon which symptoms the clinician aims to treat. These drugs certainly carry side effects, which vary to some degree but all patients on SGAs should be routinely monitored for TD, EPS, and metabolic disorders.

There are a few areas of SGA off-label prescription use that are worth discussing that were not included in the paragraphs above in order to alert the reader to some trends in psychopharmacological practice. Delirium is a neuropsychiatric disorder involving an acute alteration in mental status that is characterized by a disturbance of consciousness, attention, cognition and perception. These symptoms often fluctuate in a hallmark fashion during the course of the day and often peak in the evening (sundowning) [102]. Delirium occurs in 20 - 50 % of hospitalized elderly patients, [103] and patients receiving palliative care often possess multiple risk factors and predisposing conditions for delirium [104]. The American Psychiatric Association has developed a practice guideline for the treatment of patients with delirium, where psychiatric consultation may help to optimize treatment and decrease hospital lengths of stay [105]. Antipsychotics have been the mainstay of pharmacological treatment and have been shown to be effective in treating symptoms of delirium by improving agitation, cognition, executive functioning and alleviating psychosis when present. Haloperidol is considered to be the first-line treatment when an antipsychotic is needed for treating delirum. It is a FGA that has high potency D2 receptor blockade with a minimum of antihistamine or anticholinergic potential, thus avoiding any artificial alterations to the patient's mental state. Potential benefits of the SGAs in treating delirium have been noted since the mid-1990s. The single key benefit of the SGA in treating delirium is that there is less of a risk for akathisia. Developing akathisia while delirous may be misinterpreted as a worsening agitation of delirium and the FGA may be uptitrated perpetuating the akathisia. The SGA tend to have less EPS and especially akathisia risk [106]. Risperidone and olanzapine have been used widely in the treatment of delirium. [102]

A Comparative efficacy study of haloperidol, olanzapine and risperidone at a flexible dose regimen (haloperidol -0.25 to 10 mg; risperidone -0.25 to 4 mg; olanzapine -1.25 to 20 mg) demonstrated that risperidone and olanzapine were as effective as haloperidol in the treatment of delirium [107]. Data from a controlled pilot study has also shown that quetiapine used as an adjunct to haloperidol at a dose of 50mg every 12hrs resulted in faster delirium resolution and less agitation compared to placebo.

Interestingly, adding low dose quetiapine to haloperidol would pharmacodynamically allow the FGA haloperidol to appear atypical. The quetiapine would add 5HT-2a receptor antagonism thus lowering EPS risk, even if the quetiapine itself was not lending antipsychotic D2 receptor blockade potential. Aripiprazole is also mentioned in a number of case reports. Dosages varied from 5 to 30 mg/day [108]. Recently an open label trial of aripiprazole dosed 5-30mg in hospitalized cancer patients revealed its effectiveness in resolving delirium symptoms [109].

A case report on ziprasidone in patient with delirium showed ziprasidone at a dose of 20-100mg helped cleared delirium to a significant degree, as evidenced by improvement in patient's thought process, better ability to focus and shift attention, and a decrease in paranoia

[110]. In summary, it appears that the use of SGA in the treatment of delirium is widespread and likely becoming the standard of care in many consultation-liaison practices.

Attention deficit hyperactivity disorder (ADHD) is a heterogeneous psychiatric syndrome that is characterized primarily by symptoms of inattention, impulsivity, and/or hyperactivity that are judged to be developmentally inappropriate [111]. The gold standard of treatment is to make an accurate diagnosis and the evidence supports the judicious use of stimulant-based medications, all of which have a supportive evidence base with large effect sizes. Approvals for norepinephrine reuptake inhibitors and noradrenergic alpha-2 receptor agonists have also garnered ADHD indications for use. It has become increasingly clear that ADHD continues to impair many domains of functioning in adulthood and more adults are seeking psychopharmacologic treatment here as well [112].

Fullerton et al. [113] found that the percentage of children with ADHD treated with medication from 1996-2005 increased from 60% to 63%, and specifically, the percentage taking antipsychotics more than doubled, from 8% to 18%. A MEDLINE search revealed few, if any controlled trials for ADHD treatment of SGA despite the statistic of its escalating off-label use. Aripiprazole has an open-label trial in 14 adolescents showing statistical improvement in ADHD scale scores while dosed on average at 6-7mg/d. [114] A small randomized and controlled trial found modest ADHD symptom improvement (30%ADHD improvement in 100% of risperidone patients) at an average of 1mg/d [115]. This ADHD cohort was singled out as being associated with high aggression scores.

On the surface, a controversy exists in that children that are hyperactive are being sedated or tranquilized by the SGA medications to control their behavior. These are expensive medications with the potential for severe side effects (EPS, TD, metabolic, suicidality, etc.) that have very little, if any large, controlled trials to support their use.

After reading this article, the reader should be able to formulate an SGA pharamcodynamic theory to support SGA use for treating ADHD especially when other, mainstream treatments have failed to yield efficacy. For example, high doses of SGA seem unwarranted as antagonizing D2 receptors lowers mania and psychosis which are typically not associated with ADHD. Higher doses may also tranquilize patients, but this might more adequately be used in acute, transient situations where the ADHD might be comorbid with conduct disorder or pervasive development disorder where tranquilization might lower combativeness and protect patients, caregivers, or providers. Lower doses of the SGA might have beneficial properties. Those SGA that antagonize 5HT-2c receptors (for example olanzapine, quetiapine) will ultimately allow greater fronto-cortical dopamine and norepinephrine activity to occur, perhaps improving cognition.

Many ADHD treatments facilitate these two transmitters in the same fashion to improve attention, vigilance, concentration and executive functioning. The SGA's 5HT-2c mechanism is different but with a net effect of monoamine facilitation and in certain patients might prove to be directly beneficial in lowering ADHD symptoms. Other SGA's frankly possess NRI mechanisms identical to the approved ADHD atomoxetine product's NRI abilities. Quetiapine and ziprasidone have noradrenergic potential that may be helpful in more refractory ADHD cases.

In conclusion, the SGA are multi-modal in that they possess pharmacodynamic properties that may be utilized to treat a myriad of psychiatric symptoms. There is excellent data supporting their use for the treatment of schizophrenia, mania, bipolar and unipolar depression, and autism. Less stringent data is emerging regarding their use in anxiety disorders, delirium, dementia, and ADHD. These latter condition warrant scrutiny prior to prescribing, however when typical, guideline-based treatments fail, the SGA may be employed to lessen patients' symptoms based upon pharmacodynamic theory, rationale, and clinical practice.

CONFLICT OF INTEREST

Thomas L. Schwartz, MD, is an associate professor of psychiatry at Upstate Medical University and has served as a Consultant to PamLab. He has served on speakers bureaus for Pfizer Inc; Wyeth Pharmaceuticals, AstraZeneca, and Merck pharmaceuticals and received research and/or grant support from Cephalon, Forest, Cyberonics.

Umar Siddiqui, MD has no conflicts of interest to declare.

Stephen M. Stahl, MD, PhD, is an adjunct professor of psychiatry at the University of California, San Diego School of Medicine and an honorary visiting senior fellow at the University of Cambridge, UK and has served as a Consultant to Allergan, Astra Zeneca, BioMarin, BioVail, Boehringer Ingelheim, Bris tol Myers-Squibb, Cenerex, Covance, Cypress Bioscience, Dianippon, Eisai, Eli Lilly, Forest, GlaxoSmith Kline, Labopharm, Lund- beck, Marinus, Meda Corp, Meiji, Merck, Novartis, Pfizer, Pfizer Canada, Pierre Fabre, PamLab, Prexa Pharmaceuticals, Propagate Pharma, Royalty Pharma, Sanofi, Schering Plough Corporation, Shire, SK Corporation, Soffinova, Solvay, Vanda and Wyeth. He has served on speakers bureaus for Pfizer Inc; Wyeth Pharmaceuticals and Schering Plough Corporation and has received research and/or grant support from Astra Zeneca, Boehringer Ingelheim, Bristol Myers-Squibb, Cephalon, Dainippon, Eli Lilly, Forest, Lundbeck, Novartis, PamLabs, Pfizer, Pfizer Canada, Pharmasquire, Sanofi Aventis, Schering Plough, Shire and Wyeth.

ACKNOWLEDGMENTS

The authors would like to thank Kelly Canfield at SUNY Upstate Medical University for her time in logistical support and preparation of this manuscript.

REFERENCES

[1] Citrome, L., Jaffe, A., Levine, J. Dosing of second generation antipsychotic medication in a state hospital system. *J. Clin. Psychopharm.* 2005;25:388–390.
[2] Citrome, L., Volavka, J. Optimal dosing of atypical antipsychotics in adults: A review of the current evidence. *Harv. Rev. Psychiatry* 2002;10:280–291.
[3] Olanzapine (ZyprexaTM) FDA Package Insert.
[4] Quetiapine (SeroquelTM) FDA Package Insert.
[5] Aripiprazole (AbilifyTM) FDA Package Insert.

[6] Marcus, R. N., McQuade, R. D., Carson, W. H., Hennicken, D., Fava, M., Simon, J. S., et al. The efficacy and safety of aripiprazole as adjunctive therapy in major depressive disorder: Second multicenter, randomized, double-blind, placebo-controlled study. *J. Clin. Psychopharmacol.* 2008;28:156–165.

[7] Weisler, R., Joyce, M., McGill, L., Lazarus, A., Szamosi, J., Eriksson, H., et al. Extended release quetiapine fumarate monotherapy for major depressive disorder: Results of a double-blind, randomized, placebo-controlled study. *CNS spectr.* 2009;14:299–313.

[8] Sadock, B. J., Sadock, V. A., editors. *Kaplan and Sadock's synopsis of Psychiatry,* 9th ed. Philadelphia: Lippincott Williams and Wilkins, 2003.

[9] Eltanaihi-Furtm¨uller, N., Hummer, M., Fleischhacker, W. W. Switching between second-generation antipsychotics: Why and how? *CNS Drugs* 2005;19:27–42.

[10] Stahl, S. M. Stahl's essential psychopharmacology: *Neuroscientific basis and practical applications*, 3rd ed. Cambridge: Cambridge University Press, 2008.

[11] Zhang, W., Bymaster, F. P. The in vivo effects of olanzapine and other antipsychotic agents on receptor occupancy and antagonism of dopamine D1, D2, D3, 5HT2A and muscarinic receptors. *Psychopharmacology* 1999; 141:267–278.

[12] Seeger, T. F., Seymour, P. A., Schmidt, A. W., Zorn, S. H., Schulz, D. W., Lebel, L. A., et al. Ziprasidone (CP-88,059): A new antipsychotic with combined dopamine and serotonin receptor antagonist activity. *J. Pharmacol. Exp. Ther.* 1995;275:101–113.

[13] Arnt, J., Skarsfeldt, T. Do novel antipsychotics have similar pharmacological characteristics? A review of the evidence. *Neuropsychopharmacology* 1998;18:63–101.

[14] Schmidt, C. J., Sorensen, S. M., Kehne, J. H., Carr, A. A., Palfreyman, M. G. The role of 5-HT2A receptors in antipsychotic activity. *Life Sci.* 1995;56:2209–2222.

[15] Akhondzadeh, S., Malek-Hosseini, M., Ghoreishi, A., Raznahan, M., Rezazadeh, S. A. Effect of ritanserin, a 5HT2A/2C antagonist, on negative symptoms of schizophrenia: A double-blind randomized placebo-controlled study. *Prog. Neuropsychopharmacol. Biol. Psychiatry* 2008;32:1879–1883.

[16] Haas, M., Unis, A. S., Armenteros, J., Copenhaver, M. D., Quiroz, J. A., Kushner, S. F. A 6-week, randomized, double-blind, placebo-controlled study of the efficacy and safety of risperidone in adolescents with schizophrenia. *J. Child Adolesc. Psychopharmacol.* 2009;19:611–621.

[17] Khanna, S., Vieta, E., Lyons, B., Grossman, F., Eerdekens, M., Kramer, M. Risperidone in the treatment of acute mania: Double-blind, placebo-controlled study. *Br. J. Psychiatry* 2005;187:229–234.

[18] Scott, L. J., Dhillon, S. Risperidone: A review of its use in the treatment of irritability associated with autistic disorder in children and adolescents. *Paediatr. Drugs* 2007;9:343–354.

[19] Keitner, G. I., Garlow, S. J., Ryan, C. E., Ninan, P. T., Solomon, D. A., Nemeroff, C. B., et al. A randomized, placebo-controlled trial of risperidone augmentation for patients with difficult-to-treat unipolar, non-psychoticmajor depression. *J. Psychiatr. Res.* 2009;43:205–214.

[20] Yoshimura, R., Umene-Nakano, W., Ueda, N., Ikenouchi-Sugita, A., Hori, H., Nakamura, J. Addition of risperidone to sertraline improves sertraline-resistant refractory depression without influencing plasma concentrations of sertraline and desmethylsertraline. *Human Psychopharmacol.* 2008;23:707–713.

[21] Reeves, H., Batra, S., May, R. S., Zhang, R., Dahl, D. C., Li, X. Efficacy of risperidone augmentation to antidepressants in the management of suicidality in major depressive disorder: A randomized, double-blind, placebo-controlled pilot study. *J. Clin. Psychiatry* 2008;69:1228–1336.

[22] Sen, S., Duman, R., Sanacora, G. Serum brain-derived neurotrophic factor, depression, and antidepressant medications: Meta-analyses and implications. *Biol. Psychiatry* 2008;64:527–532.

[23] Meltzer, H. Y., Bobo, W. V., Nuamah, I. F., Lane, R., Hough, D., Kramer, M., et al. Efficacy and tolerability of oral paliperidone extended-release tablets in the treatment of acute schizophrenia: Pooled data from three 6-week, placebo-controlled studies. *J. Clin. Psychiatry* 2008;69:817–829.

[24] Paliperidone(Invega TM), FDA Package Insert, 2008.

[25] Yang, F. W., Liang, C. S. Paliperidone augmentation for treatment-resistant depression: a case report. *J. Clin. Psychopharmacol.* 2011;31:245-6

[26] Kowalski, J. L., Wink, L. K., Blankenship, K., Habenicht, C. D., Erickson, C. A., Stigler, K. A., et al. Paliperidone palmitate in a child with autistic disorder. *J. Child Adolesc. Psychopharmacol.* 2011;21:491-3.

[27] Stigler, K. A., Erickson, C. A., Mullett, J. E., Posey, D. J., McDougle, C. J. Paliperidone for Irritability in Autistic Disorder. *J. Child Adolesc. Psychopharmacol.* 2010 Feb.;20:75-8.

[28] Stigler, K. A., Mullett, J. E., Erickson, C. A., Posey, D. J., McDougle, C. J. Paliperidone for irritability in adolescents and young adults with autistic disorder. *Psychopharmacology*. 2012 May 3.

[29] Stahl SM. Stahl's essential psychopharmacology: Neuroscientific basis and practical applications, 4th ed. Cambridge:Cambridge University Press, In Press 2012

[30] McEvoy, J. P., Lieberman, J. A., Stroup, T. S., Davis, S. M., Meltzer, H. Y., Rosenheck, R. A., et al. CATIE Investigators. Effectiveness of clozapine versus olanzapine, quetiapine, and risperidone in patients with chronic schizophrenia who did not respond to prior atypical antipsychotic treatment. *Am. J. Psychiatry* 2006;163:600–610.

[31] Kryzhanovskaya, L., Schulz, S. C., McDougle, C., Frazier, J., Dittmann, R., Robertson-Plouch, C., et al. Olanzapine versus placebo in adolescents with schizophrenia: A 6-week, randomized, double-blind, placebo-controlled trial. *J. Am. Acad. Child Adolesc. Psychiatry* 2009;48:60–70.

[32] Tohen, M., Kryzhanovskaya, L., Carlson, G., Delbello, M., Wozniak, J., Kowatch, R., et al. Olanzapine versus placebo in the treatment of adolescents with bipolar mania. *Am. J. Psychiatry* 2007;164:1547–1556.

[33] Citrome, L., Kantrowitz, J. T. Olanzapine dosing above the licensed range is more efficacious than lower doses: Fact or fiction? *Expert Rev. Neurotherapeutics* 2009;9:1045–1058.

[34] Citrome, L., Stauffer, V. L., Kinon, B. J., Kinon, B. J., Kurtz, D. L., Jacobson, J. G., et al. Olanzapine plasma concentrations after treatment with 10,20,40mg/d in patients with schizophrenia: An analysis of correlations with efficacy, weight gain, and prolactin concentration. *J. Clin. Psychopharmacology* 2009;29:278–283.

[35] Kinon, B. J., Volvaka, J., Stauffer, V., Edwards, S. E., Liu-Seifert, H., Chen, L., et al. Standard and higher dose of olanzapine in patients with schizophrenia or schizoaffective disorder: A randomized, double-blind, fixed dose study. *J. Clin. Psychopharmacology* 2008;28:392–400

[36] Mathews, J., Garcia, K. S., Mintun, M. A., Sheline, Y. I. Antidepressant efficacy of olanzapine as monotherapy in major depressive disorder, without psychosis: A pilot study. *Psychiatry Res.* 2006;146:149–155. Epub. 2006 Mar. 3.

[37] Barnett, S. D., Kramer, M. L., Casat, C. D., Connor, K. M., Davidson, J. R. Efficacy of olanzapine in social anxiety disorder: A pilot study. *J. Psychopharmacol.* 2002;16:365–368.

[38] Corya, S. A., Perlis, R. H., Keck, P. E. Jr., Lin, D. Y., Case, M. G., Williamson, D. J., et al. A 24-week open-label extension study of olanzapine-fluoxetine combination and olanzapine monotherapy in the treatment of bipolar depression. *J. Clin. Psychiatry* 2006;67:798–806.

[39] Croxtall, J. D., Scott, L. J. Olanzapine/fluoxetine: A review of its use in patients with treatment-resistant major depressive disorder. *CNS Drugs* 2010;24:245–262.

[40] Cutler, A., Ball, S., Stahl, S. M. Dosing Atypical antipsychotics. *CNS Spectr.* 2008;135:1–16.

[41] Holt, R. I., Peveler, R. C. Obesity, serious mental illness and antipsychotic drugs. *Diabetes Obes. Metab.* 2009;11:665–679.

[42] Treuer, T., Hoffmann, V. P., Chen, A. K., Rimia, V., Ocampo, M., Wang, G., et al. Factors associated with weight gain during olanzapine treatment in patients with schizophrenia or bipolar disorder: Results from a six-month prospective, multinational, observational study. *World J. Biol. Psychiatry* 2009;10 (4 Pt 3):729–740.

[43] Reynolds, G. P., Kirk, S. L. Metabolic side effects of antipsychotic drug treatment–pharmacological mechanisms. *Pharmacol. Ther.* 2010;125:169–179.

[44] Monteleone, P., Martiadis, V., Maj, M. Management of schizophrenia with obesity, metabolic, and endocrinological disorders. *Psychiatr. Clin. N Am.* 2009;32:775–794.

[45] Nguyen, D., Brakoulias, V., Boyce, P. An evaluation of monitoring practices in patients on second generation antipsychotics. *Austral. Asian. Psychiatry* 2009;17:295–299.

[46] Newcomer, J. W. Comparing the safety and efficacy of atypical antipsychotics in psychiatric patients with comorbid medical illnesses. *J. Clin. Psychiatry* 2009;70:30–36.

[47] Patel, J. K., Buckley, P. F., Woolson, S., Hamer, R. M., McEvoy, J. P., Perkins, D. O., et al. Metabolic profiles of second-generation antipsychotics in early psychosis: Findings from the CAFE study. *Schizophr. Res.* 2009;111:9–16.

[48] Peuskens, J., Trivedi, J. K., Brecher, M., Miller, F. Study 4 Investigators. Long-term symptomatic remission of schizophrenia with once-daily extended release quetiapine fumarate: Post-hoc analysis of data from a randomized withdrawal, placebo-controlled study. *Int. Clin. Psychopharmacol.* 2010;25:183–187.

[49] Vieta, E., Mullen, J., Brecher, M., Paulsson, B., Jones, M. Quetiapine monotherapy for mania associated with bipolar disorder: Combined analysis of two international, double-blind, randomised, placebo-controlled studies. *Curr. Med. Res. Opin.* 2005;21:923–934.

[50] Stahl, S. M. *Essential psychopharmacology: The prescriber's guide.* 3rd ed. Cambridge University Press:Cambridge, 2009.

[51] Citrome, L., Jaffe, A., Levine, J. The ups and downs of dosing second generation antipsychotics. *Psychiatr. Serv.* 2007;58:11.

[52] Citrome, L., Jaffe, A., Levine, J., Lindenmayer, J. P. Dosing of quetiapine in schizophrenia: How clinical practice differs from registration studies. *J. Clin. Psychiatry* 2005;66:1512–1516.

[53] Suppes, T., Datto, C., Minkwitz, M., Nordenhem, A., Walker, C., Darko, D. Effectiveness of the extended release formulation of quetiapine as monotherapy for the treatment of acute bipolar depression. *J. Affect. Disord.* 2010;121:106–115.

[54] Bauer, M., Pretorius, H. W., Constant, E. L., Earley, W. R., Szamosi, J., Brecher, M. Extended-release quetiapine as adjunct to an antidepressant in patients with major depressive disorder: Results of a randomized, placebo-controlled, double-blind study. *J. Clin. Psychiatry.* 2009;70:540–549.

[55] Bandelow, B., Chouinard, G., Bobes, J., Ahokas, A., Eggens, I., Liu, S., et al. Extended-release quetiapine fumarate (quetiapine XR): A once-daily monotherapy effective in generalized anxiety disorder. Data from a randomized, double-blind, placebo- and active-controlled study. *Int. J. Neuropsychopharmacol.* 2010;13:305–320.

[56] Gao, K., Sheehan, D. V., Calabrese, J. R. Atypical antipsychotics in primary generalized anxiety disorder or comorbid with mood disorders. *Expert. Rev. Neurother.* 2009;9:1147–1158.

[57] Wang, H. N., Peng, Y., Tan, Q. R., Chen, Y. C., Zhang, R. G., Qiao, Y. T., et al. Quetiapine ameliorates anxiety-like behavior and cognitive impairments in stressed rats: Implications for the treatment of posttraumatic stress disorder. *Physiol. Res.* 2010;59:263–271.

[58] Merideth, C., Cutler, A. J., She, F., Eriksson, H. Efficacy and tolerability of extended release quetiapine fumarate monotherapy in the acute treatment of generalized anxiety disorder: a randomized, placebo controlled and active-controlled study. *Int. Clin. Psychopharmacol.* 2012;27:40-54.

[59] Altamura, A. C., Serati, M., Buoli, M., Dell'Osso, B. Augmentative quetiapine in partial/nonresponders with generalized anxiety disorder: a randomized, placebo-controlled study. *Int. Clin. Psychopharmacol.* 2011;26:201-5.

[60] Nyberg, S., Widzowski, D. Translational pharmacology of quetiapine and norquetiapine: Preclinical findings support multifunctional psychotropic properties. *Eur. Psychiatry* 2010;25:1446.

[61] Scharf, M., Rogowski, R., Hull, S., Cohn, M., Mayleben, D., Feldman, N., et al. Efficacy and safety of doxepin 1 mg, 3 mg, and 6 mg in elderly patients with primary insomnia: A randomized, double-blind, placebo-controlled crossover study. *J. Clin. Psychiatry* 2008;69:1557–1564.

[62] Jahanshahi, A., Lim, L. W., Steinbusch, H. W., Visser-Vandewalle, V., Temel, Y. Buspirone-induced changes in the serotonergic and non-serotonergic cells in the dorsal raphe nucleus of rats. *Neurosci. Lett.* 2010;473:136–140.

[63] Shajahan, P., Taylor, M. The uses and outcomes of quetiapine in depressive and bipolar mood disorders in clinical practice. *J. Psychopharmacol.* 2010;24:565–572.

[64] McIntyre, A., Gendron, A., McIntyre, A. Quetiapine adjunct to selective serotonin reuptake inhibitors or venlafaxine in patients with major depression, comorbid anxiety, and residual depressive symptoms: A randomized,placebo-controlled pilot study. *Depress Anxiety* 2007;24:487–494.

[65] Keck, P. E. Jr., McElroy, S. L., Arnold, L. M. Ziprasidone: A new atypical antipsychotic. *Expert Opin. Pharmacother.* 200 1;2: 103 3–1042.

[66] Warrington, L., Lombardo, I., Loebel, A., Ice, K. Ziprasidone for the treatment of acute manic or mixed episodes associated with bipolar disorder. *CNS Drugs* 2007;21:835–849.

[67] Ziprasidone (Geodon™) FDA Package Insert, Pfizer. 2001.

[68] Citrome, L., Reist, C., Palmer, L., Montejano, L. B., Lenhart, G., Cuffel, B., et al. Impact of real-world ziprasidone dosing on treatment discontinuation rates in patients with schizophrenia or bipolar disorder. *Schizophr. Res.* 2009;115:115–120.

[69] Citrome, L., Jaffe, A., Levine, J. How dosing of ziprasidone in a state hospital system differs from product labeling. *J. Clin. Psychiatry* 2009;70:975–982.

[70] Stahl, S. M., Shayegan, D. The psychopharmacology of ziprasidone: Receptor-binding properties and real-world psychiatric practice. *J. Clin. Psychiatry* 2003;64:6–12.

[71] Shayegan, D. K., Stahl, S. M. Atypical Antipsychotics: Matching receptor profile to individual patient's clinical profile. *CNS Spectrums* 2003;9:6–14.

[72] Stahl, S. M., Lombardo, I., Loebel, A., Mandel, F. Efficacy of Ziprasidone in Dysphoric Mania: Pooled analysis of 2 double blind studies. *J. Affect. Disord.* 2010;122:

[73] Cutler, A., Ball, S., Stahl, S. M. Expert review supplement dosing atypicals antipsychotics.*CNS Spectrums* 2008;13:1–14.

[74] Liebowitz, M. R., Salman, E., Mech, A., Dunner, D., Johnson, A. E., Akhtar, J., et al. Ziprasidone monotherapy in bipolar II depression: An open trial. *J. Affect. Disord.* 2009;118:205–208.

[75] Rosa, A. R., Franco, C., Torrent, C., Comes, M., Cruz, N., Horga, G., et al. Ziprasidone in the treatment of affective disorders: A review. *CNS Neurosci. Ther.* 2008;14:278–286.

[76] Papakostas, G. I., Petersen, T. J., Nierenberg, A. A., Murakami, J. L., Alpert, J. E., Rosenbaum, J. F., et al. Ziprasidone augmentation of selective serotonin reuptake inhibitors (SSRIs) for SSRI-resistant major depressive disorder. *J. Clin. Psychopharmacol.* 2004;65:217–221.

[77] Snyderman, S. H., Rynn, M. A., Rickels, K. Open-label pilot study of ziprasidone for refractory generalized anxiety disorder. *J. Clin. Psychopharmacol.* 2005;25:497–499.

[78] Dunner, D. L., Amsterdam, J. D., Shelton, R. C., Loebel, A., Romano, S. J. Efficacy and tolerability of adjunctive ziprasidone in treatment-resistant depression: A randomized, open-label, pilot study. *J. Clin. Psychiatry* 2007;68:1071–1077.

[79] Edwards, S. J., Smith, C. J. Tolerability of atypical antipsychotics in the treatment of adults with schizophrenia or bipolar disorder: A mixed treatment comparison of randomized controlled trials. *Clin. Ther.* 2009; (Pt 1):1345–1359.

[80] Stip, E., Tourjman, V. Aripiprazole in schizophrenia and schizoaffective disorder: A review. *Clin. Ther.* 2010;32 :S3–S20.

[81] Young, A. H., Oren, D. A., Lowy, A., et al. Aripiprazole monotherapy in acute mania: 12-week randomized placebo- and haloperidol-controlled study. *Br. J. Psychiatry* 2009;194:40–48.

[82] Arbaizar, B., Dierssen-Sotos, T., Gomez-Acebo, I., Llorca, J. Aripiprazole in major depression and mania: Meta-analyses of randomized placebo-controlled trials. *Gen. Hosp. Psychiatry* 2009;31:478–483.

[83] Nelson, J. C., Mankoski, R., Baker, R. A., Carlson, B. X., Eudicone, J. M., Pikalov, A., et al. Tran QV. Effects of aripiprazole adjunctive to standard antidepressant treatment on the core symptoms of depression: A post-hoc, pooled analysis of two large, placebo-controlled studies. Berman RM. *J. Affect. Disord.* 2010;120:133–140.

[84] Marcus, R. N., Owen, R., Kamen, L., Manos, G., McQuade, R. D., Carson, W. H., et al. A placebo-controlled, fixed-dose study of aripiprazole in children and adolescents with irritability associated with autistic disorder. *J. Am. Acad. Child Adolesc. Psychiatry* 2009;48:1110–1119.

[85] Hoge, E. A., Worthington, J. J. 3rd., Kaufman, R. E., Delong, H. R., Pollack, M. H., Simon, N. M. Aripiprazole as augmentation treatment of refractory generalized anxiety disorder and panic disorder. *CNS Spectrums* 2008;13:522–527.

[86] Menza, M. A., Dobkin, R. D., Marin, H. An open-label trial of aripiprazole augmentation for treatment-resistant generalized anxiety disorder. *J. Clin. Psychopharmacol.* 2007;27:207–210.

[87] Asenapine (Saphris ^{TM}) FDA Package Insert. 2009.

[88] McIntyre, R. S., Cohen, M., Zhao, J., Alphs, L., Macek, T. A., Panagides, J. Asenapine in the treatment of acute mania in bipolar I disorder: A randomized, double-blind, placebo-controlled trial. *J. Affect. Disord.* 2010;122:27–38.

[89] Tarazi, F. I., Shahid, M. Asenapine maleate: A new drug for the treatment of schizophrenia and bipolar mania. *Drugs of Today* 2009;45:865–876.

[90] Potkin, S. G., Cohen, M., Panagides, J. Efficacy and tolerability of asenapine in acute schizophrenia: A placebo- and risperidone-controlled trial. *J. Clin. Psychiatry* 2007;68:1492–1500.

[91] Franberg, O., Marcus, M. M., Ivanov, V., Schilstrom, B., Shahid, M., Svensson, T. H. Evidence for activation of cortical and subcortical dopamine systems by different mechanisms. *Psychopharmacology* 2009;204:251–264.

[92] Iloperidone (Fanapt TM) FDA Package Insert. Vanda Pharmaceuticals. 2009.

[93] Potkin, S. G., Litman, R. E., Torres, R., Wolfgang, C. D. Efficacy of iloperidone in the treatment of schizophrenia: Initial phase 3 studies. *J. Clin. Psychopharmacol.* 2008;28: S4–S 11.

[94] Kalkman, H. O., Feuerbach, D., Lotscher, E., Schoeffter, P. Functional characterization of the novel antipsychotic iloperidone at human D2, D3, alpha 2C, 5-HT6, and 5-HT1A receptors. *Life Sci.* 2003;73:1 151–1159.

[95] Kantrowitz, J.T., Citrome L. Lurasidone for schizophrenia: what's different?. *Expert Review of Neurotherapeutics.* 2012;12(3):265-73.

[96] http://clinicaltrials.pharmaceutical- accessed 7/8/12)

[97] Seneca, N., Finnema, S. J., Laszlovszky, I., Kiss, B., Horváth, A., Pásztor, G., et al. Occupancy of dopamine D_2 and D_3 and serotonin $5\text{-}HT_1A$ receptors by the novel antipsychotic drug candidate, cariprazine (RGH-188), in monkey brain measured using positron emission tomography. *Psychopharmacology* (Berl.). 2011 Dec.;218(3):579-87.

[98] Laszlovszky István, Bose, Anjana; Andor, György; Németh, György; Werner, Peter. The efficacy and tolerability of cariprazine in acute mania associated with bipolar I disorder: a phase II trial. *International Clinical Psychopharmacology*: September 2011 - Volume 26 - Issue - p e15. doi: 10.1097/01.yic.0000405646. 66223.c0

[99] Gründer, G. Cariprazine, an orally active D2/D3 receptor antagonist, for the potential treatment of schizophrenia, bipolar mania and depression. *Curr. Opin. Investig. Drugs*. 2010;11:823-32.

[100] http://clinicaltrials.govict2/results?term=0PC-34712, accessed 7/8/12

[101]Stahl, S. M. Multifunctional drugs: A novel concept for psychopharmacology. *CNS Spectrums* 2009;14:71–73.

[102] Kim, S. W., Yoo, J. A., Lee, S. Y., Kim, S. Y., Bae, K. Y., Yang, S. J., Kim, J. M., Shin, I. S., Yoon, J. S. Risperidone versus olanzapine for the treatment of delirium. *Hum. Psychopharmacol*. 2010 Jun.;25(4):298-302.

[103] Dtsch Med. Wochenschr. 2011 Apr.;136(14):681-4. Epub. 2011 Mar. 29. [Delirium in the elderly] [Article in German] Singler, K., Singler, B., Heppner, H. J.

[104] Zimmerman, K., Rudolph, J., Salow, M., Skarf, L. M. Delirium in palliative care patients: focus on pharmacotherapy *Am. J. Hosp. Palliat. Care*. 2011;28:501-10. doi: 10.1177/1049909111403732. Epub. 2011 Mar. 30.

[105] Schwartz, T. L., Masand, P. S. The Role of Atypical Antipsychotics in the Treatment of Delirium. *Psychosomatics* 2002;43:3.

[106] Briskman, I., Dubinski, R., Barak, Y. Treating delirium in a general hospital: a descriptive study of prescribing patternsand outcomes. *Int. Psychogeriatr*. 2010 ;22:328-31.

[107] Grover, S., Kumar, V., Chakrabarti, S. Comparative efficacy study of haloperidol, olanzapine and risperidone in delirium. *J. Psychosom. Res*. 2011;71:277-81.

[108] Attard, A., Ranjith, G., Taylor, D. Delerium and its treatment. *CNS Drugs* 2008; 22 (8): 631-644.

[109] Boettger, S., Breitbart, W. An open trial of aripiprazole for the treatment of delirium in hospitalized cancer patients. *Palliat Support Care*. 2011;9:351-7.

[110] Leso, L., Schwartz, T. L. Ziprasidone treatment of delirium. *Psychosomatics* 2002; 43:1; 61.

[111] Katz, L. J. ADHD in adults: The syndrome and its reconceptualization. Goldstein, Gerald (Ed.); Incagnoli, Theresa, M. (Ed.); Puente, Antonio, E. (Ed.). (2011). *Contemporary neurobehavioral syndromes*. (pp. 71-109). xi, 311 pp. New York, NY, US: Psychology Press; US.

[112] Scott, C. W. Adult attention deficit hyperactivity disorder. *Journal of Men's Health* 2011;8:299-305.

[113] Fullerton, C. A., Epstein, A. M., Frank, R. G., Normand, S. L., Fu, C. X., McGuire, T. G. Medication use and spending trends among children with ADHD in Florida's Medicaid program, 1996-2005 *Psychiatr. Serv*. 2012 ;63:115-21.

[114] Findling, R. L., Short, E. J., Leskovec, T., Townsend, L. D., Demeter, C. A., McNamara, N. K., et al. Aripiprazole in children with attention-deficit/hyperactivity disorder. *Journal of Child and Adolescent Psychopharmacology* 2008; 18:347-54.

[115] Armenteros, J. L., Lewis, J. E., Davalos, M. Risperidone augmentation for treatment-resistant aggression in attention-deficit/hyperactivity disorder: a placebo-controlled pilot study. *Journal of the American Academy of Child and Adolescent Psychiatry* 2007;46:558-65.

In: Antipsychotic Drugs
Editors: T.L. Schwartz, J. Megna and M.E. Topel
ISBN: 978-1-62100-071-6

Chapter 6

DEPOT ANTIPSYCHOTICS

Nisha Warikoo[1], Thomas L. Schwartz[1] and Leslie Citrome[2*]
[1]SUNY Upstate Medical University, Department of Psychiatry, Syracuse, NY, US
[2]New York Medical College, Valhalla, NY, US

ABSTRACT

Introduction: Schizophrenia is a chronic mental disorder generally treated with antipsychotic medications. A major determinant of outcome is treatment adherence, with partial or complete non-adherence to treatment commonly interfering with recovery. Nonadherence has very serious consequences that include exacerbation of psychotic symptoms, substance use, increased aggression toward self and others; poor prognosis, increased hospital and emergency room use and higher health care costs. One clinical approach to the problem of non-adherence is the use of long-acting injectable "depot" formulations of antipsychotic medication instead of, or in addition to, oral preparations.

Conclusion: Depot antipsychotics have several advantages compared to oral antipsychotics that include early detection of nonadherence, increased adherence, stable plasma concentrations, controlled administration, patient convenience, reduced relapse rates and improved global functioning. Despite the high rates of nonadherence in the community, depot antipsychotics are underutilized. This chapter will review the different depot antipsychotics available in the United States.

INTRODUCTION

Schizophrenia is a chronic mental disorder generally treated with antipsychotic medications. A major determinant of outcome is treatment adherence, with partial or complete non-adherence to treatment commonly interfering with an optimal recovery.

[*] Thomas L. Schwartz, MD, SUNY Upstate Medical University, Department of Psychiatry, 750 East Adams Street, Syracuse, NY 13210, 315 464-3100, Fax 315-464-3163.
Leslie Citrome, MD, MPH, Clinical Professor of Psychiatry and Behavioral Sciences, New York Medical College, Valhalla, NY, US.

Reported rates of non-adherence (noncompliance) to antipsychotics range from 20–89%, with an average rate of approximately 50% [1].

Nonadherence has very serious consequences. These include exacerbation of psychotic symptoms, increased aggression toward self and others, poor prognosis [2, 3], increased hospital and emergency room visits [4, 5] and higher health care costs [6]. Studies have shown clinically relevant symptom exacerbation in 75% of patients who stopped taking antipsychotic medication over the course of a year [7]. The estimated relapse rate because of nonadherence is as high as 50% during the year following discharge [8]. Frequent and multiple psychotic relapses are associated with an increased risk of homelessness [5], the likelihood of aggression toward self and others, damage to property [9,10] and may result in treatment resistance to antipsychotic medications, to the development of chronic psychotic symptoms [3] and overall long term poorer prognosis [2,11].

Finally, psychotic relapse resulting from non-adherence to medication increases health care costs associated with schizophrenia because of a greater need for hospitalization and emergency room care [5]. Research suggests that about 40% of the costs of hospitalization for persons who have schizophrenia are attributable to nonadherence to medication; the remaining 60% results from lost efficacy of antipsychotic medication [6]. Nonadherence has also been associated with other adverse outcomes such as, suicide, arrests, violence, victimizations, poor mental functioning, poor life satisfaction, greater substance use, and greater alcohol-related problems [12].

Additionally, if nonadherence goes unrecognized, it may lead to a faulty impression that a medication regimen is ineffective, leading to unnecessary changes in medication [13], increases in monotherapy drug dose [13,14], increases in polypharmacy [13], and the inaccurate categorization of patients as being treatment-resistant rather than non-adherent.

One clinical approach to the problem of non-adherence is the use of long-acting injectable "depot" formulations of antipsychotic medication instead of, or in addition to, oral preparations. This chapter will focus on this antipsychotic formulation.

History of Depot Antipsychotics

Depot antipsychotics have been available for use in the US since 1967 when fluphenazine enanthate was approved, which was followed in 1972 by fluphenazine decanoate. Haloperidol decanoate was approved in 1986. Other first-generation antipsychotics are available in a depot formulation (for example perphenazine) but these have not been commercialized in the US. In 2003 the first second-generation antipsychotic (SGA), risperidone long-acting injectable was approved by US Food and Drug Administration (FDA) [15].

Other SGA depot preparations have followed. Paliperidone palmitate received FDA approval in 2009 [16], which was shortly followed by olanzapine palmoate [17]. Depot formulations of aripiprazole [18] and ilioperidone [19] are in development.

ADVANTAGES OF DEPOT ANTIPSYCHOTICS

See also table I. The main advantage of depot antipsychotic formulations is that it overcomes the problem of covert nonadherence. The depot form's guaranteed injectable delivery eliminates covert noncompliance and should lead to greater effectiveness [20]. Patients who refuse their injection, miss their injection appointment, or do not receive it for any other reason can be immediately identified and clinically managed thus thwarting any ongoing nonadherence.

Additionally, if the patient does relapse despite receiving routine depot antipsychotics, it is then clear that other reasons for psychotic relapse need to be considered and explored. Stable plasma concentrations can be achieved over long periods of time, allowing for injections every few weeks [21]. This eliminates the patient's need to take the oral medication daily, thus enhancing patient convenience and also it may save staff a considerable amount of time in the inpatient setting [22].

In a recent meta-analysis that included ten studies with 1700 participants, depot formulations significantly reduced relapses with relative and absolute risk reductions of 30% and 10%, respectively. Initiation of depot antipsychotic therapy was associated with a decline in hospitalization rates and costs [23]. In a recent nation-wide cohort study of 1588 patients diagnosed with schizophrenia following a first hospitalization, the risk of re-hospitalization for patients receiving depot medications was about one-third of that for patients receiving oral medications [24]. This reduction in hospitalization translates into significant cost savings [25]. Not only can the use of depot antipsychotics prevent or delay relapse [26,27], but early detection of nonadherence and improved adherence associated with their use, may lead to improved global functioning [28]. Although brand name depot medication can cost significantly more than oral forms, these costs may be insignificant when compared with the time saved by staff (when administering medication biweekly or monthly rather than daily), by shortening hospital stays, rates of re-hospitalization and improving patient outcomes [22]. During the critical inpatient-to-outpatient transition period, depot antipsychotics may be advantageous in getting patients to better attend outpatient clinic programs [29]. Use of depot preparations alone is also advantageous in that it reduces the availability of medications for overdose or abuse [30].

The remainder of the chapter will review and focus on the first and second-generation depot antipsychotic preparations available in the US.

Table 1. Advantages of Depot Antipsychotics

Early detection of nonadherence
Increased adherence
No oral absorption problems
Stable plasma concentrations
Controlled administration
Patient convenience
Reduced relapse rates, resulting in cost savings
Clearer attribution of the cause of relapse or nonresponse
Improved global functioning
Regular contact with doctors or nurses

FIRST-GENERATION DEPOT ANTIPSYCHOTICS

Fluphenazine Decanoate and Enanthate

Fluphenazine was one of the first antipsychotics made available in a depot form and is a phenothiazine compound. Fluphenazine enanthate was approved for marketing in the US in 1967. In 1972 fluphenazine decanoate became available for use and generally replaced the use of the enanthate formulation. The cost of generic fluphenazine decanoate (25 mg/ml) is approximately $68 for a 5-ml vial (local state-operated psychiatric center pharmacy cost February 25, 2012).

Formulation and Pharmacokinetics

Fluphenazine decanoate and enanthate are esters formed between the alcohol group of fluphenazine and the long chain of fatty acid- decanoic acid and enanthic acid respectively. Esterification with enanthic acid, a seven-carbon fatty acid imparts fluphenazine enanthate dissimilar properties compared to the decanoate formulation [31]. Fluphenazine enanthate and decanoate are dissolved in sesame oil. Esterification increases the fat solubility of the antipsychotic a thousand fold, causing the ester to be released from the oil phase by slow diffusion into the body water phase. Upon release from the oil, the ester is hydrolyzed immediately or following distribution to the tissues. This process helps maintain a constant serum level of the antipsychotic in between injections [32]. Fluphenazine from the enanthate formulation is released more rapidly into the bloodstream than from the decanoate formulation, thus requiring more frequent administration and is intrinsically shorter acting [33].

The elimination half-lives of enanthate and decanoate are 3.5-4 days [34,35] and 6.8-9.6 days [36] respectively after a single dose of 25 mg. For this reason, more clinicians are likely to prefer the decanoate form, which as noted can be administered less frequently as compared to the enanthate form [37]. The mean apparent half-life of fluphenazine decanoate has been calculated to be 14.3+-2.2 days, suggesting that the time to reach steady state level is 4-6 weeks. The higher apparent half-life is due to re-distribution from tissue storage sites or due to absorption of residual drug from multiple depot injection sites. Fluphenazine, and 7-hyroxyfluphenazine have been found in the urine and their conjugated forms in the feces [38]. Cerebrospinal fluid concentrations were measured to be 38% of the plasma concentrations in six patients with schizophrenia [39]. In studies evaluating fluphenazine concentrations following withdrawal, detectable levels have been observed in some patients at week 24. The decline in the plasma concentration of the drug occurs in a slow, non-linear fashion [40]. The mechanism of slow plasma concentration clearance following withdrawal has been explained by several mechanisms including slow absorption or multi-compartment tissue binding and injection technique [38,41].

Smoking has been noted to increase the clearance of fluphenazine decanoate by a factor of 2.33 [42].

Dosing and Administration

For most patients, a dose of fluphenazine decanoate12.5-25 mg should be given to initiate treatment. The usual dose range is 12.5 mg-50 mg every two weeks by deep intramuscular injection in the deltoid or gluteal muscle. Dose should not exceed 100 mg and if doses greater than 50 mg are deemed necessary, the next and succeeding doses should be increased cautiously in increments of 12.5 mg. Fluphenazine decanoate is available as 5 ml multiple dose vial (USP 25 mg/ml), is to be stored at controlled room temperature (59 to 86 F) and needs to be protected from light.

Dose response studies of fluphenazine decanoate have demonstrated that doses less than 2.5 mg and between 2.5-10 mg were significantly less effective than dose of 25 mg or greater every two weeks. While some patients were successfully maintained at a dose of 2.5 -10 mg, many patients require doses of 12.5-50 mg every two weeks [11, 43, 44]. In a recent study of inpatients with schizophrenia, the average dose of fluphenazine decanoate was 37.84±13.70 usually every two weeks [22]. Collectively, studies indicate that doses of fluphenazine decanoate as low as 5–10 mg every two weeks have been shown to be effective, and some patients may respond to even lower doses, but the risk of relapse can increase significantly with these lower doses. However, consideration should be given to judicious reduction in the long-acting injectable dose over time, especially for patients with adverse side effects, in order to evaluate the optimal dose and lower TD and EPS risks [44-46]. 10 mg of fluphenazine decanoate every two weeks has been estimated to be equivalent to 100 mg chlorpromazine a day [21]. The depot-oral conversion ratio is 0.5 ml (12.5 mg) of decanoate every 3 weeks for every 10 mg of fluphenazine hydrochloride daily [47].

Efficacy

With few exceptions [48-50], the bulk of the evidence supports the efficacy of depot fluphenazine. A longer-term study of two years duration comparing fluphenazine decanoate with placebo found that relapse was significantly reduced in the fluphenazine arm (n=54, RR 0.35, CI 0.2 to 0.6, NNT 2 CI 2 to 4) [51,52]. Across studies as described in a review [51], fluphenazine decanoate did not reduce relapse more than oral antipsychotics (n=419, 6 RCTs, RR relapse 26- 52 weeks 1.46 CI 0.8 to 2.8) [51,53-58]. It did not reduce relapse more than other depot antipsychotics (n=581, 11 RCTs, RR relapse 26-52 weeks 0.82 CI 0.6 to 1.2) [51, 56, 59-67]. Relapse rates over six months to one year were not significantly different between standard dosage of fluphenazine decanoate and a low dose group (n= 523, 4 RCTs, RR 2.09 CI 0.6 to 7.1) [44, 51, 68-70]. Studies have reported no significant difference in relapse scores (medium term) between either high or standard dose depot groups (n=184, RR 2.11, CI 0.3 to 14.9) [51, 71, 72].

Limited data is available for fluphenazine enanthate. There was no significant difference in global change (0 to 5 weeks) in subjects on fluphenazine enanthate when compared with oral antipsychotics (n=31, 1 RCTs, RR 0.67 CI 0.3 to 1.7) [51, 73] and in relapse rates over 6-26 weeks between fluphenazine enanthate and other depots [51, 74-76]. Studies have shown no significant difference in relapse rate between the fluphenazine decanoate group and the fluphenazine enanthate group at five to six months (n=30, RR 2.29 CI 0.7 to 7.5) and over medium term (six months to one year) (n=39, RR 2.43 CI 0.7 to 8.3) [51, 77].

Safety

Long-term studies tend to favor fluphenazine decanoate over oral antipsychotics for movement disorders (n=259, RR 0.47 CI 0.2 to 0.9, NNT 14 CI 10 to 82) [51, 78, 79] except for one longer-term study that found no significant difference in the incidence of movement disorders (n=44, RR 0.40 CI 0.1 to 1.3) [51,57]. Akathisia was significantly lower in the oral fluphenazine group (n=51, RR 20.54 CI 1.3 to 338) [50,51]. No significant differences emerged between fluphenazine decanoate and oral agents in regards to Simpson Angus Scale scores [51,57], general adverse effects, tremor and blurred vision. [51,80,81]. Studies also found no significant difference with movement disorders, dry mouth, tardive dyskinesia, parkinsonism, tremor, blurred vision between fluphenazine decanoate and other depot neuroleptics [51,61,62,64,66]. General adverse effects – tremors, extrapyramidal side-effects (short term data)[51,63] favored other depot neuroleptics (n=88, RR 1.36 CI 1.1 to 1.7). However, medium term data (n=249, six months to one year) were equivocal. In comparison with newer depot formulations, fluphenazine decanoate has been reported to cause greater extrapyramidal adverse effects [51,82].

The number of people needing anticholinergic drugs in short term studies was found in one study to be significantly lower for the fluphenazine decanoate group compared to enanthate group (n=33, RR 0.29 CI 0.1 to 0.70 [51,83,84]. For longer term studies (six weeks to one year) there were no significant differences in the number of people requiring anticholinergic drugs [51,77].

Haloperidol Decanoate

Haloperdol decanoate was approved for use in the US in 1986. It is the decanoate ester of the butyrophenone, haloperidol. It is available as haloperidol decanoate 50 and 100, containing 50 mg haloperidol (present as haloperidol decanoate 70.52 mg) and 100 mg haloperidol (present as haloperidol decanoate 141.04 mg) respectively. The cost of 1 ml vials of haloperidol depot 50 mg/ml and 100 mg/ml is approximately \$18 and \$34 respectively. The cost of 5 ml vials of haloperidol depot 50 mg/ml and 100 mg/ml is approximately \$92 and \$169 respectively (local state-operated psychiatric center pharmacy cost February 25, 2012).

Formulation and Pharmacokinetics

Haloperidol decanoate is dissolved in sesame oil. It has been suggested that haloperidol decanoate may have a more stable bond and slower hydrolysis resulting in a longer duration of action, compared to fluphenazine decanoate and enanthate [85]. Dissolution in sesame oil makes the ester highly lipophilic.

After an intramuscular injection, haloperidol decanoate is cleaved by the esterases in the muscle and the blood and the active moiety is released. The release and availability of the free drug from the oily site is the rate-limiting step, since the hydrolysis by esterases occurs fairly rapidly. Hence, the rate of elimination is controlled not by the rate of hepatic metabolism, but by the rate of systemic peripheral absorption. Intramuscular haloperidol provides nearly 100% bioavailability, as opposed to the oral formulation where the bioavailability is approximately 60-70% [86].

Peak plasma concentrations are reached between three to nine days following injections, with fewer plasma level fluctuations than fluphenazine decanoate or enanthate [85]. The elimination half-life of haloperidol decanoate is three weeks, suggesting that the steady state level is reached in three months. A correlation for dose and plasma level has been suggested; haloperidol decanoate 100 mg every four weeks for three consecutive months results in plasma concentrations ranging from 3-10 ug/L [87]. Haloperidol is metabolized to less active metabolites, which may bind to dopamine receptors. Reduced clearance has been noted in geriatric patients, thus necessitating a dosage reduction [88].

Dosing and Administration

Haloperidol decanoate should be administered intramuscularly in the deltoid or gluteal muscle by a "Z track technique" [85]. After selection of the injection site, the patient is to be positioned so the muscle at the injection site relaxes. The nondominant hand should be used to pull the skin downward or laterally to displace the tissue about 1 inch (2.54 cm). With the needle at a 90-degree angle to the site, the skin should be pierced using a smooth, steady motion. After ensuring that a blood vessel has not been entered by aspiration, the drug should be injected slowly at a rate of 10 mL/second of medication. Once the drug is completely instilled, the needle should be withdrawn after a 10 second wait with a smooth, steady motion and the skin should be released to its original position. Gentle pressure should be applied at the injection site [85]. Conversion from oral haloperidol to haloperidol decanoate can be achieved by using an initial dose of haloperidol decanoate that is 10 to 20 times the previous daily dose in oral haloperidol equivalents. In patients who are elderly, debilitated, or stable on low doses of oral haloperidol (e.g. up to the equivalent of 10 mg/day oral haloperidol), a range of 10 to 15 times the previous daily dose in oral haloperidol equivalents is appropriate. In patients previously maintained on higher doses of antipsychotics for whom a low dose approach risks recurrence of psychiatric decompensation, 20 times the previous daily dose in oral haloperidol equivalents should be considered for initial conversion, with downward titration on succeeding injections. The initial dose of haloperidol decanoate should not exceed 100 mg regardless of previous antipsychotic dose requirements and some have recommended a test dose of 50 mg IM initially [21]. The usual maintenance range is 10 to 15 times the previous daily dose in oral haloperidol equivalents dependent on the clinical response of the patient. The recommended dose range is 50-300 mg every four weeks. 30 mg every two weeks of haloperidol decanoate is equivalent to 100 mg/day of chlorpromazine [21]. Haloperidol decanoate is to be stored at controlled room temperature (15°–30° C, 59°–86° F) and should be protected from light.

Efficacy

Numerous uncontrolled and nonblinded studies have helped in establishing the efficacy of haloperidol decanoate [89]. A systematic review and meta-analysis is available [90]. In a haloperidol decanoate versus placebo comparison, two small studies reported that significantly fewer people on depot left treatment early (OR 0.09 CI 0.03-0.21, NNT 2 CI 1-3) or experienced no important improvement in mental state (OR 0.04 CI 0.01-0.15) [90, 91]. Data from a small study suggested that those taking haloperidol decanoate would need less additional oral antipsychotic medication (OR 0.14 Cl 0.04-0.55, NNT 2 CI 1-5) [90,92]. Haloperidol decanoate was compared to oral haloperidol in a single trial that showed no differences in global impression or mental state (n=22). Compliance with medication was not reported in this study [90,93]. Trials have compared haloperidol decanoate to other depot neuroleptics and again no differences were found for the outcomes of mortality, global impression, mental state or behavior [n=371, OR 0.92 CI 0.52-1.6) [90,94-96].

Safety

A study comparing haloperidol decanoate to placebo, reported significantly more people in the placebo group experiencing blurred vision and no difference between groups for tremors [90,92]. In a trial that compared depot with oral haloperidol, no significant differences in numbers needing anticholinergic drugs were found [90,93]. Trials that compared haloperidol decanoate to other first-generation depot antipsychotics found no differences for dyskinesias, tremor or need for anticholinergic medication [90, 94, 96].

SECOND-GENERATION DEPOT ANTIPSYCHOTICS

Risperidone Long Acting Injection

In 2003, the US FDA approved a long-acting injectable formulation of [15,97]. The cost of risperidone long-acting injection (LAI) 12.5 mg, 25 mg, 37.5 and 50 mg (1 injection) is approximately $128, $257, $385 and $514 respectively (local state-operated psychiatric center pharmacy cost February 25, 2012). In addition to the indication for schizophrenia, risperidone long-acting injection is also approved for as monotherapy or as adjunctive therapy to lithium or valproate for the maintenance treatment of Bipolar I Disorder.

Formulation and Pharmacokinetics

Risperidone is a benzisoxazole derivative with selective balanced antagonism of D_2 and HT_2 receptors. Risperidone LAI is an extended release microsphere formulation of risperidone encapsulated in polyglactin given as an intramuscular injection. Encapsulation in polymeric microspheres of D, L polyactide coglycolide, a biodegradable polymer allows the microspheres to gradually break down over a period of several weeks, thus enabling delivery of predictable and stable plasma levels of risperidone. Unlike most first-generation antipsychotic (FGA) depots, risperidone lacks a free hydroxyl group and hence esterification with a long-chain fatty acid to allow delivery in a viscous oil medium is not possible [98].

After a single intramuscular injection of this drug, a small initial amount (<1%) is released from the surface of the microsphere. The main release of the drug does not begin until 3 weeks after the administration and therapeutic serum plasma levels are attained within four to six weeks, subsiding by week seven. The elimination phase that occurs by hydrolysis is complete by week seven to eight. It is rapidly metabolized to 9-hydroxy risperidone (paliperidone) by CYP450 2D6. The pharmacokinetics of long-acting risperidone is linear in the dose range of 25 to 50 mg.

Following extensive first-pass metabolism of risperidone by the liver, 90% is bound in plasma to albumin and alpha-1 acid glycoprotein prior to elimination via the kidneys. Plasma levels are essentially no different in patients with hepatic insufficiency, but may be raised by 60% in patients with renal impairment [99]. Aging is associated with decreased rates of renal blood flow, glomerular filtration, renal clearance, reduced levels of synthesis and activity of hepatic microsomal enzymes and a fall in total body water may result in higher plasma concentrations of risperidone LAI, increasing both its activity and the potential for adverse effects.

Additionally, with age, loss of ascending dopaminergic neurons and postsynaptic dopamine receptors can halve the levels of striatal dopamine by age 65 years, resulting in more parkinsonism and tardive dyskinesia given risperidone's high affinity for dopaminergic D2 receptors [100,101].

Dosing and Administration

Risperidone LAI is to be administered by intramuscular injection in the deltoid or gluteal muscle. It is available as 25, 37.5 and 50 mg dose packages. It must be reconstituted by mixing the LAI powder with solvent by shaking vigorously for at least few seconds. Risperidone LAI is administered every two weeks using the safety needle provided in the package. It is recommended to begin treatment with risperidone LAI using the minimum effective dose, 25 mg every two weeks, with maximum dose not to exceed 50 mg every two weeks. For those already stabilized on an oral dose of risperidone for two weeks or more, the following conversion guidelines have been suggested. Patients on 4 mg/day or less of oral risperidone may be prescribed 25 mg IM risperidone LAI every two weeks; persons being treated with higher doses should receive risperidone LAI 37.5 mg IM every two weeks. Any further increases in dose may be considered after a trial on the previous dose for at least four weeks. Supplementation with oral risperidone should be provided for three weeks after initiating risperidone LAI and after any dose increase in order to ensure adequate plasma levels. The dosage recommendations for the elderly are 25 mg IM every two weeks. In patients with hepatic, or renal impairment or drug interactions that increase risperidone plasma concentrations, dose reduction as low as 12.5 mg may be appropriate, keeping in mind that the efficacy of the 12.5 mg dose has not been investigated fully in clinical trials [102,103,104].

Risperidone LAI should be stored in a refrigerator at 2-8°C and protected from light. If refrigeration is unavailable, it can be stored at temperatures not exceeding 25°C for no more than 7 days prior to administration[102].

Efficacy

Substantial evidence supports the effectiveness of long acting risperidone in patients with schizophrenia [105-114]. In risperidone LAI versus placebo comparisons, treatment with risperidone LAI resulted in significant improvements in Positive and Negative Syndrome Scale (PANSS) total scores, compared with placebo ($p < 0.01$) [105,106]. Various studies have reported that long-acting risperidone is effective in patients switching from oral antipsychotic therapy [107,113] and long-acting FGA treatments [110, 113,115,116]. In 188 patients receiving first-generation depot antipsychotic monotherapy at entry, Positive and Negative Syndrome Scale (PANSS)-total scores improved significantly after receiving long-acting risperidone [110].

In another study of 182 subjects, sustained, significant improvement in symptom control, and functioning was seen in stable patients treated with RLAI over 6 months following a switch from previous FGA (long acting) [116]. Studies comparing oral versus risperidone LAI have shown no significant difference for the PANSS total, negative and general psychopathology score [117-118]. Risperidone LAI has been shown to improve patient functioning, health-related quality of life (QOL) and patient satisfaction in recent studies [109, 113, 114, 119].

A recent international, long-term, prospective, observational study in patients who were commencing long-acting risperidone treatment including 1232 patients from six countries, evaluated the effectiveness of long-acting risperidone on personal and social functioning. At six months, the mean Personal and Social Performance scale scores had significantly improved compared to baseline on LAI [120].

Safety

Recent reviews and multiple studies have highlighted the short- term and long-term safety and tolerability profile of risperidone LAI [121, 122-124]. In a review, five studies were identified including patients were treated with Risperidone LAI 25 - 75 mg every 2 weeks (n = 928) and a low incidence of extrapyramidal symptoms was found and changes in lipids and glucose were of no clinical relevance. The most commonly reported adverse effects with risperidone LAI versus placebo in a representative 12-week trial included headache (20 vs 12%), agitation (15 vs 26%), insomnia (15 vs 14%), psychosis (12 vs 24%) and anxiety (9 vs 15%) [105]. Furthermore, there were ten cases of hyperprolactinemia and one patient with dysmenorrhea. Data from three 12-week trials showed elevations in prolactin plasma, although mean prolactin plasma levels tended to decrease over time [106,111,117,119]. In a 12-week study in 141 patients switched to long-acting risperidone (25, 37.5 or 50 mg) from oral FGAs or SGAs, mean (± SD) serum prolactin levels increased from 23.5 (± 2.4) ng/ml at baseline to 52.2 (± 3.7) ng/ml at end point [108]. Tardive dyskinesia (TD) was reported for 4 of 166 patients treated with RLAI in one of these 12-week trials [117]. A recent 12-week clinical trial including fifty hospitalized stable schizophrenic patients who had been treated with oral risperidone for three months and were then randomized during their hospitalization to oral risperidone or risperidone LAI reported similar efficacy with both risperidone formulations, although tolerability was better with RLAI [118]. Recently, 3-year follow-up data were published for 211 consecutive patients treated with RLAI in routine clinical practice. Over the 3 years, 37 patients discontinued RLAI due to an AE (17.5%), including parkinsonism, sexual dysfunction, injection site pain, akathisia/agitation, sedation, weight gain and peripheral edema. Similar to short-term data, serious side effects occurred infrequently with risperidone LAI and only 4 (1.9%) of 211 patients had discontinued treatment due to injection site pain [125].

Overall, risperidone LAI has demonstrated good safety and tolerability in both short and long-term studies, with an estimated total patient exposure of about 678,000 patient-years [121,126].

Paliperidone Palmitate

Paliperidone palmitate, whose active moiety is the 9- hydroxyrisperidone, the major active metabolite of risperidone, received FDA approval in 2009. The approximate cost of 1 injection of paliperidone palmitate 234, 156, 117, 78 and 39 mg is $1542, $1028, $771, $513 and $256 respectively (local state-operated psychiatric center pharmacy cost February 25, 2012).

Formulation and Pharmacokinetics

Paliperidone palmitate is a benzisoxazole derivative; it is hydrolyzed to the active moiety paliperidone. Its therapeutic efficacy is thought to be mediated via its combined antagonist activity towards central dopamine D2 and 5-HT2A receptors. Paliperidone also acts as an antagonist at alpha1 - and alpha2 -adrenergic receptors and histamine (H1) receptors and has no affinity for beta1 and beta2 -adrenergic or cholinergic muscarinic receptors [127]. Paliperidone palmitate has very low water solubility and dissolves slowly after intramuscular injection before being hydrolysed to paliperidone and absorbed into the systemic circulation. The rate-limiting factor is the dissolution of paliperidone palmitate at the injection site [128]. Following a single dose, plasma concentrations rise to reach maximum plasma concentrations at thirteen days. The release of the drug starts as early as day one and lasts for as long as 126 days. The median apparent half-life of paliperidone following a single intramuscular dose of 39–234 mg (injection site not specified) ranged from 25 to 49 days [129]. In single [130] and multiple dose [131,132] studies, maximum plasma paliperidone concentration (Cmax) values were higher (28%) after injection in the deltoid muscle than after injection in the gluteal muscle, and may be explained by the different distribution of muscle and adipose tissue at these sites. [129]. It is recommended that paliperidone palmitate be initiated by two initial deltoid injections spread one week apart to achieve therapeutic concentrations rapidly. At a steady state, little difference has been found in plasma paliperidone concentrations between the deltoid and gluteus sites for a given dose. Area under the concentration-time curve is dose proportional across the dose range of 39–234 mg, but peak concentrations are somewhat less than dose proportional for the higher doses. This has been attributed to the prolonged half-life for the higher doses explained by a slower absorption rate here [128]. The mean steady-state peak: trough ratio for paliperidone was 2.2 and 1.8 following deltoid or gluteal administration of 156 mg respectively [133].

The apparent volume of distribution of paliperidone is 391 L [128]. Approximately 74% of racemic paliperidone is bound to plasma proteins [133]. Animal studies have suggested that Paliperidone is excreted in breast milk; hence female patients receiving intramuscular paliperidone palmitate should not breastfeed [133]. Paliperidone is primarily excreted renally and is not extensively metabolized in the liver. No relationship has been found between CYP450 2D6, CYP450 3A4 / 5 genotype and paliperidone PK parameters [129]. Body mass index (BMI), creatinine clearance, injection site and volume, and needle length were all found to be important predictors of the pharmacokinetic profile of intramuscular paliperidone palmitate[128].

Renal impairment reduces the clearance of paliperidone. It is not recommended in patients with moderate or severe renal impairment but may be administered after dosage adjustment in patients with mild renal impairment [133].

Dosing and Administration

A trial of oral paliperidone or oral risperidone is recommended to establish tolerability prior to using paliperidone palmitate, in those patients who have never been on this drug [129]. Prefilled syringes of containing 39, 78, 117, 156 or 234 mg of paliperidone palmitate are available. The recommended dosage regimen is 234 mg on day one followed by 156mg on day eight, both administered in the deltoid muscle, and then 117 mg every four weeks thereafter, administered in the deltoid or gluteal muscle [133]. The maintenance dose of 117mg every four weeks (±7 days) may be adjusted monthly within a 39–234 mg range, depending on individual patient' tolerability or efficacy [133]. Those patients with a one-month to six-week interval since their last dose of intramuscular paliperidone palmitate should recommence therapy with one intramuscular paliperidone palmitate injection (at the previously stabilized dose), in the deltoid muscle, followed by monthly injections, whereas those with a > 6-week to < 6-month interval since their last dose should recommence therapy with two intramuscular paliperidone palmitate injections (at the previously stabilized dose unless the patient was initially stabilized with the 234 mg dose, in which case the 156 mg dose should be utilized) one week apart, in the deltoid muscle, followed by monthly injections. In those in whom greater than six months has elapsed since the last intramuscular injection, therapy should commence with 234 mg on day one followed by 156mg on day eight, both administered in the deltoid muscle [129]. In patients switching from other depot preparations, it has been suggested that Paliperidone palmitate may be administered in place of the next scheduled injection and then monthly.

A 1.5-inch, 22-gauge needle is recommended for patients whose weight is at least 90 kg (200 lb) and a 1-inch, 23 gauge for those who weigh < 90 kg (< 200 lb). For gluteal muscle injection, the recommended needle size for administration is a 1.5-inch 22-gauge [129]. As noted, paliperidone palmitate is not recommended for patients with moderate or severe renal impairment. For those with mild renal impairment, the recommended initiation is with a dose of 156 mg on day one and 117 mg one week later, with subsequent monthly injections of 78 mg. No dose adjustment is required in patients with mild or moderate hepatic impairment or for the elderly people without renal impairment [129]. Paliperidone palmitate should be stored at room temperature (25°C, 77°F); excursions between 15°C and 30°C (between 59°F and 86°F) are permitted.

Efficacy

The FDA approved paliperidone palmitate for the acute treatment of schizophrenia as evaluated in four short-term (one 9-week and three 13-week) double-blind, randomized, placebo-controlled, fixed-dose studies of acutely relapsed adult inpatients who met DSM-IV criteria for schizophrenia [133-136]. In all four studies, paliperidone palmitate was administered on days 1, 8 and 36, and for the 13-week studies, also on day 64. The primary efficacy outcome measure for the acute efficacy studies was the PANSS. In one 13-week study, all three paliperidone palmitate dose groups (39, 156 and 234 mg) showed a statistically significant improvement over placebo in the change in PANSS total score [136]. In another thirteen-week study, among the three dosage strengths of paliperidone palmitate tested (78, 156, and 234 mg), only the 156 mg group was superior to placebo in improving the PANSS total score [133]. In the third 13-week study comparing three fixed doses (39 mg/4 weeks, 78 mg/4 weeks, and 156 mg/4 weeks) to placebo, all three doses were superior to placebo in improving the PANSS total score. In the 9-week study (n=197) comparing two fixed doses of (78 mg/4 weeks and 156 mg/4 weeks) to placebo, both doses of were superior to placebo in improving PANSS total score.

Paliperidone palmitate injection was compared with risperidone long-acting injection (RLAI) in a 53-week non-inferiority study [137]. Although both agents resulted in decreases in PANSS total score, paliperidone was not shown to be non-inferior to RLAI. The authors concluded that non-inferiority was not established because patients had been initiated with suboptimal initial dosing of paliperidone and had been administered paliperidone in the gluteal muscle. Another non-inferiority study between paliperidone palmitate and RLAI was performed, which was a randomized (1:1), double-blind, double-dummy, active- controlled, parallel-group, 13-week comparative Phase III study, Paliperidone was shown to be non-inferior to RLAI [138]. Another open-label, rater-blinded, parallel-group study in Chinese adult patients with schizophrenia established the non-inferiority of paliperidone (50-150 mg eq., flexibly dosed, without oral paliperidone supplementation) to risperidone-LAI (25-50 mg, flexibly dosed, with oral risperidone supplementation) [139].

Safety

Paliperidone palmitate was reasonably well tolerated in the short-term efficacy studies. The incidence of extrapyramidal symptoms with paliperidone was generally low. However, in the 9-week study [135] 21% of the patients receiving paliperidone palmitate 156 mg used medications to treat extrapyramidal symptoms, with a number needed to harm (NNH) vs. placebo of 8 (95% CI 4–40) [140]. Orthostatic changes were infrequently encountered. Prolactin elevation is noted but very few prolactin-related adverse events were reported among the study participants in these short-term studies. Mean weight gain was generally low (1.5 kg or less); the proportion of patients with a body weight gain of at least 7% was as high as 11% for the 156 mg group in one study [134] and 13% for the 234 mg group in another study [136] with NNH vs. placebo of 12 (95% CI 7–33) and 13 (95% CI 8–54) respectively [140]. Injection site problems were infrequent; in one study they were more common with the paliperidone palmitate 156 and 234 mg groups than with placebo [133], and in other studies injection site problems occurred at similar rates with paliperidone palmitate as for placebo [134-136]. Cardiac tolerability appeared to be safe, with no patients experiencing QT_c prolongation or a $QT_c > 450$ msec.

Findings from the long-term relapse prevention study [141] showed that weight increase occurred more frequently in patients treated with paliperidone palmitate (7%) than placebo (1%), as did increased blood glucose levels (3%) versus placebo (1%). Mean weight, from transition baseline to the double-blind endpoint, increased by 1.9 kg for paliperidone-treated patients, but remained unchanged for placebo patients. In accordance with other studies, prolactin levels increased for the paliperidone group, again more in women than in men, while levels decreased in the placebo group. There were no clinically relevant changes from transition baseline to the double-blind end-point in extrapyramidal symptom rating scales and no reports of orthostatic hypotension or ECG changes during the double-blind phase.

The safety and tolerability of initiating treatment with paliperidone palmitate via either deltoid or gluteal injections were investigated in a crossover study of 252 stable outpatients comparing the two routes [132]. This trial randomly assigned 1:1:1 to three dose groups of paliperidone and two treatment sequences including deltoid muscle injection (13 weeks), followed by gluteal muscle injection (12 weeks), or the reverse. The proportion of patients with injection-site pain appeared to be higher after deltoid administration compared with gluteal administration, but the overall incidence of adverse effects did not differ significantly between deltoid injections and gluteal injections and there was no dose-dependent increase in the incidence of adverse effects. In the three non-inferiority studies of paliperidone palmitate and RLAI, the overall rates of adverse effects were found to be similar between the two groups [137-139].

Olanzapine Pamoate

The FDA approved olanzapine LAI in 2009. Use of olanzapine LAI is governed by a Risk Evaluation and Mitigation Strategy (REMS) program that requires a post-injection monitoring period. The cost of 1 injection of olanzapine LAI 210 mg, 300 mg and 405 mg is approximately $540, $772 and $1042 respectively (local state-operated psychiatric center pharmacy cost February 15, 2012).

Formulation and Pharmacokinetics

The depot intramuscular formulation of olanzapine is a crystalline salt formulation, olanzapine pamoate monohydrate, composed of olanzapine and pamoic acid [142]. The individual crystals are micron-sized and suspended in water. When injected into the muscle, the salt slowly dissolves and, in solution, dissociates into separate molecular entities of olanzapine and pamoic acid, which then enter into systemic circulation. Absorption of olanzapine occurs over a period of several weeks, owing to the slow dissolution rate of the crystalline salt formulation. When the olanzapine pamoate monohydrate crystalline salt comes into contact with a substantial amount of blood or plasma, the salt dissolves more quickly, resulting in the release of a large amount of olanzapine. Thus accidental injection into vasculature can lead to potentially very high plasma levels of olanzapine within a matter of minutes to hours, explaining the need for post injection monitoring. The pharmacokinetics of multiple doses of olanzapine LAI has been described in an open-label study in 282 symptom-stabilized patients with schizophrenia [142] Patients were stabilized on daily oral olanzapine, then received multiple olanzapine depot injections at doses of 100, 150, 160, 200 and 300 mg every two weeks, and 200, 255, 300 and 405 mg every four weeks for 24 weeks. Plasma olanzapine concentrations accumulated two to threefold upon multiple dosing and reached steady-state conditions after three months of dosing. Peak-to-trough fluctuation in concentrations averaged 51% for the 2-week injection interval and 75% for the 4-week interval. Maximum concentration and area under the curve for olanzapine were proportionate to depot dose. Time to peak concentration after injection was 4 days, half-life ~ 26 days, corresponding to 6 h for the time to peak concentration and 29-h half-life, respectively, for oral olanzapine [143].

Dosing and Administration

To determine the dose correspondence relative to oral olanzapine, periodic sampling of plasma olanzapine concentrations was performed in a subset of 346 patients who had participated in the 24-week maintenance of response study [144-146]. Olanzapine LAIdoses of 150 mg every two weeks, 405 mg every four weeks and 300 mg every two weeks produced 10th–90th percentile steady-state plasma concentrations (5–41, 8–51 and 7–73 ng / ml) similar to those for 10, 15 and 20 mg/ day oral olanzapine (13–48, 21–63 and 21–85 ng/ml), with steady state concentrations achieved after approximately three months of depot treatment. The authors recommended the following switching strategies in order to minimize the risk for exacerbation of psychosis: for patients stabilized on oral olanzapine 10 mg/ day, the starting olanzapine LAI dose should be 210 mg every two weeks or 405 mg every four weeks, and then if clinically indicated, patients can be evaluated two months later for a reduction to a maintenance dose of 150 mg every two weeks or 300 mg every four weeks; for patients stabilized on oral olanzapine 15 mg/ day, the starting olanzapine LAI dose should be

300 mg every two weeks, and then if clinically indicated, patients can be evaluated two months later for a reduction to a maintenance dose of 210 mg every two weeks or 405 mg every four weeks; for patients stabilized on oral olanzapine 20 mg/ day, the recommended starting and maintenance dose is 300 mg every two weeks.

Olanzapine LAI should only be administered as a deep intramuscular gluteal injection using a 19-gauge, 1.5 inch needle (2 Hypodermic Needle-Pro needles with protection device are included). For obese patients a 2-inch, 19-guage or larger needle can be used for administration (not included). Olanzapine LAI is not to be administered intravenously or subcutaneously. There is a warning for Post-Injection Delirium/Sedation Syndrome (PDSS), which is believed to occur following inadvertent partial intravascular administration, and is the reason behind the REMS program mandated for the use of this product. Injection technique recommendations [146] include the aspiration of the syringe to ensure that no blood is visible, and to not proceed with injection if blood is visible. In these circumstances, the syringe is discarded, a new vial reconstituted and injection placed into the alternate buttock, deep into the gluteal muscle. Additional risk management recommendations include that after each injection, clinicians observe the patient for at least 3 hours at a healthcare facility for symptoms of PDSS. Olanzapine LAI has not been studied in sufficient number of persons age 65 and older to determine if this population responds differently. Starting older patients on a low dose should be considered. There are no dosing recommendations for patients with kidney or hepatic impairment.

Olanzapine LAI should be stored at room temperature not to exceed 30°C [146]. When the drug product is suspended in the solution, it may be held at room temperature for 24 hours. The vial should be agitated immediately prior to product withdrawal. Once the suspension is withdrawn into the syringe, it should be used immediately.

Efficacy

In a double blind, placebo-controlled, 8-week study of olanzapine pamoate, in-patients with acute schizophrenia were treated with 210 mg every two weeks, 300 mg every two weeks, 405 mg every four weeks or placebo in a randomized design [147]. Olanzapine LAI separated significantly from placebo on the PANSS total score as early as Day 3 after injection. Oral antipsychotics were not required nor allowed.

In a 24-week double-blind trial, olanzapine LAI was compared with oral olanzapine to assess maintenance of antipsychotic treatment in stable schizophrenia outpatients [148]. Patients were randomized to receive olanzapine LAI 405 mg every four weeks, 300 mg every two weeks, 150 mg every two weeks, 45 mg every four weeks, or 10, 15 or 20 mg/ day oral olanzapine. Patients had maintained stability on an oral dose of olanzapine (10, 15 or 20 mg/day for 4 -8 weeks) before randomization. Each of the therapeutic olanzapine LAI doses was statistically superior to the 45 mg every four weeks dose with respect to time to exacerbation of symptoms. In addition, the three active olanzapine LAI dose groups showed effective maintenance as measured by PANSS scores compared with the 45-mg group, which showed a statistically significant worsening. Mean baseline to end point change in PANSS total score for the oral olanzapine group was not significantly different from the high olanzapine pamoate dose group, but superior to the other LAI doses. The pooled 150 mg and 300 mg every two weeks olanzapine LAI groups were non-inferior to the oral olanzapine group in nonexacerbation rate over 24 weeks. Also, the three active olanzapine LAI groups showed non-inferiority compared with the oral olanzapine group in exacerbation of symptoms.

In a 2-year, open-label trial, comparing patients with schizophrenia on olanzapine LAI versus oral dosing [149], no significant difference emerged in all-cause discontinuation rates or in any other efficacy or safety variables.

Safety

In an acute study [147], discontinuation rates because of adverse events were low for all groups. Sedation and increased appetite were significantly higher for the highest dose of olanzapine LAI relative to placebo. Mean weight gain (3.2–4.8 kg vs. 0.3 kg) and incidence of weight gain at least 7% of baseline (23.6–35.4% vs. 12.4%) were significantly greater for olanzapine LAI vs. placebo. In addition, significant differences between all olanzapine LAI groups and placebo were observed regarding mean baseline-to-end-point changes in fasting total cholesterol and fasting triglycerides. There were no differences between the olanzapine LAI groups and placebo regarding motor side effects. No significant between-group differences were observed in the incidence of anticholinergic use or mean anticholinergic daily dose between the two groups.

Similarly low were treatment-related adverse events leading to discontinuation in the maintenance trial [148] in the four olanzapine LAI groups. No significant differences in motor side effects were reported between the olanzapine LAI groups and oral olanzapine. Clinically relevant weight gain (‡ 7%) was 21% for oral olanzapine compared with 21, 15, 16 and 8% for the high, medium, low and very low olanzapine LAI dose. Total cholesterol and fasting LDL cholesterol decreased significantly less in the three higher-dosed LAI groups compared with the very low dose of 45 mg every four weeks, while no significant group differences were seen in fasting triglyceride and glucose levels. Incidence of a local injection site reaction was low (2.8%).

In an analysis of PDSS events following assessment of data on 45,000 olanzapine pamoate injections given to 2054 patients, PDSS occurred in 0.07% injections or in 1.4% of patients and symptoms were consistent with olanzapine overdose. 80% of the PDSS events occurred within 1 h of injection and symptom onset ranged from immediate to 5 hour post-injection (median 25 min). Most events occurred after patients had received several months of injections (PDSS ranged from 1st injection to 40th injection). All patients recovered within 1.5 to 72 hours and most patients continued olanzapine LAI treatment. No clinically relevant declines in vital signs were observed [150].

In general, tolerability and safety of olanzapine LAI is similar to that for oral olanzapine aside from injection site reactions and PDSS.

CONCLUSIONS

Disadvantages of Depot Antipsychotic Medication

Since the depot antipsychotics are usually administered once every 2 weeks or once monthly, this prevents the dosing flexibility that is usually present with oral medications.

Moreover, patients may be reluctant to accept injections and have a sense of being overly controlled [31].

In the event of side effects, slow distribution from deep tissue compartments may lead to accumulation, making management of side effects challenging, in addition to possible requirement of dose reduction after several months of treatment [151]. Additionally, there have been reports of injection site reactions- pain, erythema, swelling and discomfort. Haloperidol decanoate is particularly notorious for these reactions and the manufacturer has recommended injection volume not to exceed 3 ml. Some of these reactions may be avoided by alternating the injection site, using a Z technique to avoid leakage of the drug. With olanzapine LAI, there is the risk of PDSS thus requiring a REMS program.

In addition, the acquisition cost of SGA LAIs are substantially higher than other options including generic oral SGAs.

Why use Depot Antipsychotics?

Nonadherence to antipsychotic medication has received increasing attention. It generally is agreed that roughly half of patients with schizophrenia do not adhere to their prescribed oral medication regimen. Studies have documented substantial cost increases associated with nonadherence among these patients and it is generally accepted that the depot formulations offer a distinct advantage in the ability to document and observe non-adherent behavior, thus increasing adherence rates. Hence, it would seem clinically logical to select non-adherent patients for depot formulations. But the paradox is that "depot antipsychotics play a relatively minor role in the treatment of schizophrenia," [152] and American clinicians appear to use these formulations less often than many non-US counterparts [153]. Indeed, a recent prospective, observational study of the treatment for schizophrenia in the US conducted by Shi et al [154] found that only 26% of patients (569/2,186) were treated with depot formulations of typical antipsychotics at least once during the designated three-year period. A recent study examining the utilization rates of depot antipsychotics in hospitals operated by the New York State Office of Mental Health for patients requiring immediate and long-term care showed that the percentage of patients receiving depot antipsychotic medication has ranged from 21.2% (first quarter of 1999) to 34.1% (third quarter of 2008) [155]. There can be negative attitudes regarding the use of depot antipsychotics: a recent systemic review that examined the attitude of patients and staff to long-acting injections suggested that depot antipsychotics continue to have an “image” problem [156]. The introduction of better-tolerated LAIs and better education of both staff and patients may encourage individuals to re-examine their attitudes. The most positive attitudes among patients were seen in those already prescribed an LAI [156].

There is the potential for improved tolerability (particularly in terms of motoric side effects) with the SGA LAIs. This can lead to greater acceptance of the newer depot antipsychotics over haloperidol or fluphenazine decanoate. In addition to risperidone, paliperidone and olanzapine LAI, aripiprazole LAI is also expected to be commercialized in the near term. Head-to-head controlled clinical trials may help differentiate the optimal populations of patients that would benefit more from one or the other option. Additional health-economic studies may also be helpful in encouraging the use of this therapeutic modality.

REFERENCES

[1] Byerly, M., Nakonezny, P., Lescouflair, E. Antipsychotic medication adherence in schizophrenia. *Psychiatr. Clin. North Am.* 2007; 30: 427-452.

[2] Wyatt, R. J. Neuroleptics and the natural course of schizophrenia. *Schizophr. Bull.* 1991; 17: 325–351.

[3] Lieberman, J. A., Sheitman, B., Chakos, M., et al. The development of treatment resistance in patients with schizophrenia: a clinical and pathophysiologic perspective. *J. Clin. Psychopharmacol.* 1998; 18: 20S–24S.

[4] Fenton, W. S., Blyler, C. R., Heinssen, R. K. Determinants of medication compliance in schizophrenia: empirical and clinical findings. *Schizophr. Bull.* 1997; 23: 637–51.

[5] Olfson, M., Mechanic, D., Hansell, S., et al. Predicting medication noncompliance after hospital discharge among patients with schizophrenia. *Psychiatr. Serv.* 2000; 51: 216–22.

[6] Weiden, P. J., Olfson, M. Cost of relapse in schizophrenia. *Schizophr. Bull.* 1995; 21: 419–429.

[7] Ayuso-Gutierrez, J. L., del Rio Vega, J. M. Factors influencing relapse in the long-term course of schizophrenia. *Schizophr. Res.* 1997; 28: 199–206.

[8] Stefen, L., Stephen, H. Epidemiology, clinical consequences and psychosocial treatment of nonadherence in schizophrenia. *J. Clin. Psychiatry* 2006; 67: S3-8.

[9] Steadman, H. J., Mulvey, E. P., Monahan, J., et al. Violence by people discharged from acute psychiatric inpatient facilities and by others in the same neighborhoods. *Arch. Gen. Psychiatry* 1998; 55: 393–401.

[10] Swartz, M. S., Swanson, J. W., Hiday, V. A., et al. Taking the wrong drugs: the role of substance abuse and medication noncompliance in violence among severely mentally ill individuals. *Soc. Psychiatry Psychiatr. Epidemiol.* 1998; 33: S75–S80.

[11] Johnson, D. A. W., Pasterski, J. M., Ludlow, J. M., et al. The discontinuance of maintenance neuroleptic therapy in chronic schizophrenic patients: drug and social consequences. *Acta Psychiatr. Scand.* 1983; 67: 339–352.

[12] Fenton, W. Schizophrenia: Integrative treatment and functional outcomes. Sadock, B. J., Sadock, V. A. *Comprehensive textbook of psychiatry* 8th ed. Philadelphia: Williams and Wilkins; 2004.

[13] Velligan, D. I., Wang, M., Diamond, P., et al. Relationships among subjective and objective measures of adherence to oral antipsychotic medications. *Psychiatr. Serv.* 2007;58:1187–1192.

[14] Velligan, D. I., Lam, Y. W., Glahn, D. C., et al. Defining and assessing adherence to oral antipsychotics: a review of the literature. *Schizophr. Bull.* 2006;32:724–742.

[15] Harrison, T. S., Goa, K. L. Long-acting risperidone: a review of its use in schizophrenia. *CNS Drugs* 2004; 18 : 113–132.

[16] Johnson and Johnson, 2009. FDA Approves Invega Sustenna for the Acute and Maintenance Treatment of Schizophrenia. Press release, 31 July 2009. Available at: http://www.jnj.com/connect/news/all/ 20090731_153000. Accessed 2 September 2009.

[17] Citrome, L. Olanzapine pamoate: a stick in time? A review of the efficacy and safety profile of a new depot formulation of a second generation antipsychotic. *Int. J. Clin. Pract.* 2009; 63: 140–150.

[18] Otsuka Pharmaceutical Development and Commercialization, Inc., 2008. Intramuscular Depot Formulation of Aripiprazole as Maintenance Treatment in Patients with Schizophrenia (ASPIRE). Registry entry, 7 Aug 2008. Available at: http://clinicaltrials.gov/ct2/show/ NCT00731549. Accessed 31 Oct. 2008.

[19] Citrome, L. Iloperidone for schizophrenia: a review of the efficacy and safety profile for this newly commercialised second-generation antipsychotic. *Int. J. Clin. Pract.* 2009; 63: 1237–1248.

[20] Levine, J., Schooler, N. R., Cassano, G. B. The role of depot neuroleptics in the treatment of schizophrenic patients. *Psychol. Med.* 1979; 9:383–386.

[21] Barnes, T. R., Curson, D. A. Long-term depot antipsychotics. A risk-benefit assessment. *Drug Saf.* 1994;10:464-479.

[22] Citrome, L., Jaffe, A., Levine, J. Treatment of schizophrenia with depot preparations of fluphenazine, haloperidol, and risperidone among inpatients at state-operated psychiatric facilities. *Schizophr. Res.* 2010;119:153-159.

[23] Leucht, C., Heres, S., Kane, J. M., et al. Oral versus depot antipsychotic drugs for schizophrenia--a critical systematic review and meta-analysis of randomised long-term trials. *Schizophr. Res.* 2011;127:83-92.

[24] Tiihonen, J., Haukka, J., Taylor, M., et al. A nationwide cohort study of oral and depot antipsychotics after first hospitalization for schizophrenia. *Am. J. Psychiatry* 2011;168:603-609.

[25] Peng, X., Ascher-Svanum, H., Faries, D., et al. Decline in hospitalization risk and health care cost after initiation of depot antipsychotics in the treatment of schizophrenia. *Clinicoecon. Outcomes Res.* 2011;3:9-14.

[26] Davis, J. M., Metalon, L., Watanabe, M. D. Depot antipsychotic drugs: place in therapy. *Drugs* 1994; 47:741-773.

[27] Mentschel. 156th mtg of APA; San Francisco, May 17-22, 2003. *Abstract book*, page 71.

[28] Adams, C. E., Fenton, M. K., Quraishi, S., et al. Systematic meta-review of depot antipsychotic drugs for people with schizophrenia. *Br. J. Psychiatry* 2001; 179:290-299.

[29] Weiden, P., Rapkin, B., Zygmunt, A. Postdischarge medication compliance of inpatients converted from an oral to a depot neuroleptic regimen. *Psychiatr. Serv.* 1995;46:1049–1054.

[30] Barnes, T. R. Depot antipsychotic drugs and prevention of psychotic relapse. *Clin. Neuropharmacol.* 1991;14: S1-6.

[31] Pollack, S. L., Tourlentes, T. T., Zocchi, A. F. Clinical Trial of Fluphenazine Enanthate-- a Long-Acting Injectable Tranquilizer. *Am. J. Psychiatry* 1964;121:73-74.

[32] Kane, J. M., Aguglia, E., Altamura, A. C., et al. Guidelines for depot antipsychotic treatment in schizophrenia. European Neuropsychopharmacology Consensus Conference in Siena, Italy. *Eur. Neuropsychopharmacol.* 1998;8:55-66.

[33] Pandarakalam, J. P. Atypical and conventional depot medications. *Hosp. Med.* 2003;64:658-663.

[34] Bucci, L., Fuchs, M., Simeon, J., et al. Depot fluphenazine in the treatment of psychosis in a community mental health clinic. *Dis. Nerv. Syst.* 1970;31:28-31.

[35] Caffey, E. M. Jr, Diamond, L. S., Frank, T. V., et al. Discontinuation Or Reduction of Chemotherapy in Chronic Schizophrenics. *J. Chronic Dis.* 1964;17:347-358.

[36] Ereshefsky, L., Saklad, S. R., Jann, M. W., et al.Future of depot neuroleptic therapy: pharmacokinetic and pharmacodynamic approaches. *J. Clin. Psychiatry* 1984;45:50-59.

[37] Marder, S. R., Van Putten, T., Aravagiri, M., et al. Fluphenazine plasma levels and clinical response. *Psychopharmacol. Bull.* 1990;26:256-259.

[38] Jann, M. W., Ereshefsky, L., Saklad, S. R. Clinical pharmacokinetics of the depot antipsychotics. *Clin. Pharmacokinet.* 1985;10:315-333.

[39] Wiles, D. H., Gelder, M. G. Plasma fluphenazine levels by radioimmunoassay in schizophrenic patients treated with depot injections of fluphenazine decanoate. *Adv. Biochem. Psychopharmacol.* 1980;24:599-602.

[40] Wistedt, B., Wiles, D., Kolakowska, T. Slow decline of plasma drug and prolactin levels after discontinuation of chronic treatment with depot neuroleptics. *Lancet* 198; 23:1163.

[41] Amdisen, A., Thomsen, N. J. Drug levels after withdrawal of long-term depot neuroleptics. *Lancet* 1981;1:1425.

[42] Ereshefsky, L., Jann, M. W., Saklad, S. R., et al. Effects of smoking on fluphenazine clearance in psychiatric inpatients. *Biol. Psychiatry* 1985;20:329-332.

[43] Kane, J. M., Rifkin, A., Woerner, M., et al. Low-dose neuroleptic treatment of outpatient schizophrenics. I. Preliminary results for relapse rates. *Arch. Gen. Psychiatry* 1983;40:893-896.

[44] Hogarty, G. E., McEvoy, J. P., Munetz, M., et al. Dose of fluphenazine, familial expressed emotion, and outcome in schizophrenia. Results of a two-year controlled study. *Arch. Gen. Psychiatry* 1988;45:797-805.

[45] Schooler, N. R., Keith, S. J., Severe, J. B., et al. Relapse and rehospitalization during maintenance treatment of schizophrenia: the effects of dose reduction and family treatment. *Arch. Gen. Psychiatry* 1997; 54:453–463.

[46] Kane, J. M., Woerner, M., Sarantakos, S.: Depot neuroleptics: a comparative review of standard, intermediate, and low-dose regimens. *J. Clin. Psychiatry* 1986; 47:30–33.

[47] Schooler, N. R., Levine, J. The initiation of long-term pharmacotherapy in schizophrenia: dosage and side effect comparisons between oral and depot fluphenazine. *Pharmakopsychiatr. Neuropsychopharmakol.* 1976;9:159-169.

[48] Hirsch, S. R. The interaction between depot-phenothiazines and the social and clinical manifestations of behavior in patients with stabilised chronic schizophrenia. In: Van Praag, H. M. editor(s). On the origin of schizophrenic psychoses. *De Erven. Bohn BV*, 1975:209–222.

[49] Odejide, O. A., Aderounmu, A. F. Double-blind placebo substitution: Withdrawal of fluphenazine decanoate in schizophrenic patients. *Psychopharmacology* 1982;43:195–206.

[50] Rifkin, A., Quitkin, F., Kane, J., et al. Fluphenazine decanoate, oral fluphenazine, and placebo in the treatment of remitted schizophrenics II. Rating scale data. *Psychopharmacol. Bull.* 1977;13:40–50.

[51] David, A., Adams, C. E., Eisenbruch, M., et al. Depot fluphenazine decanoate and enanthate for schizophrenia. *Cochrane Database Syst. Rev.* 2005;(1)(1):CD000307.

[52] Jolley, A. G., Hirsch, S. R., Morrison, E., et al. Trial of brief intermittent neuroleptic prophylaxis for selected schizophrenic outpatients: clinical and social outcome at two years. *Brit. Med. J.* 1990;301: 837–842.

[53] Barnes, T. R. E., Milavic, G., Curson, D. A., et al. Use of the social behaviour assessment schedule (SBAS) in a trial of maintenance antipsychotic therapy in schizophrenic outpatients: pimozide versus fluphenazine. *Soc. Psychiatr.* 1983; 18:193–9.

[54] Curry, S. H., Adamson, L. Double-blind trial of fluphenazine decanoate. *Lancet* 1972;2:543–4.
[55] Fallon, I., Watt, D. C., Shepherd, M. The social outcome of patients in a trial of long-term continuation therapy in schizophrenia: pimozide vs fluphenazine. *Psychol. Med.* 1978;8:265–74.
[56] Simon, P., Fermanian, J., Ginestet, D., et al. Standard and long-acting depot neuroleptics in chronic schizophrenics. *Arc. Gen. Psychiat.* 1978; 35:893–7.
[57] Shu, L. Double-blind study of domestic penfluridol and fluphenazine decanoate. Zhonghua Shen Jing Jing Shen Ke Za Zhi. 1983;16:141-5. Chinese. No abstract available.
[58] Schooler, N. R., Levine, J., Severe, J. B. Depot fluphenazine in the prevention of relapse in schizophrenia: Evaluation of a Treatment Regimen. *Psychopharmacol. Bull.* 1979;15:44–7.
[59] Chouinard, G., Annable, L., Campbell, W., et al. A double-blind, controlled clinical trial of haloperidol decanoate and fluphenazine decanoate in the maintenance treatment of schizophrenia. *Psychopharmacol. Bull.* 1984;20:108–9.
[60] Cookson, J. C., Kennedy, N. M., Gribbon, D. Weight gain and prolactin levels in patients on long-term antipsychotic medication: a double-blind comparative trial of haloperidol decanoate and fluphenazine decanaote. *International Clin. Psychopharmacol.* 1986;1:41–51.
[61] Dencker, S. J., Frankenberg, K., Lepp, M., et al. Three years' maintenance neuroleptic treatment in schizophrenia - before and beyond. *Act. Psychia. Scand.* 1978;57:103–114.
[62] Feng, L. Double blind controlled trial of haloperidol decanoate and fluphenazine decanoate in chronic schizophrenia. *Chinese Journal of Nervous and Mental Disorders* 1990;16:299.
[63] Frangos, H., Zississ, N. P., Leontopoulos, I., et al. Double blind therapeutic evaluation of fluspirilene compared with fluphenazine decanoate in chronic schizophrenics. *Act. Psychiat. Scand.* 1978;57:436–446.
[64] Leong, O. K., Wong, K. E., Tay, W. K., et al. A comparative study of pipothiazine palmitate and fluphenazine decanoate in the maintenance of remission of schizophrenia. *Singapore Medical Journal* 1989;30:536–540.
[65] McKane, J. P., Robinson, A. D. T., Wiles, D. H., et al. Haloperidol decanoate versus fluphenazine decanoate as maintenance therapy in chronic schizophrenic in-patients. *Brit. J. Psych.* 1987;151:333–336.
[66] McLaren, S., Cookson, J. C., Silverstone, T. Postive and negative symptoms, depression and social disability in chronic schizophrenia: a comparative trial of bromoperidol and fluphenazine decanoates. *Int. Clin. Psychopharm.* 1992;7:67–72.
[67] Schlosberg, A., Shadmi, M. A comparative controlled study of two long-acting phenothiazines: Pipothiazine palmitate and fluphenazine decanoate. *Curr. Ther. Res.* 1978;23:642–54.
[68] Asarnow, R. E., Marder, S. R., Mintz, J., et al. Differential effect of low and conventional doses of fluphenazine on schizophrenic outpatients with good or poor information-processing skills. *Arch. Gen. Psychiat.* 1988;45:822–827.
[69] Marder, S. R., Van Putten, T., Mintz, J., et al. Low and conventional dose maintenance therapy with fluphenazine decanoate. *Arch. Gen. Psychiat.* 1987;44:518–521.

[70] Marder, S. R., Van Putten, T., Mintz, J., McKenzie, J., Lebell, M., Faltico, G., May, P. R. A. Costs and benefits of two doses of fluphenazine. *Arch. Gen. Psychiat.* 1984;41: 1025–1029.
[71] McClelland, H., Farquharson, R. G., Leyburn, P., et al. Furness, J. A., Schiff, A. A. Very high dose fluphenazine decanoate. *Arch. Gen. Psychiat.* 1976;33:1435–1449.
[72] Kreisman, D., Blumenthal, R., Borenstein, M., et al. Family attitudes and patient social adjustment in a longitudinal study of outpatient schizophrenics receiving low-dose neuroleptics: the family's view. *Psychiatry* 1988;51:3–13.
[73] Chien, C. P., Cole, J. O. Depot phenothiazine treatment in acute psychosis: A sequential comparative clinical study. *Am. J. Psych.* 1973;130:13–17.
[74] Albert, J. M., Elie, R., Cooper, S. F. Long term double-blind evaluation of pipotiazine palmitate and fluphenazine decanoate. *Curr. Ther. Res.* 1980;27: 897–907.
[75] Chouinard, G., Annable, L., Kropsky, M. A double-blind controlled study of pipothiazine palmitate in the maintenance treatment of schizophrenic outpatients. *J. Clin. Psychopharmacol.* 1978;148–154.
[76] Malm, U., Perris, C., Rapp, W., et al. A Multicentre Trial of Flusperilene and Fluphenazine Enanthate in Chronic Schizophrenic syndromes. *Acta Psychiat. Scand. Supplementum* 1974;249:94–116.
[77] Donlon, P. T., Rada, R. T., Arora, K. K. Depression and the reintegration phase of acute schizophrenia. *Am. J. Psych.* 1976;133:1265–8.
[78] McCreadie, R. G., McKane, J. P., Mackie, M. Weekly pimozide versus fluphenazine decanoate in schizophrenic out and day patients. *Brit. J. Psych.* 1983;143:97–98.
[79] McCreadie, R. G., McKane, J. P., Robinson, A. D. T., et al. Depot neuroleptics as maintenance therapy in chronic schizophrenic in-patients. *Inter. Clin. Psychopharmacol.* 1986;1:13–14.
[80] Adamson, L., Currey, S. H., Bridges, P. K., Firestone, A. F., Lavin, N. I., Lewis, D. M., Watson, R. D., Xavier, C. M., Anderson, J. A. Fluphenazine decanoate trial in chronic inpatient schizophrenics failing to absorb oral chlorpromazine. *Dis. Nervous. System* 1973;34:181–191.
[81] McCreadie, R., Mackie, M., Morrison, D., Kidd, J. Once weekly pimozide versus fluphenazine decanoate as maintenance therapy in chronic schizophrenia. *Brit. J. Psych.* 1982;140:280–286.
[82] Knights, A., Okasha, M. S., Salih, M. A., et al Depressive and extrapyramidal symptoms and clinical effects: a trial of fluphenazine versus flupenthixol in maintenance of schizophrenic out-patients. *Br. J. Psychiatry* 1979;135:515-523.
[83] Van Praag, H. M., Dols, L. C. Fluphenazine enanthate and fluphenazine decanoate: a comparison of their duration of action and motor side effects. *Am. J. Psychiatry* 1973;130:801-804.
[84] Kurland, A. A., Dim, B. M., Olssen, J. E. The effectiveness of parenteral administration of fluphenazine decanoate in the treatment of chronic schizophrenics. *Dis. Nervous System* 1970;31:18–23.
[85] Beresford, R., Ward, A. Haloperidol decanoate. A preliminary review of its pharmacodynamic and pharmacokinetic properties and therapeutic use in psychosis. *Drugs* 1987;33:31-49.
[86] Forsman, A., Ohman, R. Studies on serum protein binding of haloperidol. *Curr. Ther. Res. Clin. Exp.* 1977;21:245-255.

[87] Reyntigens, A. J., Heykants, J. J., Woestenborghs, R. J et al. Pharmacokinetics of haloperidol decanoate. A 2-year follow-up. *Int. Pharmacopsychiatry* 1982;17:238-246.

[88] Viukari, M., Salo, H., Lamminsivu, U., et al. Tolerance and serum levels of haloperidol during parenteral and oral haloperidol treatment in geriatric patients. *Acta Psychiatr. Scand.* 1982;65:301-308.

[89] Hemstrom, C. A., Evans, R. L., Lobeck, F. G. Haloperidol decanoate: a depot antipsychotic. *Drug Intell Clin. Pharm.* 1988;22:290-295.

[90] Quraishi, S., David, A. Depot haloperidol decanoate for schizophrenia. *Cochrane Database Syst. Rev.* 2000;(2):CD001361.

[91] Eklund, K., Forsman, A. Minimal effective dose and relapse - double blind trial: haloperidol decanoate versus placebo. *Clin. Neuropharmac.* 1991;14:7–15.

[92] Zissis, N. P., Psaias, M., Lykctsos, G. Haloperidol decanoate, a new long actiing antipsychotic in chronic schizophrenics: Double blind comparison with placebo. *Curr. Ther. Res.* 1982;31: 650-655.

[93] Zuardi, A. W., Giampietro, A. C., Grassi, E. R., et al. Double-blind comparison between two forms of haloperidol: an oral preparation and a new depot decanoate in the maintenance of schizophrenic inpatients. *Curr. Ther. Res.* 1983;34:253-261.

[94] Bechelli, L. P. C., Lecco, M. C., Pontes, M. C. A double-blind trial of haloperidol decanoate and pipothiazine palmitate in the maintenance treatment of schizophrenics in a public out-patient clinic. *Curr. Ther. Res.* 1985;37:662–71.

[95] Guy, W. Early clinical drug evaluation (ECDEU) assessment manual for psychopharmacology. Washington, DC: US Government Printing Office, 1976. [: National Institute of Mental Health Publication No. 76–338]

[96] Wistedt, B., Koskinen, T., Thelander, S., et al. Zuclopenthixol decanoate and haloperidol decanoate in chronic schizophrenia: a double-blind multicentre study. *Acta Psychiatr. Scand.* 1991;84:14-21.

[97] Ehret, M. J., Fuller, M. A. Long-acting injectable risperidone. *Ann. Pharmacother.* 2004; 38 : 2122–2127.

[98] Lasser, R. A., Ramstack, J. M., Grandolfi, G. M., et al. Long-acting risperidone (Risperidone Microsphere): manufacture using Medisorb microsphere, technology, pharmacokinetics and injection-site assessments. Presented at the 155th Annual Meeting of the American Psychiatric Association 2002, May 18-23, 2002;Philadelphia, PA. US.

[99] MIMS Australia. Risperdal Consta. MIMS online. 2009. [Accessed May 21, 2009]. Available from: http://www.mims.com.au/

[100] Volkow, N. D., Wang, G. J., Fowler, J. S., et al. Parallel loss of presynaptic and post synaptic dopamine markers in normal ageing. *Ann. Neurol.* 1998;44:143–147.

[101] Eerdekens, M., Van Hove, I., Remmerie, B., et al. Pharmacokinetics and tolerability of long-acting risperidone in schizophrenia. *Schizophr. Res.* 2004;70:91–100.

[102] Janssen Pharmaceuticals Inc. Risperidal consta (risperidone long-acting injection): prescribing information [online]. Available from URL: http://www.janssencns.com/ risperdal-prescribing-information. Revised 12/2012.

[103] Singh, D., O'Connor, D. W. Efficacy and safety of risperidone long-acting injection in elderly people with schizophrenia. *Clin. Interv. Aging* 2009;4:351-355.

[104] Chue, P. Risperidone long-acting injection. *Expert Rev. Neurother.* 2003 Jul.;3:435-446.

[105] Kane, J. M., Eerdekens, M., Lindenmayer, J. P. Long-acting injectable risperidone: efficacy and safety of the first long-acting atypical antipsychotic. *Am. J. Psychiatry* 2003; 160: 1125–1132.
[106] Fleischhacker, W., Eerdekens, M., Karcher, K. Treatment of schizophrenia with long-acting injectable risperidone: a 12 month evaluation of the first long-acting 2nd generation antipsychotic. *J. Clin. Psychiatry* 2003: 64: 1250–1257.
[107] Van, O. S. J., Bossie, C., Lasser, R. Improvements in stable patients with psychotic disorders switched from oral conventional antipsychotics therapy to long-acting risperidone. *Int. Clin. Psychopharmacol.* 2004; 19: 229–232.
[108] Lindenmayer, J. P., Eerdekens, E., Berry, S. A., Eerdekens, M. Safety and efficacy of long-acting risperidone in schizophrenia: a 12-week, multicenter, open-label study in stable patients switched from typical and atypical oral antipsychotics. *J. Clin. Psychiatry* 2004; 65:1084–1089.
[109] Gastpar, M., Masiak, M., Latif, M. A. Sustained improvement of clinical outcome with risperidone long-acting injectable in psychotic patients previously treated with olanzapine. *J. Psychopharmacol.* 2005; 19: 32–38.
[110] Lasser, R., Bossie, C., Gharabawi, G., et al. Patients with schizophrenia previously stabilized on conventional depot antipsychotics experience significant clinical improvements following treatment with long-acting risperidone. *Eur. Psychiatry* 2004; 19: 219–225.
[111] Turner, M., Eerdekens, E., Jacko, M., et al. Long-acting injectable risperidone: safety and efficacy in stable patients switched from conventional depot antipsychotics. *Int. Clin. Psychopharmacol.* 2004;19: 241–249.
[112] Lasser, R., Bossie, C., Gharabawi, G., et al. Clinical improvement in 336 stable chronically psychotic patients changed from oral to long-acting risperidone: a 12-month open trial. *Int. J. Neuropsychopharmacol.* 2005; 8: 1–12.
[113] Marinis, T. D., Saleem, P. T., Glue, P. Switching to long-acting injectable risperidone is beneficial with regard to clinical outcomes, regardless of previous conventional medication in patients with schizophrenia. *Pharmacopsychiatry* 2007; 40: 257–263.
[114] Schmauss, M., Sacchetti, E., Kahn, J. P., et al. Efficacy and safety of risperidone long-acting injectable in stable psychotic patients previously treated with oral risperidone. *Int. Clin. Psychopharmacol.* 2007; 22: 85–92.
[115] Hawley, C., Turner, M., Latif, M. A., et al. Switching stable patients with schizophrenia from depot and oral antipsychotics to long-acting injectable risperidone: reasons for switching and safety. *Hum. Psychopharmacol.* 2010;25:37-46.
[116] Lloyd, K., Latif, M. A., Simpson, S., et al. Switching stable patients with schizophrenia from depot and oral antipsychotics to long-acting injectable risperidone: efficacy, quality of life and functional outcome. *Hum. Psychopharmacol.* 2010;25:243-252.
[117] Chue, P., Eerdekens, M., Augustyns, I. Comparative efficacy and safety of long-acting risperidone and risperidone oral tablets. *Eur. Neuropsychopharmacol.* 2005; 15: 111–117.
[118] Bai, Y. M., Chen, T. T., Wu, B. A comparative efficacy and safety study of long-acting risperidone injection and risperidone oral tablets among hospitalized patients: 12-week randomized, single-blind study. *Pharmacopsychiatry* 2006; 39: 135–141.

[119] Möller, H., Llorca, P. M., Sachetti, E., et al. Efficacy and safety of direct transition to risperidone long-acting injectable in patients treated with various antipsychotic therapies. *Int. Clin. Psychopharmacol.* 2005; 20: 121–130.

[120] Pecenak, J., Tuma, I., de Groot-Stam, L. Improvement in personal and social functioning in schizophrenia patients treated with risperidone long-acting injectable: 6-month results from E-STAR. Presented at: The *American Psychiatric Association Annual Meeting*. Washington, DC, US, 3–8 May 2008.

[121] Canas, F., Moller, H. J. Long-acting atypical injectable antipsychotics in the treatment of schizophrenia: safety and tolerability review. *Expert Opin. Drug Saf.* 2010;9:683-697.

[122] Möller, H. J. Long-acting risperidone: focus on safety. *Clin. Ther.* 2006; 28: 633–651.

[123] Kapur, S., Zipursky, R. B., Remington, G. Clinical and theoretical implications of 5-HT2 and D2 receptor occupancy of clozapine, risperidone, and olanzapine in schizophrenia. *Am. J. Psychiatry* 1999;156:286–293

[124] Kapur, S., Zipursky, R., Jones, C., et al. Relationship between dopamine D(2) occupancy, clinical response, and side effects: a double-blind PET study of first-episode schizophrenia. *Am. J. Psychiatry* 2000;157: 514–520.

[125] Taylor, D. M., Fischetti, C., Sparshatt, A. Risperidone long-acting injection: a prospective 3-year analysis of its use in clinical practice. *J. Clin. Psychiatry* 2009;70:196-200.

[126] Martinez, G., Schreiner, A. Risperidone long-acting injectable and olanzapine pamoate: review of short- and long-term safety data. Presented at the 9th World Federation of Societies of Biological Psychiatry; 29 June -- 2 July 2009; Paris, France.

[127] Yang, L. P., Plosker, G. L. Paliperidone extended release. *CNS Drugs* 2007; 21: 417-425.

[128] Samtani, M. N., Vermeulen, A., Stuyckens, K. Population pharmacokinetics of intramuscular paliperidone palmitate in patients with schizophrenia: a novel once-monthly, long-acting formulation of an atypical antipsychotic. *Clin. Pharmacokinet.* 2009; 48: 585–600.

[129] Janssen, Division of Ortho-McNeil-Janssen Pharmaceuticals, Inc. Invega Sustenna (paliperidone palmitate) Extended-Release Injectable Suspension. Accessed at URL http://www.janssencns.com/sustenna-prescribing-information (October 2011).

[130] Cleton, A., Rossenu, S., Hough, D., et al. Assessment of the dose proportionality of paliperidone palmitate 25, 50, 100 and 150 mg eq., a new long-acting injectable antipsychotic following administration in the deltoid or gluteal muscles [abstract no. PI-74]. *Clin. Pharmacol. Ther.* 2008 Mar.; 83 Suppl. 1: S31. Plus poster presented at the American Society for Clinical Pharmacology and Therapeutics; 2008 Apr. 2-5; Orlando (FL).

[131] Cleton, A., Rossenu, S., Hough, D., et al. Evaluation of the pharmacokinetic profile of gluteal versus deltoid intramuscular injections of paliperidone palmitate 100mg equivalent in patients with schizophrenia [abstract no. PI-75]. *Clin. Pharmacol. Ther.* 2008 Mar.; 83 Suppl. 1: S31. Plus poster presented at the American Society for Clinical Pharmacology and Therapeutics; 2008 Apr. 2-5; Orlando (FL).

[132] Hough, D., Lindenmayer, J.-P., Gopal, S. Safety and tolerability of deltoid and gluteal injections of paliperidone palmitate in schizophrenia. *Prog. Neuropsychopharmacol. Biol. Psychiatry* 2009; 33: 1022-31.

[133] Gopal S, Hough DW, Xu H, Lull JM, Gassmann-Mayer C, Remmerie BM, et al. Efficacy and safety of paliperidone palmitate in adult patients with acutely symptomatic schizophrenia: a randomized, double-blind, placebo-controlled, dose-response study. Int Clin Psychopharmacol 2010; 25(5):247-256.

[134] Nasrallah HA, Gopal S, Gassmann-Mayer C, Quiroz JA, Lim P, Eerdekens M, et al. A controlled, evidence-based trial of paliperidone palmitate, a long-acting injectable antipsychotic, in schizophrenia. Neuropsychopharmacology 2010 ;35(10):2072-2082.

[135] Kramer M, Litman R, Hough D, Lane R, Lim P, Liu Y, et al. Paliperidone palmitate, a potential long-acting treatment for patients with schizophrenia. Results of a randomized, double-blind, placebo-controlled efficacy and safety study. Int J Neuropsychopharmacol 2010 Jun;13(5):635-647.

[136] Pandina GJ, Lindenmayer JP, Lull J, Lim P, Gopal S, Herben V, et al. A randomized, placebo-controlled study to assess the efficacy and safety of 3 doses of paliperidone palmitate in adults with acutely exacerbated schizophrenia. J Clin Psychopharmacol 2010;30(3):235-244.

[137] Fleischhacker, W. W., Gopal, S., Lane, R., et al. A randomized trial of paliperidone palmitate and risperidone long-acting injectable in schizophrenia. *Int. J. Neuropsychopharmacol.* 2011; 22:1-12.

[138] Pandina, G., Lane, R., Gopal, S., et al. A double-blind study of paliperidone palmitate and risperidone long-acting injectable in adults with schizophrenia. *Prog. Neuropsychopharmacol. Biol. Psychiatry* 2011; 15;35:218-226.

[139] Li, H., Rui, Q., Ning, X., et al. A comparative study of paliperidone palmitate and risperidone long-acting injectable therapy in schizophrenia. *Prog. Neuropsychopharmacol. Biol. Psychiatry* 2011;35:1002-1008.

[140] Citrome L. Paliperidone palmitate - review of the efficacy, safety and cost of a new second-generation depot antipsychotic medication. Int J Clin Pract 2010 Jan;64(2):216-239.

[141] Hough D, Gopal S, Vijapurkar U, Lim P, Morozova M, Eerdekens M. Paliperidone palmitate maintenance treatment in delaying the time-to-relapse in patients with schizophrenia: a randomized, double-blind, placebo-controlled study. Schizophr Res 2010 Feb;116(2-3):107-117.

[142] Kurtz, D., Bergstrom, R., McDonnell, D. P., et al. Pharmacokinetics (PK) of multiple doses of olanzapine long-acting injection (OLAI), an intramuscular (IM) depot formulation of olanzapine (OLZ) in stabilized patients with schizophrenia. *Biol. Psychiatry* 2008;63: abstract 909.

[143] Callaghan, J. T., Bergstrom, R. F., Ptak, L. R., et al. Olanzapine, pharmacokinetic and pharmacodynamic profile. *Clin. Pharmacokinet.* 1999;37:177-193.

[144] Gulliver, A., McDonnell, D. P., Kryzhanovskaya, L. A., et al. Comparison of metabolic parameters during treatment for schizophrenia with olanzapine intramuscular longacting injection versus olanzapine oral formulation [abstract]. *Int. J. Neuropsychopharmacol.* 2008; 11: 152.

[145] Gulliver, A., Detke, H. C., McDonnell, D. P., et al. Olanzapine long-acting injection: Pharmacokinetic and dose correspondence data relative to oral Olanzapine [abstract]. *Int. J. Neuropsychopharmacol.* 2008; 11: 152–153.

[146] Eli Lilly and Company. Zyprexa Olanzapine Pamoate (OP) Depot. Accessed at URL http://pi.lilly.com/us/zyprexa_relprevv.pdf (revised 07/2011).

[147] Lauriello, J., Lambert, T., Andersen, S., et al. An 8-week, double-blind, randomized, placebo-controlled study of olanzapine long-acting injection in acutely ill patients with schizophrenia. *J. Clin. Psychiatry* 2008;69:790-799.
[148] Kane, J. M., Detke, H. C., Naber, D., Sethuraman, G., Lin, D. Y., Bergstrom, R. F., McDonnell, D. Olanzapine long-acting injection: a 24-week, randomized, double-blind trial of maintenance treatment in patients with schizophrenia. *Am. J. Psychiatry* 2010;167:181-189.
[149] Detke, H. C., Weiden, P. J., Lambert, T. Olanzapine long-acting injection vs oral olanzapine in schizophrenia outpatients: a 2-year, randomized, open-label study. *Eur. Neuropsychopharmacol.* 2010;20 (Suppl. 3):464.
[150] McDonnell, D. P., Detke, H. C., Bergstrom, R. F. Post-injection delirium/sedation syndrome in patients with schizophrenia treated with olanzapine long-acting injection, II: investigations of mechanism. *BMC Psychiatry* 2010;10:45.
[151] Remington, G. J., Adams, M. E. Depot neuroleptic therapy: clinical considerations. *Can. J. Psychiatry* 1995;40:S5-11.
[152] Heres, S., Hamann, J., Kissling, W., et al. Attitudes of psychiatrists toward antipsychotic depot medication. *J. Clin. Psychiatry* 2006;67:1948-1953.
[153] Glazer, W. M., Kane, J. M. Depot neuroleptic therapy: An underutilized treatment option. *J. Clin. Psychiatry* 1992;53:426-433.
[154] Shi, L., Ascher-Svanum, H., Zhu, B., et al. Characteristics and use patterns of patients taking first-generation depot antipsychotics or oral antipsychotics for schizophrenia. *Psychiatr. Serv.* 2007;58:482-488.
[155] Citrome, L., Jaffe, A., Levine, J. Datapoints: depot antipsychotic use in New York State hospitals, 1994 to 2009. *Psychiatr. Serv.* 2010;61:9.
[156] Waddell, L., Taylor, M. Attitudes of patients and mental health staff to antipsychotic long-acting injections: systematic review. *Br. J. Psychiatry* Suppl. 2009 ;52:S43-50.

Part III: Atypical Antipsycholtic Use

Adverse Effects

In: Antipsychotic Drugs
Editors: T.L. Schwartz, J. Megna and M.E. Topel
ISBN: 978-1-62100-071-6

Chapter 7

ATTITUDES TOWARD PSYCHIATRIC DRUG TREATMENT IN SCHIZOPHRENIA: SOCIO DEMOGRAPHIC AND ILLNESS-RELATED FACTORS

Maria Francesca Pantusa [*] ***and Serena Paparo***
Department of Mental Health, ASP CS – Rogliano, Italy

ABSTRACT

Introduction: Schizophrenia is a chronic disease that requires long-term treatment. Adherence to antipsychotic medications is not only determined by the drug's pharmacological profile but through the interaction of different factors, including patients' attitudes toward their prescribed medications. A study was developed to evaluate attitudes toward medication and associated factors for patients with schizophrenia and related disorders, and a total of 76 outpatients were assessed using standardized tools.

Conclusion: Attitudes toward medication did not vary with age, sex, educational status, illness duration, nor duration of the last drug treatment. Drug attitudes were no different between patients taking first- or second-generation antipsychotics or mixed treatment. Factors significantly associated with poor attitudes toward medication include elevated symptom severity and lower psychosocial functioning.

INTRODUCTION

Schizophrenia is a chronic disease that needs long-term therapeutic treatments. Rates of medication non adherence among schizophrenic outpatients have been observed in approximately 50% of cases during the first year and 75% during second year after discharge from inpatient care units [1]. A 2008 analysis of Medicaid prescription records for 5898

[*] Corresponding author: Maria Francesca Pantusa. Distretto di Rogliano, Via E. Altomare, 87054- Rogliano (CS) Italy. Tel: 347/6045458. Fax: +39-0984/987123. E mail: pantusa.csm@libero.it.

patients with schizophrenia revealed that more than 90% of patients discontinued treatment within a year of filling their first prescriptions [2].

Previous studies reported that schizophrenic patients' attitude toward antipsychotic medication exerts a significant impact on adherence and clinical outcomes. Liu-Sefert et al., [3], reported that a positive attitude toward medication was significantly associated with greater clinical improvement on the Positive and Negative Syndrome Scale and lower discontinuation rates. Conversely, poor adherence with antipsychotic medications increases the risk of relapse and readmission to hospital [4]. Research data have revealed that several variables, including patient characteristics, pharmacological treatment and the treating clinician, could predict drug attitude responses.

Certain demographic characteristics have been linked to treatment adherence. Women tend to be more compliant than men [5]. Fleischhacker et al. [6] reported that problems with adherence may increase with age. Older patients, especially males, have been found to be poor compliers, because they have more complex medication regimens due to physical comorbidities and they have more difficulties with cognition. In a study by Jeste et al. [7], cognitive functions, like conceptualization and memory, were the strongest patient-related predictors of medication adherence.

Adewuya et al. [8], reported that the factors significantly associated with poor attitude towards medication (as assessed by DAI) include presence of symptoms and presence of side-effects, like dyskinesia and sedation, lack of insight into the illness, and being employed. In a study by Mohamed et al., [9] more positive medication attitudes were significantly associated with both lower symptom levels and better community functioning. Barbui et al. [10], in a study of 409 schizophrenic patients, found that a poor subjective tolerability of antipsychotics and unemployment status were significantly associated with low levels of patient ratings of adherence.

Freudenreich et al. [11], in a cross-sectional study of 81 DSM-IV-diagnosed schizophrenia outpatients, found that less awareness of current symptoms, the presence of deficit symptoms, and employment status predicted a negative attitude toward psychiatric medications as well. Drug attitudes were no different among patients taking first- or second-generation antipsychotics.

With regard to pharmacological treatment numerous studies have found that different types of medication may influence treatment non adherence. In some studies, the use of atypical antipsychotics was seen to be associated with greater treatment adherence relative to typical neuroleptics. However, other studies report no difference and suggest that patients' gender and dose frequency may be responsible for differences in treatment adherence rather than the type of antipsychotic used [12].

In a study by Sajatovic *et al.* [13], insight into illness and attitudes towards medications were explored among in-patients with schizophrenia. The patients were evaluated before and after treatment with first-generation drugs (FGA), second-generation drugs (SGA), or mixed antipsychotic medications. They found that symptoms improved significantly in all three treatment groups, while the Drug Attitude Inventory scores improved only among those patients who had received first-generation antipsychotics.

Pollice et al., in a 2008 [14] study, found that patients receiving SGAs show better subjective responses compared with patients undergoing FGA treatment, although the adherence to pharmacotherapy and clinical improvement do not differ between the groups.

On the contrary, in a study by Rocca et al. [15], patients taking second-generation antipsychotics showed more positive attitudes toward treatment than patients treated with neuroleptics.

Besides, they found that lack of insight, a more severe psychopathology, and a later age at the onset of schizophrenia correlated with a worse medication attitude.

As for the other variables associated with drug attitude, Day et al., [16] reported that negative attitudes toward treatment were predicted by poor relationship with the prescriber, experience of coercion during admission, and low insight.

Similarly, in a cross-sectional study by Dassa et al. [17], the most important features associated with non-adherence were therapeutic alliance, insight, duration of untreated psychosis (DUP), and prescription of typical antipsychotics.

After examining the literature data, the goal of this study was to analyze the correlations of attitudes toward antipsychotics drugs with demographic and clinical variables in outpatients with a diagnosis of schizophrenia and related disorders, according to DSM-IV TR classification.

Method

This is an observational study conducted in a community-based psychiatric service in Southern Italy (Rogliano-CS, Italy).

During the first half of 2010 76 outpatients (Males 39, mean age 46.7±12.1, r 22-77) were recruited.

The study protocol was approved by the institutional ethics review board at ASP of Cosenza before implementation.

The inclusion criteria for patients enrolled in the present research were:

1 Aged 18 or older
2 Affected by schizophrenia and related disorders according to DSM-IV TR diagnostic criteria
3 Taking antipsychotic medication continuously for at least 12 months with a second-generation antipsychotic and/or first-generation antipsychotic.
4 Written informed consent to participate in this study

Data on socio-demographic background, (age, gender, educational status, marital status, occupation), illness related variables (total duration of illness, severity of illness), and prescribed medication were collected.

All patients were assessed using standardized tools:

- DAI- 10 (Drug Attitude Inventory), abbreviated version to evaluate their attitudes toward medications. The Italian version has been validated by Rossi et al. [18].
- Brief Psychiatric Rating Scale (BPRS) 24 item to evaluate psychosis. The Italian version was translated and validated by de Girolamo et al. [19].
- GAF (Global Assessment of Functioning) to evaluate functional level (Endicott et al.) [20].

Statistical Analysis

Analyses were conducted using SPSS for Windows version 8.0. Quantitative variables were expressed as mean (SD), and categorical variables as percentages. The Student '*t*' test and analysis of variance (ANOVA) were used for continuous data, with Bonferroni correction if required. The *Chi square* test or Fisher's exact test was used for categorical data. Pearson correlation analysis was used to evaluate relationships between two variables. All statistical tests were two-tailed. The significance level was set at $P < 0.05$.

Results

Table 1. Demographic and clinical variables distribution

	Patients enrolled n. 76	
	N (%)	Mean±SD
Sex: Males Females	 39 (51.3) 37 (48.7)	
Mean age		46.7±12.1
Mean years of education		10.3±4.1
Marital status:		
married	20 (26.3)	
never married	56 (73.7)	
Patient's occupation (YES)	31 (40.8)	
Mean age at onset of illness:		
- males		23.1±7.2*
- females		30.6±9.2
Mean duration of illness (years)		20.6±12.5
Mean duration of psychopharmacological treatment (months).		64.2±46.2
Diagnosis:		
Schizophrenia	56 (73.7)	
Schizoaffective disorder	20 (26.3)	
Antipsychotic treatment:		
-FGA	15 (19.7)	
-SGA	49 (64.5)	
-FGA e SGA	12 (15.8)	
DAI		6.9±2.4
GAF		52.7 ± 14.4
BPRS (1-14 item)		30.2 ± 9.9
BPRS (15-24 item)		23.4±8.2
BPRS Total		53.5±16.9

Abbreviations: DAI: Drug Attitude Inventory; GAF: Global Assessment of Functioning; BPRS: Brief Psychiatric Rating Scale; FGA: First Generation Antipsychotics; SGA: Second Generation Antipsychotics; *p .001.

Demographic and clinical characteristics of the sample are displayed in Table 1. Seventy-six patients (M 39 - [51.3%], mean age 46.7 ± 12.1, r 22-77) were enrolled in the study. The educational status of the sample was 10.3±4.1 years. Thirty-one (40.8%) patients were employed or were involved in the family business. Fifty-six patients (73.7%) had schizophrenia, and 20 (26.3%) had schizoaffective disorder. The age at onset of schizophrenia was earlier in males than females (M 23.1 vs F 30.6, F = . 434, t = -3.568, p = .001).

The mean duration of illness was 20.6 ± 12.5 years, and for males it was significantly longer (M 22.5 ± 13.7 vs. F 18.5 ± 10.8, F = 4.186, t = 1.403, p = .044). At the time of recruitment the mean duration of psychopharmacological treatment was 64.2±46.2 months.

Forty-nine (64.5%) patients were treated with second generation antipsychotics, fifteen (19.7%)) with first generation antipsychotics, and twelve (15.8%) with mixed medication regimens. The DAI scores of the total sample were 6.9 ± 2.4, the BPRS scores were 53.5 ± 16.9 and the GAF scores were 52.7 ± 14.4. No differences among the DAI scores were evident in gender, pharmacological treatment, duration of treatment, and duration of illness.

The Pearson correlation test (Table 2) indicates that the attitude toward drugs was negatively associated with the severity of the psychosis, as measured by the BPRS, and positively associated with the Global Assessment of Functioning.

Discussion

This is a sample of 76 outpatients, middle aged on average, with a low mean education level, mostly suffering from schizophrenia, with a long history of illness and several previous psychopharmacological treatments. At study entry, the majority of subjects were receiving second generation antipsychotics. In agreement with that found in literature [13], the mean score reported on the DAI from the total sample was 6.9 ± 2.4 and the 64.5% recorded a score > 6, demonstrating a positive attitude toward pharmacologic treatment. We found no consistent relationship between the DAI total score and demographic characteristics (age, sex, education level, employment status). On the contrary, in the published literature some demographic characteristics correlate with the attitude to treatment. Females, especially those younger, have a more positive attitude than males or older females. The extreme ends of the age distribution, very young or very old age, are associated with a lower adherence to drug treatment, [5-21]. As for the employment status, several studies show that being in employment is correlated with a worse attitude toward drug treatment. A consideration might be that such patients are less tolerant to side effects or have difficulty taking a regular drug regimen [22]. With regard to clinical variables, the results of the present study show that a more severe psychopathology, as indicated by the BPRS total score and a greater presence of positive symptoms (BPRS items 1-14), is associated with a more negative attitude toward drug treatment. This finding is in agreement with that reported by Hofer et al. 2006 [22], and by Freudenreich et al. [11], and is easily understandable. It is certainly more difficult to convince patients suffering from grandiose delusions or manic symptoms to comply with pharmacological treatment, compared with patients with negative symptoms, who tend to have a passive attitude toward drug treatment [23]. However, the influence of negative symptoms in schizophrenic patients is controversial, since motivational deficits also may have a negative impact on compliance with medication [24].

Table 2. Correlation Matrix

		DAI	Mean duration of illness (years)	Mean Duration of treatment (months)	GAF	BPRS (item 1-14)	BPRS (item 15-24)	BPRS total
DAI	Pearson Correlation	1.000	-.011	.041	.252*	-.269*	-.160	-.237*
	Sig. (2-tailed)	.	.926	.730	.028	.019	.167	.040
Mean duration of illness (years)	Pearson Correlation	-.011	1.000	.344**	-.293*	.157	.185	.182
	Sig. (2-tailed)	.926	.	.003	.011	.180	.113	.118
Mean Duration of treatment (months)	Pearson Correlation	.041	.344	1.000	-.304**	.148	.305**	.235*
	Sig. (2-tailed)	.730	.003	.	.008	.207	.008	.044
GAF	Pearson Correlation	.252*	-.293	-.304**	1.000	-.801**	-.800**	-.864**
	Sig. (2-tailed)	.028	.011	.008	.	.000	.000	.000
BPRS (item 1-14)	Pearson Correlation	-.269*	.157	.148	-.801**	1.000	.719**	.941**
	Sig. (2-tailed)	.019	.180	.207	.000	.	.000	.000
BPRS (item 15-24)	Pearson Correlation	-.160	.185	.304**	-.800**	.719**	1.000	.912**
	Sig. (2-tailed)	.167	.113	.008	.000	.000	.	.000
BPRS total	Pearson Correlation	-.237*	.182	.235*	-.864**	.941**	.912**	1.000
	Sig. (2-tailed)	.040	.118	.044	.000	.000	.000	.

Note: Significant Correlation shown in boldface; *Correlation is significant at the 0.05 level (2-tailed). **Correlation is significant at the 0.01 level (2-tailed).

Confirming the data in the literature [25], in our study a better global functioning, as assessed with the GAF, is associated with a more positive attitude to pharmacologic treatment. In the multicenter study of Puschner et al. [26], the global social functioning represented, together with psychopathology and side effects, a strong predictor of adherence to drug treatment. In the study of Rossi et al. [27], too, a better global functioning and fewer positive symptoms correlated with a better attitude to drug treatment. We have found no correlation between DAI score and illness duration. In other studies [28] a longer duration of illness was associated with a more favorable attitude to drug treatment.

Regarding medication administered treatment we found no differences between the class of antipsychotic used and the DAI score. The small sample size did not allow us to compare the different molecules used, however. Antipsychotic drugs have an important role in the treatment of schizophrenia. The first-generation antipsychotics are very effective on positive symptoms, but they are burdened with heavy side effects. The second generation antipsychotics are better tolerated subjectively, although they aren't free from side effects, especially metabolic ones. The literature data are inconclusive.

Although it is a fairly widespread belief that SGA antipsychotics, less burdened with side effects, are associated with greater adherence to treatment, there are very few comparative studies. Freudenreich et al. [11] found no difference in relation to the class of antipsychotic agents used or to the presence of extra pyramidal side effects. Fleischhacker et al. [6] found no correlation between side effects and adherence to treatment as well. In a study by Hofer et al. 2007 [29], the correlations between antipsychotic-induced side effects and drug attitude tended to be weak. Similarly,Meier et al. [30] in their study, revealed that treatment adherence was unrelated to the class of drug, formulation, or side effect of antipsychotic medication used.

On the contrary, Menzin et al. [31], in a sample of outpatients with schizophrenia, have found, after one year of treatment, a better adherence in patients treated with SGAs. These conflicting results confirm the necessity of rigorous comparative studies not only between first-generation and second-generation antipsychotics but also between different molecules (within and between classes).

In fact, Garcia-Cabeza et al. [32], in a naturalistic study conducted in Spain that compared olanzapine, risperidone and haloperidol monotherapy, revealed that olanzapine treated subjects achieved significantly higher DAI positive attitude scores than those treated with either risperidone or haloperidol. These results are similar to the data of another naturalistic study conducted by Chengappa et al. [33] that evaluated the attitudes of psychiatric patients receiving either olanzapine or first-generation antipsychotic agents. Subjects switched to olanzapine treatment improved attitudes toward taking medication as compared to those who were treated with first generation agents.

In a randomized, double-blind, parallel-group, multi-centre study [34], sertindole and risperidone were similarly effective in improving Clinical Global Impression (Severity and Improvement), Drug Attitude Inventory and Global Assessment of Functioning scores. Obviously, these data require replication in a controlled, random-assignment, longer-term clinical trial with specific adherence measures.

Our study has some limitations that should be considered. First of all, it is possible that the small size of the sample prevented the detection of a significant difference among the variables examined. Future studies are needed in order to replicate our results making use of a greater number of patients.

Secondly, this is a sample composed predominantly of individuals with a long clinical history and several previous psychopharmacological treatments. Finally, the patients treated with SGA are clearly prevalent. Notwithstanding these limitations, the study has the advantage of examining a sample of patients with schizophrenic spectrum disorders (in chronic course) who belong to the real world of community mental health services.

Conclusion

Our results confirm some data in the literature. The majority of patients examined show a positive attitude toward drug treatment and certain clinical variables (psychopathology, psychosocial functioning) influence this response while demographic characteristics are less relevant.

We have found no significant differences among the three groups of patients who were treated either with second-generation antipsychotics, first generation antipsychotics, or mixed medication regimens. It does not mean that the three types of treatment are equivalent. Again, it is possible that our use of a small sample may have prevented the detection of significant differences.

ACKNOWLEDGMENTS

No grants have been provided to the Authors for the execution of this study, for the analysis of the data or for the writing of this paper. The authors report no conflicts of interest in this work.

REFERENCES

[1] Gray, R., Wykes, T., Gournay, K. From compliance to concordance: A review of the literature on interventions to enhance compliance with antipsychotic medication. *J. Psychiatr. Ment. health Nurs.* 2002; 9:277-284.

[2] Mullins, C. D., Obeidat, N. A., Cuffel, B. J., et al. Risk of discontinuation of atypical antipsychotic agents in the treatment of schizophrenia. *Schizophr. Res.* 2008;98:8–15

[3] Liu-Seifert, H., Osuntokun, O. O., Godfrey, J. L., et al. Feldman PD Patient perspectives on antipsychotic treatments and their association with clinical outcomes. *Patient Prefer Adherence.* 2010 Oct. 5; 4:369-77.

[4] Ascher-Svanum, H., Faries, D. E., Zhu, B., et al. Ernst, F. R., Swartz, M. S., Swanson, J. W. Medication adherence and long-term functional outcomes in the treatment of schizophrenia in usual care. *J. Clin. Psychiatry* 2006; 67:453–460.

[5] Riecher-Rössler, A. *Geschlechtsunterschiede bei Schizophrenien.* Presented at the 3rd Congress "Psychiatrische Erkrankungen bei Frauen"; Nov. 4–6, 1999; Basel, Switzerland

[6] Fleischhacker, W. W., Meise, U., Günther, V., et al. Compliance with antipsychotic drug treatment: influence of side-effects. *Acta Psychiatr. Scand. Suppl.* 1994;382:11–15

[7] Jeste, S. D., Patterson, T. L., Palmer, B. W., Dolder, C. R., Goldman, S., Jeste, D. V. Cognitive predictors of medication adherence among middle-aged and older outpatients with schizophrenia. *Schizophr. Res.* 2003; 63:49-58.

[8] Adewuya, A. O., Ola, B. A., Mosaku, S. K., et al. Attitude towards antipsychotics among outpatients with schizophrenia in Nigeria. *Acta Psychiatr. Scand.* 2006; 113: 207–211.

[9] Mohamed, S., Rosenheck, R., McEvoy, J., et al. Cross-sectional and longitudinal relationships between insight and attitudes toward medication and clinical outcomes in chronic schizophrenia. *Schizophr. Bull.* 2008;35:336-46.

[10] Barbui, C., Kikkert, M., Mazzi, M. A., et al. Comparison of patient and clinician perspectives in the assessment of antipsychotic medication adherence. *Psychopathology* 2009; 42:311-7.
[11] Freudenreich, O., Cather, C., Evins, A. E., et al. Henderson DC, Goff DC. Attitudes of schizophrenia outpatients toward psychiatric medications: relationship to clinical variables and insight. *J. Clin. Psychiatry* 2004; 65: 1372–1376.
[12] Diaz, E., Neuse, E., Sullivan, M. C., et al. Adherence to conventional and atypical antipsychotics after hospital discharge. *J. Clin. Psychiatry* 2004; 65:354–360.
[13] Sajatovic, M., Rosch, D. S., Sivec, H. J., et al. Insight Into Illness and Attitudes Toward Medications Among Inpatients With Schizophrenia. *Psychiatr. Serv.* 2002; 53:1319-1321.
[14] Pollice, R., Tomassini, A., Malavolta, M., et al. Subjective and psychopathological response in patients under different antipsychotic treatments: are there differences in real clinical practice? *J. Biol. Regul. Homeost. Agents* 2008; 22:83-91.
[15] Rocca, P., Crivelli, B., Marino, F., et al. Correlations of attitudes toward antipsychotic drugs with insight and objective psychopathology in schizophrenia *Comprehensive Psychiatry* 2008; 49:170-176.
[16] Day, J. C., Bentall, R. P., Roberts, et al. Attitudes toward Antipsychotic Medication. The Impact of Clinical Variables and Relationships with Health Professionals. *Archives of General Psychiatry* 2005; 62: 717-724.
[17] Dassa, D., Boyer, L., Benoit, M., et al. Factors associated with medication non-adherence in patients suffering from schizophrenia: a cross-sectional study in a universal coverage health-care system. *Aust. NZJ Psychiatry*. 2010; 44:921-8.
[18] Rossi, A., Arduini, L., De Cataldo, S., et al. Subjective response to neuroleptic medication: a validation study of the Italian version of the Drug Attitude Inventory (DAI). *Epidemiologia e Psichiatria Sociale* 2001; 10: 107-114.
[19] De Girolamo, G., Bellini, M., Bocchia, S., et al. Brief Psychiatric Rating Scale versione 4.0 ampliata (BPRS 4.0). *Epidemiologia e Psichiatria Sociale* 1994; 4: 69-85.
[20] Endicott, J., Spitzer, R. L., Fleiss, J. L., et al. The Global Assessment Scale: A procedure for measuring overall severity of psychiatric disturbance. *Arch. Gen. Psychiatry* 1976; 33:766–771.
[21] Di Matteo, M. R., Di Nicola, D. D. Achieving Patient Compliance. New York, NY: Pergamon Press; 1982
[22] Hofer, A., Fleischhacker, W. Attitudes towards medication in patients with schizophrenia. *Acta Psychiatrica Scandinavica* 2006;113: 161–162.
[23] Miner, C. R., Rosenthal, R. N., Hellerstein, D. J., et al. Prediction of compliance with outpatient referral in patients with schizophrenia and psychoactive substance use disorders. *Arch. Gen. Psychiatry* 1997; 54:706–712.
[24] Tattan, T. M., Creed, F. H. Negative symptoms of schizophrenic patients and compliance with medication. *Schizophr. Bull.* 2001; 27:149–155.
[25] Lambert, M., Naber, D., Eich, F. X., et al. Remission of severely impaired subjective wellbeing in 727 patients with schizophrenia treated with amisulpride. *Acta Psychiatrica Scandinavica* 2007; 115,106-113.
[26] Puschner, B., Born, A., Giessler, A., et al. Adherence to medication and quality of life in people with schizophrenia: results of a European multicenter study. *J. Nerv. Ment. Dis.* 2006; 194:746-52.

[27] Rossi, A., Pacifico, R., Stratta, P. Attitudes toward medication and the clinical variables in schizophrenia: Structural equation models. *Patient Preference and Adherence* 2009:305-309.
[28] Naoaki Kuroda, Shiyou Sun, Chih-Kuang Lin et al. Attitudes toward taking medication among outpatients with schizophrenia: cross-national comparison between Tokyo and Beijing. *Environ. Health Prev. Med.* 2008; 13: 288–295.
[29] Hofer, A., Rettenbacher, M. A., Edlinger, M., et al. Subjective response and attitudes toward antipsychotic drug therapy during the initial treatment period: a prospective follow-up study in patients with schizophrenia. *Acta Psychiatr. Scand.* 2007;116:354-61.
[30] Meier, J., Becker, T., Patel, A., et al. Effect of medication-related factors on adherence in people with schizophrenia: a European multi-centre study. *Epidemiol. Psichiatr. Soc.* 2010;19:251-9.
[31] Menzin, J., Boulanger, L., Friedman, M., et al. Treatment adherence associated with conventional and atypical antipsychotics in a large state medicaid program. *Psychiatr. Serv.* 2003; 54:719-723.
[32] Garcia-Cabeza, I., Gomez, J. C., Sacristan, J. A., et al. Subjective response to antipsychotic treatment and compliance in schizophrenia. A naturalistic study comparing olanzapine, risperidone and haloperidol (EFESO Study). *BMC Psychiatry*.2001; 1:7.
[33] Chengappa, N. R., Parepally, H., Brar, J. S., et al. Attitudes towards taking Medicine among those patients who either received Olanzapine or First Generation Antipsychotic Agents. *Indian. J. Psychiatry*. 2003;45:151-4.
[34] Azorin, J. M., Strub, N., Loft, H. A double-blind, controlled study of sertindole versus risperidone in the treatment of moderate-to-severe schizophrenia *International Clinical Psychopharmacology* 2006, 21:49–56

In: Antipsychotic Drugs
Editors: T.L. Schwartz, J. Megna and M.E. Topel

ISBN: 978-1-62100-071-6

Chapter 8

APPLYING ABSTINENCE, ANTICIPATION, REDUCTION, AND TREATMENT (AART) FOR THE MANAGEMENT OF ATYPICAL ANTIPSYCHOTIC SIDE EFFECTS

Annette Kennedy*
Sheridan VA Medical Center, Sheridan, WY, US

ABSTRACT

In contemporary clinical settings where pharmacotherapy and psychotherapy are typically provided by different clinicians, patients often bring their concerns about their antipsychotic medications to their psychotherapy providers. Thus, the author has first learned about many of the side effects associated with antipsychotic medications based upon patient report. Drawing upon her experience as a psychodynamically-oriented psychologist and clinical researcher, the author discusses a relational approach to the management of antipsychotic side effects. The steps in AART are hierarchical, yet also overlapping and reflective, levels of risk prevention and minimization. The author discusses key issues relevant to each level of intervention, providing examples of how AART might be integrated into clinical work.

AUTHOR NOTE

This article is a revision and expansion of an earlier article that introduced the concept of Abstinence, Anticipation, Reduction, and Treatment (AART) for the management of atypical antipsychotic side effects [1].

* Correspondence concerning this chapter should be directed to Annette Kennedy, Sheridan VA Medical Center, A-116, 1898 Fort Rd., Sheridan WY 82801; E-mail: Annette.kennedy2@va.gov

Antipsychotic medications, specifically the second generation or atypical agents, are the first-line treatment for psychotic disorders, including schizophrenia and schizoaffective disorder. They have also become a mainstay in the treatment of depression, both bipolar and unipolar. Atypical antipsychotics are often prescribed off-label as either the primary treatment or as an adjunctive treatment for a variety of mental health problems, including anxiety disorders, behavioral disorders, and insomnia. The convergence of a number of factors, including growing public awareness of mental illness, what initially appeared to be a superior side effect profile as compared to the typical neuroleptics, and aggressive marketing by the pharmaceutical industry, has prompted the ubiquitous prescribing of atypical antipsychotic and 2008. Of these visits, the majority involved the use of antipsychotic medications for indications without FDA approval, with the number growing from 4.4M visits in 1995 to 9.0M in 2008.

Many of the prescriptions for antipsychotic medications are written by prescribers with limited training in mental health. In an analysis of 472M prescriptions written for psychotropic drugs from August 2006 through July 2007, researchers from Thomson Reuters and the U.S. Substance Abuse and Mental Health Services Administration found that 37% of the prescriptions written for antipsychotic medications were written by family doctors [3].(2). The frequency with which antipsychotics are being prescribed by psychiatrists and other prescribers translated into $16.1Bn in sales, with the top brands Abilify® (aripiprazole), Seroquel® (quetiapine) and Zyprexa® (olanzapine) amassing a combined $1.4Bn in growth in 2010 [4].

The first-generation antipsychotic drugs are referred to as *typical* antipsychotic drugs because they typically produce extrapyramidal side effects (EPS). After extended use in vulnerable individuals, they often also produce tardive dyskinesia or dystonia as a result of blockade of D2 receptors in the dorsal striatum. In theory, clozapine and other "atypical" antipsychotic medications, to varying degrees, differed from the typical agents in six effects, (a) absence of tardive dyskinesia; (b) lack of serum prolactin elevations; (c) ability to eliminate positive symptoms without exacerbating motor symptoms in patients with Parkinson's disease who become psychotic due to exogenous dopaminergic agents such as levodopa (LDOPA); (d) ability to decrease or totally eliminate psychotic symptoms in approximately 60% of the patients with schizophrenia who fail to respond to typical neuroleptic drugs; (e) ability to improve primary and secondary negative symptoms; and (f) ability to improve some domains of cognition in patients with schizophrenia, especially secondary memory and semantic memory [5]. Although atypical antipsychotics are superior to the typical agents in regards to movement disorders, they have not consistently been shown to be superior in other domains and they are associated with a number of serious side effects, most notably metabolic disorders. Thus, regardless of whether one interprets the prevalence with which atypical antipsychotics are being prescribed as improved access to and delivery of mental health care or as a feat of marketing genius by big pharma, the prescription of all antipsychotic medications requires that clinicians be knowledgeable about their side effects and adept in the management of those side effects. This article discusses the application of a psychodynamically informed treatment approach to the management of atypical antipsychotic side effects—Abstinence, Anticipation, Reduction, and Treatment [1].

LEVEL ONE—ABSTINENCE

The only entirely effective method for the prevention of side effects associated with antipsychotics is to not prescribe them. Therefore, it is incumbent upon the prescriber to have a well-defined rationale for choosing to prescribe an antipsychotic. For clinical presentations that include significant symptoms of psychosis the prescription of an antipsychotic is often the most appropriate choice. However, for non-psychotic disorders the prescription of an antipsychotic is usually only one of several alternatives and often not the best one. Antipsychotic medications are routinely prescribed off-label for attention deficit hyperactivity disorder (ADHD), anxiety, dementia in elderly patients, depression, eating disorders, insomnia, obsessive compulsive disorder (OCD), personality disorders, post traumatic stress disorder (PTSD), substance abuse, and Tourette's syndrome; however, the evidence from randomized controlled trials (RCT's) only suggests that specific antipsychotic agents may be selectively effective for some of these conditions. The best evidence in support of the off-label use of antipsychotics is related to anxiety, dementia, depression, and OCD, with limited evidence for their use with personality disorders and no evidence for their use for substance abuse disorders. However, weight gain, other metabolic side effects, cardiovascular accidents, EPS, and sedation have been consistently associated with the off-label use of antipsychotic medications [6]. Thus, it is critical that the prescriber utilize all available means to analyze the benefits to risks ratio to determine if an atypical antipsychotic, or any antipsychotic for that matter, either as the primary agent or as an adjunctive agent, is clinically warranted.

How Prescribing Decisions Are Made

One of the ways that prescribers can increase the care they take when prescribing antipsychotic medications is by increasing their conscious awareness of their own decision making processes. In their ethnographic work on healthcare decision making, Gabbay and Le May [7] observed that primary care clinicians typically do not utilize explicit codified knowledge, such as guidelines, to make prescribing decisions, but rely on "mindlines," defined as "collectively reinforced, internalized, tacit guidelines" (p. 1013). Building on the work of Gabbay and Le May, Barley and colleagues [8] conducted qualitative research on how psychiatrists make decisions when prescribing antipsychotic medications. Barley et al. identified four types of knowledge—acquired, interpreted, individual experience, and contextual—which inform the "mindlines" that guide psychiatrists' prescribing practices. Increased awareness of the factors that contribute to each of these types of knowledge can make for more precise prescribing. *Acquired knowledge* consists of information from formal sources--summarized as ''what I have been told.'' Whereas, *interpreted knowledge* is "What I make of what I've been told." *Experiential knowledge* is acquired via personal and clinical experience, and *contextual knowledge* is gathered in a particular setting, in response to social and clinical pressures, expectations and events, often reflecting a particular prescribing culture.

Given the hierarchical structure of allopathic medicine, prescribers are taught to privilege *acquired knowledge* with an implicit expectation that acquired knowledge is empirically rather than intuitively or constructively derived and that it is acquired from another as opposed to the self. In actuality, while some acquired knowledge is indeed *scientific*, such as findings from RCT's, other acquired knowledge is much less objective, such as published case reports or information acquired from pharmaceutical company marketing campaigns. Without thoughtful interpretation of acquired knowledge, prescribers may weigh all forms of acquired knowledge equally. For example, biases in the ways in which scientific knowledge is disseminated may lead prescribers to acquire knowledge that on an individual item level may be accurate but which collectively may be inaccurate. Fountoulakis et al. (2004) found that 91 of 100 published case reports about the off-label use of antipsychotic medications reported positive effects. As noted by the authors, even approved therapies do not achieve 90% effect rates and it is likely that published case reports reflect a bias on the part of both researchers and journals to only publish positive outcomes [9]. However, taken out of the larger context of publication bias, this apparently scientific, acquired knowledge suggests that the off-label use of antipsychotics is highly effective.

The development of *contextual knowledge* involves the cultural interface of often diverse stakeholders, including the patient, the prescriber him or herself, family members, and various political and economic authorities. The contextual knowledge that a clinician applies to prescribing an antipsychotic medication for a particular patient includes the clinical history that the patient has shared with the prescriber. The clinical history that patients share with their prescribers is comprised of medical data, but equally importantly, it also includes all of the conscious and unconscious beliefs, hopes, and fears that the patient brings to treatment. Similarly, the *contextual* and *experiential knowledge* that the prescriber applies to prescribing medications to a particular patient include the clinician's professional and personal history, including all of the conscious and unconscious beliefs, hopes, and fears that the clinician brings to the case.

Choosing to Prescribe or Not Prescribe an Antipsychotic—Not a Simple Matter

The use of atypical antipsychotics for the treatment of PTSD exemplifies many of the issues faced by prescribers when considering the use of an atypical antipsychotic, particularly for an off-label indication. The only two FDA approved medications for the treatment of PTSD are the selective serotonin reuptake inhibitors (SSRI's) sertraline (Zoloft) and paroxetine (Paxil). Although these medications are considered the first-line pharmacological treatment for PTSD, they have been shown to have limited efficacy [10-12] with rates of response to SSRI's particularly low in combat-induced PTSD [13-15]. Thus, clinicians are eager to identify other pharmacological interventions [16]. It has been hypothesized that the serotonergic and noradrenergic actions of antipsychotic medications may render them useful for the treatment of depression and anxiety symptoms associated with PTSD [17,18]. *In addition, many individuals with PTSD display significant psychotic symptomology in the absence of a psychotic disorder* [19,20]. Thus, prescribing an antipsychotic for treatment-resistant PTSD appears to have a certain face value.

In a comprehensive review of the efficacy of antipsychotic medications for PTSD, the *Comparative Effectiveness Review (CER) 2011* analyzed ten controlled trials, varying in duration from 5 to 16 weeks [6]. Eight of the ten studies utilized the Clinician Administered

PTSD Scale (CAPS) as the primary outcome measure, with six studies involving risperidone, two olanzapine, and two quetiapine. Overall, the findings from these studies supported the efficacy of antipsychotic medications for PTSD.

Both of the studies utilizing quetiapine, one with quetiapine monotherapy and one with quetiapine in combination with sertraline reported quantitative improvements in CAPS scores. However, particularly convincing was the meta-analysis of the pooled data from four of the trials using risperidone and one using olanzapine, with the CAPS as the primary outcome measure. The sample sizes ranged from 19 to 65, and the risperidone dose ranged from 0.5mg to 3mg daily. The overall random effects pooled estimate for risperidone and the one olanzapine study was 7.79 (95% CI 2.40, 13.17), with an I-squared = 0.0 percent, a standard mean difference of 0.40 or a moderate effect size. However, it was also noteworthy that when these five trials were divided between those for combat-related PTSD in men and sexual abuse-related PTSD in civilian women, efficacy (also with a moderate effect size) was only seen in the male, combat group. Taken in its entirety, this meta-analysis provides moderately strong evidence to support the use of risperidone to treat combat-related PTSD in men. Thus, based upon this acquired and interpreted knowledge, it might be warranted for a clinician treating PTSD in a combat veteran with residual symptoms to prescribe a trial of risperidone.

However, in contrast, the findings, also published in 2011, from a large, multi-site trial, including data from 247 almost exclusively male veterans with SSRI-resistant, military-related PTSD did not find six months treatment with risperidone as an adjunct to treatment as usual to yield improvements on total CAPS scores or on outcomes for depression, anxiety, psychosis, and quality of life [21]. Risperidone did exhibit a small effect on re-experiencing and hyper-arousal symptoms, but the authors concluded that this change was probably not robust enough to be clinically significant. While risperidone was not associated with any serious adverse events, there were more self-reported cases of weight gain [risperidone: n=20, 15.3%; placebo: n=3, 2.3%], fatigue, somnolence, and hyper-salivation. Thus, the benefits of antipsychotics for PTSD remain in question, particularly given that there is growing evidence to suggest that individuals with PTSD are inherently at risk for the metabolic syndrome [22-24].

Individuals with PTSD who are also taking antipsychotic medications have an even higher prevalence rate of the metabolic syndrome than patients with schizophrenia taking antipsychotic medications, 72% and 60% respectively [25]. Thus, based upon this acquired and interpreted knowledge, it might be prudent for a clinician treating PTSD in a combat veteran with treatment-resistant symptoms to abstain from prescribing an antipsychotic. As can be seen, even the careful interpretation of acquired information often does not lead to unambiguous conclusions.

Prescribing clinicians often find themselves trying to make well-reasoned, ethical decisions when there is inconclusive and contradictory scientific evidence. In the face of scientific uncertainty, clinicians are apt to be more strongly influenced by contextual knowledge. As previously alluded to, contextual knowledge is often unconscious or at least not consciously evaluated. Contextual knowledge includes information authored and or legitimated by a variety of stakeholders, including the patient, the prescriber, family members, the medical institution, governmental and regulatory bodies, and economic decision makers. For example, the high rate of PTSD in soldiers returning from Iraq and Afghanistan and the associated high emotional and financial costs may be among the contextual factors influencing the prescription of antipsychotic medications for PTSD. Based upon computer-modeled projections, it has been estimated that as many as 35% of troops deployed to Iraq will experience PTSD [26]. Already in 2008, the Rand Corp. reported that about 300,000 U.S. military personnel who had deployed to Iraq or Afghanistan were suffering from PTSD or major depression [27]. The same report also estimated that the associated costs of taking care of those veterans could reach $6.2 billion in as little as two years. Given the magnitude of this problem, it is not surprising that almost 42% of veterans receiving off-label antipsychotic medications had a diagnosis of PTSD [28]. It is also not surprising that veterans with service-connected disability ratings of at least 50% were more likely to receive an antipsychotic medication off label (OR=1.75). One can only assume that prescribers are responding to extreme pressure, both external and internal, to help resolve this overwhelming healthcare crisis.

In an era of growing mental health treatment needs and shrinking resources, prescribers are certainly influenced by the prescribing cultures in which they are embedded and the political and economic exigencies of those cultures. However, they are also influenced by the contextual knowledge that emerges within the treating relationship [29-31]. A psychodynamic approach to psychopharmacology assumes the central importance of meanings that emerge in the relational matrix comprised of the patient, the illness, the prescriber, and the medications. These meanings include both conscious and unconscious mental represenations. They reflect the here and now, and they also consist of transference and counter-transference projections. They can provide the healthy satisfaction of a broad range of psychological needs, including attachment, agency, and healthy narcissism. These meanings can also come to embody the expression of pathological impulses.

Writing about the psychodynamics of psychopharmacology, Li et al [31] notes that both the prescriber and the patient may believe, either consciously or unconsciously, that "being prescribed a medication is a concrete sign that something is being done for one's distress, that one's problems are valid, and being taken seriously" (p. 658). The prescription of a potent medication, such as an antipsychotic, may be understood to mean that one's problems have been assigned the highest priority and are being aggressively addressed. Li has also noted that both the patient and the prescriber are apt to want to believe that the patient is receiving "the best and the latest" in science. The off-label use of medications is often equated with cutting edge innovation and thus satisfies the patient's desire to receive the best and latest treatment. Ideally, in this situation there is a mutual satisfaction of psychological needs. The patient feels understood and nurtured. The prescriber feels empatheric and effective.

However, in a less healthy treatment relationship, the act of prescribing may be used to fulfill the prescriber's own narcissistic needs, bolstering the prescriber's sense of status and authority. For example, the experience of trying to treat a patient who repeatedly fails to respond to one's best pharmacological interventions can leave a prescriber feeling hopeless and impotent, even damaging one's identity as a prescriber. Prescribing an antipsychotic off-label may help the prescriber to re-establish her identity as medical professional and the authority that carries. Prescribers may be prompted to prescribe an antipsychotic off-label in response to other counter-transference reactions as well. Milrod and Busch [33] observed that patients with panic disorder often trigger acute distress in their treating clinicians, prompting those clinicians to prescribe medications. Similarly, extreme emotional distress in patients with PTSD or major depression may trigger feelings of emotional distress and or pity in prescribers, prompting them to prescribe antipsychotic medications. The more that a prescriber becomes conscious of the influences of contextual knowledge the better she is able to determine whether the prescription of antipsychotic medication is truly warranted or whether she is capitulating to contextual influences.

There are several key questions that prescribers may ask to help guide their decision-making when considering prescribing an antipsychotic for the treatment of a non-psychotic psychiatric condition:

- Who and what am I treating? In other words, by prescribing this antipsychotic medication am I addressing the concerns of my patient, his or her spouse or family, myself, my colleagues, the payer, the courts, etc.? And what are the concerns and or agenda of each of these stakeholders?
- Do all stakeholders share the same treatment goals and are their treatment expectations realistic?
- Have there been at least two adequate (including dosage, duration, compliance, and agents of different classes, if applicable) trials of approved treatments?
- Are there lifestyle or psychosocial issues that may respond to non-pharmacological interventions?
- Does the severity of the presenting symptomology and associated functional impairment warrant the medical risks associated with an antipsychotic?
- Could the use of an antipsychotic potentially undermine a comprehensive treatment plan?

In many cases, the prescriber's responses to these questions indicate that electing to abstain from prescribing an antipsychotic and selecting an alternative therapy is the most prudent course of treatment for a non-psychotic disorder.

Level 2—Anticipation

The second level in a stepwise approach to the management of antipsychotic side effects is to anticipate the potential side effects that may be associated with the prescription of a particular atypical agent. This involves not only anticipating side effects that may emerge based upon the chemical properties of a particular medication, but it also involves anticipating side effects that may emerge as a result of the psychodynamic profile of a particular patient. By using anticipation to minimize the occurrence of treatment emergent side effects, prescribers are often able to prevent the problems associated with trying to reduce or treat side effects. The anticipation of side effects includes the integration of a thorough psychiatric evaluation, a thorough medical evaluation, and familiarity with the side effect profiles of the available atypical antipsychotic medications with an understanding of the psychodynamic issues in play.

Psychiatric Evaluation

The psychiatric evaluation is the clinical foundation of psychiatric treatment and includes both an assessment of presenting symptomology and a psychiatric history. Ideally, the psychiatric evaluation is the primary source of the contextual knowledge that the prescriber applies to his prescribing decisions. Specifically, the psychiatric evaluation is a rich source of information that can be applied to the anticipation of antipsychotic side effects. Patients' subjective attitudes and expectations about the benefits and side effects of medications can be associated with compliance [34,35]. ***When patients report that a certain medication didn't work for them, they may actually be saying that they experienced side effects that were unacceptable to them.*** Careful and sensitive questioning by prescribers about patients' experiences with and feelings about side effects, explanations for medication changes, and rationale for non-compliance will frequently lead to crucial information about what side effects to anticipate and potential problems with medication compliance.

Vlastelica [36] comments that the obverse of the placebo response is the nocebo response and that the nocebo response occurs when patients expect [consciously or unconsciously] to be harmed. An expectation of being harmed may predispose patients to experiencing intolerable side effects. Just as the placebo effect can contribute to the effectiveness of a medication for an individual patient, the nocebo response can contribute to the unacceptability of a medication to an individual patient. Self-report instruments, such as the Drug Attitude Inventory [37] may be helpful in identifying areas of inquiry regarding patients' expectations, beliefs, and fears about taking antipsychotics.

Medical Evaluation

A comprehensive medical evaluation, including both a patient and familial medical history and a physical examination, provides a wealth of information with which to anticipate the potential side effects of antipsychotic medications. While there are a number of rare, potentially lethal adverse events that can be caused by atypical antipsychotics, such as neuroleptic malignant syndrome [38] and myocarditis [39], our focus is on the prevention and minimization of the much more common and insidious side effects that pose a chronic health risk to patients treated with these medications. What's more, patients with mental illness have both limited access to and underutilize healthcare resources [40,41]; therefore, the treating prescriber needs to be aware of the central role he plays in the overall healthcare of the patient [42].

The Medical History

History taking can be a slow and arduous task with patients experiencing severe symptomology. Furthermore, it may be necessary to take a history more than once in order to develop a comprehensive and cohesive picture of the patient's personal and familial medical history. However, taking a thorough medical history can help to minimize side effects and to reduce the necessity for medication changes. In general, specific and probing questions, as opposed to open-ended questions, will yield a more detailed and accurate medical history:

- While patients may not know the medical diagnoses carried by their first-degree relatives, they may know the age of death, the symptoms of illness, or the medications taken by their family members.
- Questions about the meals and snacks eaten over the last few days will be more informative than questions about diet or nutrition.
- Questions about tobacco use should include the number and type of cigarettes smoked and other forms of tobacco consumption.
- Even among patients who report that they exercise regularly, in-depth questions about daily activities may reveal a predominantly sedentary lifestyle.
- Querying about the presence of specific signs and symptoms of cardiac and metabolic pathologies may uncover otherwise unrecognized risks.

Ideally, a prescriber would compile a complete profile of a patient's physical health—including metabolic, cardiac, neuromuscular, endocrine, and hematologic functioning, as well as concomitant medications—prior to prescribing an antipsychotic medication. However, frequently in clinical practice, acute symptomology precludes gathering complete medical information prior to prescribing medication. Often the prescriber is only able to accrue this information once the patient's symptoms have at least partially stabilized and the patient has begun to develop trust in the provider-patient relationship. ***Thus, the prescriber often needs to re-evaluate initially prescribed medications once the results of physical examination and laboratory tests become available.*** De Hert et al. [43] have reviewed 18 different sets of guidelines for the screening and monitoring of cardiometabolic risks in patients with schizophrenia. Based upon their review, they have developed a rigorous but practicable timetable for diagnostic procedures (Figure 1).

	Baseline	6 weeks (if starting drug treatment)	12 weeks (if starting drug treatment)	Annually (or more more frequently)
Medical History	√	√	√	√
Weight/waist/BMI	√	√	√	√
Blood Pressure	√	√	√	√
Fasting glucose	√	√	√	√
Fasting lipids	√	√	√	√
Lifestyle advice	√	√	√	√

Figure 1. Monitoring protocol for managing individuals with normal baseline values at start of an episode from De Hert et al. [43].

Anticipated Side Effects

With the exception of clozapine for treatment-refractory schizophrenia, no one atypical antipsychotic has shown superior effectiveness [44]. However, the prescriber can utilize a general knowledge of the pharmacodynamic profiles of the various agents to anticipate both efficacy and possible side effects (Table 1) [45-47]. Acquired knowledge about the pharmacodynamics of the available agents in combination with contextual knowledge about the medical and psychiatric history of the patient can inform predictions about outcome. The same pharmacodynamic action may in one patient be associated with the efficacy of a particular atypical antipsychotic and in another patient be associated with an intolerable side effect. For example, one patient may experience the sedating properties of quetiapine as soothing and attribute the experience to the benevolent intentions of the prescriber. Whereas, another patient may experience those same sedating properties as disabling and attribute the experience to the malevolent intentions of the prescriber. An understanding of what psychodynamic functions medications fill for an individual patient can help the prescriber to anticipate how different potential side effects may be experienced by the patient.

The Metabolic Syndrome.

People with mental disorders die 8.2 years sooner than the general population [51]. The increased risk of premature death for patients with schizophrenia is 2.6 times that of the general population [52], with people with schizophrenia dying around 19 years earlier on average than the general population [53]. Cardiovascular mortality is the primary cause of premature death due to natural causes and is elevated 6 fold in patients with severe mental illness [54]. Cardiovascular mortality in schizophrenia is associated with the convergence of several risk factors, including genetic predisposition, lifestyle, and the metabolic side effects of antipsychotic medications.

One of the primary cardiovascular risk factors in patients with schizophrenia is the presence of one or more components of the metabolic syndrome. The metabolic syndrome is the co-occurrence within a single individual of several metabolic abnormalities that are associated with an increased risk of cardiovascular disease. The metabolic abnormalities include abdominal or visceral obesity, dysregulation of glucose metabolism, high plasma triglycerides, low plasma high-density lipoprotein cholesterol (HDL-C), and elevated blood pressure (Table 2). The clinical significance of the co-occurrence of these risks is that the combined risk of two or more of these abnormalities is more than additive. Thus, in a patient with 5 risk factors, the global risk of coronary heart disease may be 15 to 30-fold higher than for an individual with none of these abnormalities [54]. A number of psychiatric disorders, including depression, anxiety, bipolar disorder, and, as previously noted, PTSD have been shown to be associated with metabolic abnormalities, and it is most likely that this relationship is both bi-directional and multi-determined [55]. However, antipsychotic medications are clearly a significant contributor to the high incidence of metabolic disorders in severely mentally ill patients.

Table 1. Possible Therapeutic Effects and Side Effects of Receptor Blockade by Atypical Antipsychotics

Receptor System	Therapeutic Effect	Side Effect	Receptor Blockade by Atypical Antipsychotics and Haloperidol in Descending Order
D_2-Dopaminergic	Reduction of psychotic symptoms	Extrapyramidal movement disorders, prolactin elevation	Aripiprazole, Asenapine, Lurasidone; Paliperidone, Iloperidone, Haloperidol, Ziprasidone, Olanzapine, Risperidone, Quetiapine, Clozapine
A_1-Adrenergic	Sedation	Potentiation of prazosin, postural hypotension, dizziness, reflex tachycardia	Iloperidone, Asenapine, Clozapine, Risperidone, Paliperidone, Haloperidol, Ziprasidone, Quetiapine, Aripiprazole, Lurasidone, Olanzapine
H_1-Histaminergic	Sedation	Sedation, drowsiness, weight gain, potentiation of CNS depressants	Asenapine, Olanzapine, Paliperidone, Quetiapine, Clozapine, Iloperidone, Risperidone, Aripiprazole, Ziprasidone, Lurasidone, Haloperidol
M_3-Muscarinic	Reduction of extrapyramidal side effects	Blurred vision, attack or exacerbation of narrow-angle glaucoma, dry mouth, constipation, urinary retention, sinus tachycardia, cognitive impairments	Clozapine, Olanzapine, Lurasidone, Aripiprazole, Iloperidone, Paliperidone, (Haloperidol, Quetiapine, Risperdione, Ziprasizone, all equivalent)
5-HT_{2A} Serotonergic	Reduction of negative and affective symptoms, reduction of extrapyramidal side effects, improvement in cognition	Unknown	Asenapine, Risperidone, Iloperidone, Ziprasidone, Paliperidone, Olanzapine, Lurasidone, Clozapine, Aripiprazole Haloperidol, Quetiapine

Adapted from Ishibashi et al. [48], Kroeze et al. [49], and Richelson and Souder [50].

A large multicentre, cross-sectional pharmacoepidemiological study (METEOR) of metabolic disorders in patients with schizophrenia was performed in 12 European countries [56]. Prevalence rates for the metabolic syndrome were universally high, with a 36.7% prevalence rate in patients taking atypical antipsychotics and a 30.7% prevalence rate in patients taking first generation antipsychotics. In the largest study to date collecting data on the incidence of the metabolic syndrome in schizophrenia, the Clinical Antipsychotic Trials of Intervention Effectiveness (CATIE) study found the metabolic syndrome in 41% of schizophrenia patients overall (51.6% in women, 36.0% in men), as compared to 25.1% and 19.7% in healthy women and men, respectively [57].

Atypical antipsychotics indisputably cause weight gain, often to the point of obesity [56,59-61]. Medically, weight gain increases the risk for hypertension, coronary heart disease, ischemic stroke, poor glucose tolerance, diabetes mellitus, dyslipidemia, respiratory problems, osteoarthritis, liver problems, gall bladder disease, and certain cancers. Pathological weight gain or obesityObesity is most commonly defined by the body mass index (BMI), derived by dividing the individual's weight in kilograms by his height in meters squared or by dividing the individual's weight in pounds by his height in inches squared and then multiplying by 703. Typically, an adult with a BMI between 25 and 29.9 is classified as overweight; an adult with a BMI of 30 or higher is classified as obese. Defining obesity as a BMI of 27 or higher, Allison et al. [59] found that 42% of patients with schizophrenia were obese, with women particularly affected. Clinically, measuring waist circumference can be as important as measuring BMI. Visceral abdominal obesity is the most dangerous pattern of fat deposition because of its association with hypertension, diabetes, dyslipidemia, and the metabolic syndrome [62].

Table 2. The Metabolic Syndrome as Indicated by Three or More Risk Factors

Risk Factor	Defining Level
Abdominal Obesity (waist)	
Men	> 102 cm (> 40 in)
Women	> 88 cm (> 35 in)
Fasting Triglycerides	≥ 150 mg/dL
High-Density Lipoprotein Cholesterol	
Men	< 40 mg/dL
Women	< 50 mg/dL
Blood Pressure	≥ 130/ > 85 mm Hg or on antihypertensive medication
Fasting Glucose	≥ 100 mg/dL or on insulin or hypoglycemic medication

Adapted from Grundy et al. [58].

Based upon short-term studies, the different atypical antipsychotic agents can be ranked by weight-gain potential (Table 3). With the exception of clozapine and olanzapine at the high end and ziprasizone at the low end of the weight gain continuum, data from long-term studies is more ambiguous regarding which agents pose the greatest risk [63,64]. However, the CATE study found that quetiapine and risperidone caused weight gain of approximately 0.25 kg gain per month of treatment [65]. It is also clear that apart from clozapine, olanzapine poses the greatest risk for weight gain, causing a severe weight gain (4.15 kg) after only 10 weeks of treatment [59]. Similarly, in the CATIE study, patients on olanzapine gained weight at the rate of 0.9 kg per month. The pattern of weight gain also appears to be different for clozapine and olanzapine than for risperidone and quetiapine, with weight gain due to these former agents not plateauing until months or even years after the initiation of treatment [66]. Although aripiprazole has a generally superior metabolic profile as compared to other atypical antipsychotics, a 2012 meta-analysis of head-to-head comparisons of the atypical antipsychotics found no difference between risperidone and aripiprazole on weight gain [64]. ***In addition to the metabolic risks associated with antipsychotic-induced weight gain, weight gain can be one of the main factors contributing to subjective intolerability of an antipsychotic medication and associated non-compliance [67,68].***

Table 3. Estimated weight change in pounds at 10 weeks of atypical antipsychotic treatment

Aripiprazole	0.99a
Asenapine	1.6b
Clozapine	4.45
Haloperidol	1.08
Iloperidone	3.0c
Olanzapine	4.15
Quetiapine	1.8
Risperidone	2.1
Sertindole	2.92
Ziprasidone	0.4

Adapted from Roerig, Steffen, and Mitchell [74]. Unless otherwise noted, data from Allison et al. [59].
a Over 4 weeks, Lee et al. [75].
b Over 3 weeks, McIntyre [76].
c Over 29 days,Cutler et al. [77].

Although patients with schizophrenia appear to have an increased risk for insulin resistance and type 2 diabetes mellitus apart from the effects of atypical antipsychotics [69-71], treatment with many of the first generation and most of the atypical antipsychotic agents is associated with increased risk of insulin resistance, hyperglycemia, type 2 diabetes, and dyslipidemia [72]. It has traditionally been thought that the relationship between atypical antipsychotics and dysregulation of glucose metabolism was largely mediated by weight gain. However, obesity is probably only one of several key pathways resulting in insulin resistance. Stahl et al. [73] explain that in addition to weight gain, atypical antipsychotics also produce atherogenic dyslipidemia, including elevated fasting triglyceride levels and low serum high-density lipoprotein (HDL) cholesterol. Low HDL cholesterol and high fasting triglycerides are strongly linked to insulin resistance. In turn, insulin resistance triggers compensatory hyperinsulinemia, eventually causing pancreatic b-cell failure, prediabetes and finally type 2 diabetes. Thus, insulin resistance and associated pathology can occur in the absence of weight gain. Therefore, clinicians cannot assume normal regulation of glucose metabolism in patients who are not overweight or who do not exhibit weight changes in response to antipsychotics. Laboratory assessments of metabolic outcomes provide the most reliable information about potential risks. As noted above, baseline measures of fasting glucose and lipids can signal potential metabolic side effects in response to atypical antipsychotics. The identification of a pre-existing metabolic abnormality prior to the prescription of an atypical antipsychotic may be a reason for abstaining from prescribing one. If the prescription of an antipsychotic is indeed clinically indicated, to date, aripiprazole, ziprasidone, and lurasidone appear to pose the fewest metabolic risks [72].

Prolongation and Sudden Cardiac QTC Death

Another uncommon but potentially fatal cardiac risk factor that should be considered when prescribing antipsychotic medications is prolongation of the corrected QT interval (QTc), as measured by an electrocardiogram. Prolongation of the QTc may result in torsades de pointes, an arrhythmia that can cause sudden cardiac death (SCD). The incidence rate of SCD in individuals receiving antipsychotics is approximately 15 cases per 10,000 years of drug exposure [78], but the exact association between prolonged QTc and SCD is difficult to determine [79]. Most patients who exhibit antipsychotic-associated torsade de pointes and subsequently die from SCD have other risk factors, such as older age, female gender, hypokalaemia and cardiovascular disease.

Regarding monitoring QTc, a QTc interval in the range of 450 to 500 milliseconds is considered a marker for increased risk and a QTc interval greater than 500ms is cause for discontinuation of the suspected causal agent. Almost all first and second generation antipsychotics appear to increase the risk of QTc prolongation. Thioridazine and ziprasidone cause the greatest prolongation in the QTc interval [80]. However, when compared to olanzapine, ziprasidone treatment was not associated with an increased risk of nonsuicide mortality in real-world use in patients with schizophrenia [73]. QTc prolongation in patients taking antipsychotic medications may be due to an additive effect of the combination of multiple drugs that prolong the QTc interval. Macrolide, antibacterials, lithium, and methadone are among the agents that can prolong QTc interval. With antipsychotic medications, QT interval prolongation is also often dose dependent, although these agents typically reach a plateau of maximum effect on QTc. Patients who have other cardiac risk factors, including advanced age, a known history of cardiovascular disease, an existing prescription for a QTc interval-prolonging drug, a personal or family history of syncope, or a family history of sudden death, need to be monitored most closely. Prior to initiating treatment with ziprasidone or another QTc interval-prolonging antipsychotic, these patients should receive an ECG. A second ECG should be administered once the agent reaches steady state [79].

Other Common Side Effects

EPS is categorized as either an acute syndrome (dystonia, akathisia and parkinsonism) or as a tardive syndrome (dyskinesia and dystonia), and the acute syndrome is a risk factor for the frequently irreversible tardive syndrome [81]. It was previously believed that one of the features that make atypical antipsychotic medications "atypical" is a lack of EPS [82]. In a large meta-analysis, Correll et al. [84] reported that first generation antipsychotics have a 6-fold higher incidence of tardive dyskinesia (TD) than atypical antipsychotics. However, some of the apparent superiority of the atypical agents in early efficacy trials of antipsychotics may have been due to comparisons which were made with haloperidol at relatively high doses. More recent data from large-scale effectiveness trials, such as the CATIE and the Cost Utility of the Latest Antipsychotic Drugs in Schizophrenia Study (CUTLASS), have cast doubt on the superiority of atypical antipsychotic agents as related to EPS [65,84,85]. What is certain is that there are a number of repeatedly identified risk factors for TD. These factors include pre-existing EPS, older age, brain injury or dementia, and substance abuse [84]. Thus, extra caution should be taken when considering prescribing high potency antipsychotics, particularly haloperidol, to patients with these risk factors.

Another one of the features that make atypical antipsychotic medications "atypical" is a lack of hyperprolactinemia [82]. However, like all of the typical, first generation antipsychotics, risperidone has been shown to cause elevations in plasma prolactin levels, with almost two thirds of patients exhibiting a greater than 2-fold increase above normal [86]. Hyperprolactinemia can cause galactorrhea and sexual dysfunction in both men and women, and menstrual disturbances in women. It can also induce weight gain and may be related to metabolic abnormalities [87]. Although schizophrenia itself is associated with decreased libido, many patients with schizophrenia are sexually active [88], and sexual side effects may reduce medication compliance [89]. Prescribers should inquire about symptoms of hyperprolactinemia, including galactorrhea and sexual dysfunction, prior to initiating treatment with an atypical antipsychotic and at regular intervals thereafter. If a patient develops symptoms of hyperprolactinemia, quetiapine and aripiprazole have better profiles than risperidone, olanzapine or haloperidol and may be viable alternatives [90].

Concomitant Medications

The medical evaluation should include information regarding the patient's concomitant medications. The physician should apply this knowledge to anticipate drug-drug interactions and additive side effects. The atypical antipsychotics are metabolized in the liver by cytochrome P450 isoenzymes, with each agent displaying a unique pharmacokinetic profile [91]. In general, the plasma levels of atypical antipsychotics can be influenced by agents, including nicotine, that inhibit or induce liver metabolism or strongly bind to plasma proteins. Common potent CYP2D6 and CYP3A subfamily inhibitors include cimetidine, erythromycin, fluoxetine, fluvoxamine, ketoconazole, paroxetine, and verapamil. Common potent CYP3A subfamily inducers include barbiturates, carbamazepine, and phenytoin. Potentially additive side effects of an antipsychotic medication in combination with another medication metabolized by the same cytochrome P450 isoenzymes include a decreased threshold for seizures, weight gain, and as previously noted, QTc prolongation. Age or pathology-related reduced hepatic and or renal function can impact elimination of an atypical agent or its metabolites and dose adjustment may be necessary.

Level Three—Reduction

The third level in a stepwise approach to the management of antipsychotic side effects is to reduce side effects and or their associated risks. The prescriber has the greatest leverage to reduce side effects and or their associated risks by making medication changes. If a patient is on an antipsychotic medication that is clearly causing a specific side effect or group of side effects, switching to an agent with a different side effect profile may be the best option. However, it is important to remember that switching medications is in and of itself destabilizing. Often, a reduction in dose may be a less disruptive course of action. Many side effects, such as EPS and weight gain, have a dose-response relationship, and by reducing the dose, the benefits of the medication can be maintained while minimizing the side effects. Reducing the dose of a concomitant medication, such as a mood-stabilizer, may also reduce additive side effects.

Although psychiatric polypharmacy is a common clinical practice which may be appropriate in a specific case, there is limited evidence to suggest its generalized use as a long-term treatment strategy for stable outpatients with schizophrenia [92,93]. In many cases, discontinuation of an adjunctive antipsychotic, mood stabilizer or anti-depressant may be an effective and safe strategy for the reduction of side effects, particularly obesity. However, this intervention is not without risks. In Essock's "stay or switch study," comparing participants switched to monotherapy with participants who stayed on two antipsychotics over a six month period, BMI in the switch group decreased by 0.50 points (SD=2.32), and increased by 0.28 points (SD=2.31) in the stay group. However, in that same study, patients who were switched to monotherapy also had a shorter time to discontinuation than did patients who were maintained on their established polypharmacy regimen. This finding highlights the risk for de-stabilization associated with any change; therefore, any proposed change to a patient's treatment regimen, even if it is in the interest of reducing side effects, must first be understood and agreed upon by the patient. ***Finally, as important as making medication changes, prescribers can also prescribe and support a number of lifestyle changes that will reduce the net cardiovascular risks associated with atypical antipsychotics.***

Weight Loss, Dietary Changes, and Exercise

In the 3-year observational Schizophrenia Health Outcomes Study (SOHO), 44% of patients on olanzapine, 39% of patients on risperidone, 36% of patients on an "other" atypical antipsychotic, and 17% of patients on a typical antipsychotic gained at least 7% of their body weight [94]. Since obesity is a risk factor for the other components of the metabolic syndrome, weight loss can positively influence a number of metabolic outcomes and reduce cardiovascular risk. In addition to medication-induced weight gain, lack of motivation to exercise, poor diet, cigarette smoking, and limited resources for nutritional and educational services contribute to obesity in patients with schizophrenia [95]. In non-psychiatric populations, weight loss in the range of 5% to 10% over a 6-month period can be achieved through behavioral weight loss programs that combine low-calorie diet, cognitive-behavioral therapy, and exercise. There is growing evidence to suggest that a similar rate of weight loss can be achieved in psychiatric populations.

The PORT group reviewed seven randomized, controlled investigations targeting weight loss among individuals with schizophrenia spectrum disorders [96]. Interventions were between three and 6 months and the mean weight loss across the interventions was 5.8 lbs. However, these studies provided little information regarding long-term outcomes, with only one study documenting sustained weight loss 6 months post intervention. In addition, there is not yet sufficient data to determine which psychosocial interventions work best for which subgroups of patients taking antipsychotic medications. However, the PORT group recommends weight loss interventions that are at least three months in duration. They also recommend that psychosocial interventions for weight loss include psychoeducation focused on nutritional counseling, caloric expenditure, and portion control; behavioral self-management including motivational enhancement; goal setting; regular weigh-ins; self-monitoring of daily food and activity levels; and dietary and physical activity modifications.

The hopeful news is that relatively inexpensive, easy-to-deliver interventions may have a significant impact. At the end of a year, participation in a weekly group providing lifestyle advice resulted in an average weight loss of 6.2 ± 0.6 kg [97]. Similarly, schizophrenic participants in a 24 week diabetes education intervention that provided psychoeducation and recommended simple strategies such as eating slowly showed modest but significant reductions in BMI at 12 months follow-up [98]. In addition several studies suggest that proactive interventions to prevent weight gain can help reduce the magnitude of antipsychotic-induced weight gain [99,100]. However, for people with schizophrenia, presumably due to negative symptoms, low motivation is a significant barrier to sustained participation in weight loss and exercise programs [101]. The addition of a motivational, therapeutic, or psychoeducational component that provides a high level of staff interaction and positive feedback appears to significantly improve outcomes [101-103].

Smoking Cessation

Cigarette smoking roughly triples the risk for cardiac disease, a critical fact for patients with schizophrenia and other psychiatric disordrers. In the 2007 U.S. National Health Interview Survey, smoking prevalence in adults with schizophrenia was 59% versus 18% for adults with no mental illness [104]. Many patients with schizophrenia who are smokers smoke more than 30 cigarettes per day [105], and schizophrenics extract more nicotine from cigarettes than other smokers [106]. Individuals with schizophrenia and other psychiatric disorders may smoke more than non-psychiatric populations due to differences in the pharmacokinetics of nicotine. Nicotine may produce both stronger rewards, larger cognitive improvements, and more pronounced withdrawal symptoms in the brains of people with schizophrenia [107]. So far, the usual smoking cessation aids have not been found to be particularly helpful in patients with schizophrenia. A 2010 Cochrane review of smoking cessation interventions in individuals with schizophrenia found buproprion SR as compared to placebo to be effective upon trial completion but not at 6 months follow-up [108]. The same review did not find nicotine replacement therapy to improve cessation. Among behavioral interventions, only contingency reinforcement with money showed promise as an aid in cessation. Despite the difficulty of treating tobacco dependence in individuals with schizophrenia, over a quarter of smokers with schizophrenia do quit, and just like psychiatrically normal smokers, motivation predicts smoking cessation [109]. Thus, when psychiatric prescribers are encouraging their patients to quit smoking a combination of buproprion with individualized motivational enhancement is apt to be the most effective method. ***Finally, prescribers need not wait until the emergence of side effects to discontinue or reduce problematic or redundant medications or to prescribe and support lifestyle interventions. These interventions are part of good clinical practice and prescribers should routinely screen for opportunities to introduce these changes.***

From a psychological perspective, it is very important that the prescriber share and explain his concerns about emergent side effects with the patient. It is also very important that the prescriber illicit the patient's thoughts and feelings about the overall effectiveness, including side effects, of his medication regimen. There are a variety of reasons that patients may not spontaneously share their concerns about medication side effects. Patients may find it embarrassing to discuss sexual side effects, weight gain, or disfiguring involuntary movements. Patients may also respond to non-verbal messages put forth by prescribers and not want to "rock the boat." Specifically, patients may react to a prescriber's harried presentation by under-reporting problems with their medications. Patients may unconsciously collude with a prescriber's wish to be a smart or successful clinician and deny or minimize problems with their medications. Similarly, patients may want to be perceived as agreeable, good, or obedient and fear that sharing their concerns will make them less appealing in the eyes of their prescribers.

Patients and prescribers may participate in a sort of folie-a-deux in which there is an implicit agreement to claim efficacy and discount problems. Along different lines, patients may have diminished expectations regarding the quality of their treatment and passively accept sub-standard outcomes. Or, patients may have unrealistically high expectations regarding what medications can do for them. Conversely, patients may become anxious if a medication is too effective, fearing loss of financial or emotional support or fearing their own latent impulses. Thus, it is incumbent upon the prescriber to invite all of the patients' feelings, fears, and fantasies into the therapeutic relationship itself not just into the office. Asking patients to report efficacy and side effects on paper may keep patients' concerns emotionally distant, eclipsing the strong affect that is typically associated with the need to take psychotropic medications. Often, it is only by working through these issues within the relational context of the treatment dyad that the prescriber and patient are able to identify and address the issues that impact the long-term effectiveness of a particular medication regimen.

Level Four—Treatment

The fourth and final level in a stepwise approach to the management of antipsychotic side effects involves the treatment of iatrogenic pathologies. Under ideal circumstances, the previous levels in this stepwise approach will have forestalled the need for any pharmacological treatment of side effects. However, frequently, the prescriber is required to determine the benefits to risks ratio of maintaining a treatment-resistant patient, who has failed several medication trials, on an atypical antipsychotic that is yielding a significant clinical response but is also causing medically significant side effects. In many cases, the severity of the patient's psychiatric symptomology dictates that the least harmful course of treatment is to maintain the patient on his current antipsychotic medication and to try to treat the emergent side effects. It is critical that the prescriber and the patient together identify and assess the potential risk and benefits of this course of action. Finally, in the event of severe or potentially chronic side effects, the prescriber should consider referring the patient for specialty care.

Pharmacological interventions for the metabolic syndrome include oral antidiabetic agents, statins and fibrates, anti-hypertensives, and weight loss medications. Weight loss medications may be the least effective of the pharmacological treatments for the metabolic syndrome and there are several issues regarding these medications relevant to psychiatric practice. Due to dopamine and serotonin agonism, a number of medications that are used for weight loss or control, such as sibutramine and amantadine, have the potential to exacerbate psychiatric symptoms. In contrast, orlistat is not centrally acting and is largely unabsorbed; thus, not causing psychiatric effects. In a 16 week double blind trial, orlistat did yield a weight loss of 1.29 ± 3.04 kg, (p = .007), in patients stable on olanzapine or clozapine [110]. However, orlistat can be associated with unpleasant gastrointestinal side effects, including oily stools.

In a 2010 review of the medications used to treat antipsychotic-induced weight gain, Ellinger et al. found the largest body of evidence to support the use of topiramate and metformin [112]. In three randomized trials, topiramate was found to effectively reduce weight, yielding losses in the magnitude of 5% after 12 weeks treatment at a dose of 200 mg. However, topiramate was also associated with paresthesias and increased psychiatric symptoms [112]. Ellinger et al. also reviewed six RCT's comparing metformin to placebo for weight gain in patients on antipsychotics. Two of the studies were adequately powered to provide moderately strong evidence for the efficacy of metformin; the other studies were less conclusive due to power and design limitations. The study done by Wu and colleagues included a lifestyle intervention which seems to have worked additively with metformin. Patients who received metformin and the lifestyle intervention lost an average of 4.7 kg, as compared to the average weight loss of 3.2 kg in the metformin alone group (p = 0.02). In contrast, the average weight *gain* with placebo was 3.1 kg. In the metformin and lifestyle intervention group, there were also decreases in body mass index (BMI) of 1.8 (95% confidence interval [CI], 1.3-2.3), insulin resistance index of 3.6 (95% CI, 2.7-4.5), and waist circumference of 2.0 cm (95% CI, 1.5-2.4cm). Finally, in the six RCT's reviewed, metformin was not associated with serious adverse events or increases in psychiatric symptoms. Thus, although additional research is required to irrefutably establish the efficacy of metformin for the treatment of antipsychotic-induced metabolic side effects, there is sufficient preliminary evidence to justify its off-label use in select cases.

Typically, psychiatric prescribers, as opposed to neurologists or other medical providers, treat medication-induced movement disorders. Given the high prevalence of antipsychotic-induced movement disorders, prescribers should do a baseline screening, even in neuroleptic-naïve patients, prior to prescribing an atypical antipsychotic, followed by frequent screenings during stabilization and routine screenings during maintenance treatment. Although the atypical antipsychotic medications are associated with a lower incidence of EPS, treatment-emergent dystonia, parkinsonism, and akathisia do occur [84]. In general, acute EPS can be resolved with a dose reduction or if need be a switch to a low potency agent. Dystonia involves painful muscle stiffness and postural distortion. Although its incidence rate is usually very low, young men on high doses of potent antipsychotics are particularly vulnerable. Acute dystonia typically rapidly resolves with treatment with anti-parkinsonism medication, such as benzatorpine, or an anticholinergic agent. Anticholinergic agents can also be helpful for the management of tardive dystonia. The development of drug-induced parkinsonism is dose dependent and occurs in 20 to 40 percent of patients. An anticholinergic agent or amantadine may be helpful for reducing tremor, rigidity and other parkisonian symptoms. Akathisia is also quite common, occurring in up to 90% of patients within three months, and difficult to treat. Beta-blockers such as propanolol is one of the first lines of treatment followed by medications with generalized sedative effects, including benzodiazapines and clonidine [84,113].

Prescribers can work to aggressively avoid triggering newly emergent movement disorders through the routine utilization of EPS rating scales, such as the Simpson Angus Scale (SAS) [114], Barnes Akathisia Rating Scale (BAS) [115], and the Abnormal Involuntary Movement Scale (AIMS) [116], and selection of antipsychotic agents with weak dopamine antagonism. However, even if prescribers are successful not causing new cases of TD, patients who have previously been treated with haloperidol or other high potency agents present with tardive movement disorders. A variety of classes of adjunctive medications are prescribed for tardive disorders, including dopamine depleters and agonists, cholinergic and anticholinergic medications, calcium channel blockers, and GABA agonists. There have been very few large, well-designed studies to test the efficacy of various agents, and to date, there is no one class of medication that has been shown to be both effective and well-tolerated. In many cases, the benefits to risks ratios of these treatments do not justify their use [81]. Although Vitamin E does not appear to effectively reduce tardive dyskinesia, it does appear to inhibit further neurological deterioration [117].

CONCLUSION

It has been known since the 1950's that antipsychotic medications cause significant side effects. When the second generation, "atypical antipsychotics" first came on the market, it was believed that they would produce fewer extrapyramidal side effects, such as parkinsonism, akathisia, and the frequently irreversible movement disorder—tardive dyskinesia. Initially, atypical antipsychotic medications seemed to be associated with less social stigma, better subjective tolerance, and better medication compliance. However, with time, their apparent advantage regarding EPS has come under scrutiny and it has become evident that they are strongly associated with significant weight gain and other metabolic disorders. Despite these known side effects, the use of atypical antipsychotics for both approved and off-label indications has continued to sky rocket. In clinical practice, prescribers must frequently act as both mental health provider and primary healthcare provider. Thus, the management of the physiological side effects associated with these medications is as integral to clinical practice as is the treatment of psychiatric symptomology. In addition, for the patient the act of taking an antipsychotic medication and for the clinician the act of prescribing an antipsychotic medication has psychological meanings which influence tolerability and effectiveness. In this article, the author has discussed the application of have a stepwise, holistic approach—Abstinence, Anticipation, Reduction, and Treatment (AART)—for the management of antipsychotic side effects. By working collaboratively within the context of the therapeutic dyad, the psychiatric prescriber and the patient can maximize treatment effectiveness and minimize iatrogenic harm.

REFERENCES

[1] Kennedy A, Tapp A, Kelly WS et al. Abstinence, anticipation, reduction, and treatment (AART): a stepwise approach to the management of atypical antipsychotic side effects. *Essential Psychopharmacology.* 2006;7:1-14.

[2] Alexander GC, Moloney RM, Gallagher SA et al. Increasing off-label use of antipsychotic medications in the United States 1995 -2008. *Pharmacoepidemiology and Drug Safety.* 2011;20(74):177-184.

[3] Morgan D. U.S. Family Doctors Prescribe Most Mental Health Drugs. *Reuters.com | Busines and Financial News.* 2009. http://www.reuters.com/article/2009/09/30/us-drugs. Accessed June 30, 2012.

[4] IMS Institute for Healthcare Informatics. The Use of Medicines in the United States: Review of 2010. 2011.

[5] Meltzer H Y. Mechanism of action of atypical antipsychotic drugs. In: Davis KL and American College of Neuropsychopharmacology, eds. *Neuropsychopharmacology: The Fifth Generation of Progress: An Official Publication of the American College of Neuropsychopharmacology.* Philadelphia, PA: Lippincott Williams & Wilkins; 2002:819-831.

[6] Maglione M, Ruelaz Maher A, Hu J et al. Off-Label Use of Atypical Antipsychotics: An Update. *Comparative Effectiveness Review No. 43.* AHRQ Publication No. 11-EHC087-EF. Rockville, MD: Agency for Healthcare Research and Quality; Sept. 2011.

[7] Gabbay J, le May A. Evidence based guidelines or collectively constructed "mindlines?" Ethnographic study of knowledge management in primary care. *BMJ: British Medical Journal.* 2004; 329(7473):1013.

[8] Barley M, Pope C, Chilvers R et al. Guidelines or mindlines? A qualitative study exploring what knowledge informs psychiatrists decisions about antipsychotic prescribing. *Journal of Mental Health.* 2008;17:9-17.

[9] Fountoulakis KN, Nimatoudis I, Iacovides A, Kaprinis G. Off-label indications for atypical antipsychotics: A systematic review. *Ann Gen Hosp Psychiatry.* 2004;3(1):4.

[10] David D, De Faria L, Lapeyra O et al. Adjunctive risperidone treatment in combat veterans with chronic PTSD. *Journal of Clinical Psychopharmacology.* 2004; 24(5):556-559.

[11] Stein MB, Kline NA, Matloff JL. Adjunctive Olanzapine for SSRI-Resistant Combat-related PTSD: A Double-Blind, Placebo-Controlled Study. *American Journal of Psychiatry.* 2002;159(10):1777-1779.

[12] Zohar J, Amital D, Miodownik C etal. Double-blind placebo-controlled pilot study of sertraline in military veterans with posttraumatic stress disorder. *Journal of Clinical Psychopharmacology.* 2002;22:190-195.

[13] Friedman MJ, Marmar CR, Baker DG et al. Randomized, double-blind comparison of sertraline and placebo for posttraumatic stress disorder in a Department of Veterans Affairs setting. *The Journal of Clinical Psychiatry.* 2007;68:711-720.

[14] Hertzberg MA, Feldman ME, Beckham C et al. Lack of Efficacy for Fluoxetine in PTSD: A Placebo Controlled Trial in Combat Veterans. *Annals of Clinical Psychiatry.* 2000;12:101-105.

[15] van der Kolk BA, Dreyfuss D, Michaels M et al. Fluoxetine in posttraumatic stress disorder. *The Journal of Clinical Psychiatry.* 1994;55:517-522.

[16] Ahearn EP, Juergens T, Krahn D et al. A review of atypical antipsychotic medications for posttraumatic stress disorder. *International Clinical Psychopharmacology.* 2011;26:193-200.

[17] Krystal JH, Neumeister A. Noradrenergic and serotonergic mechanisms in the neurobiology of posttraumatic stress disorder and resilience. *Brain Research.* 2009;1293:13-23.

[18] Raskind M S. Pharmacologic treatment of posttraumatic stress disorder. In: Shiromani PJ, Keane TM, LeDoux JE, eds. *Posttraumatic Stress Disorder.* New York, NY: Humana; 2009:337-361.

[19] Hamner MB, Frueh BC, Ulmer H G et al. Psychotic features and illness severity in combat veterans with chronic posttraumatic stress disorder. *Biological Psychiatry.* 1999;45:846-852.

[20] Ivezic S, Bagaric A, Oruc L et al. Psychotic symptoms and comorbid psychiatric disorders in Croatian combat-related posttraumatic stress disorder patients. *Croatian Medical Journal.* 2000;41:179-183.

[21] Krystal JH, Rosenheck R A, Cramer J et al. Adjunctive risperidone treatment for antidepressant-resistant symptoms of chronic military service-related PTSD: a randomized trial. *JAMA: the Journal of the American Medical Association.* 2011;306:493-502.

[22] Heppner PS, Crawford EF, Haji UA et al. The association of posttraumatic stress disorder and metabolic syndrome: a study of increased health risk in veterans. *BMC Medicine.* 2009;7:1.

[23] Jakovljevic M, Babic D, Crncevic Z et al. Metabolic syndrome and depression in war veterans with post-traumatic stress disorder.*Psychiatria Danubina.* 2008;20:406-410.

[24] Violanti JM, Fekedulegn D, Hartley TA et al. Police trauma and cardiovascular disease: association between PTSD symptoms and metabolic syndrome. *International Journal of Emergency Mental Health.* 2006;8:227-237.

[25] Jin H, Lanouette NM, Mudaliar S et al. Association of posttraumatic stress disorder with increased prevalence of metabolic syndrome. *Journal of Clinical Psychopharmacology.* 2009;29:210-215.

[26] Institute for Operations Research and the Management Sciences. Iraq troops' PTSD rate as high as 35 percent, analysis finds. *ScienceDaily.* Sept, 14, 2009. http://www.sciencedaily.com/releases/2009/09/090914151629.htm. Accessed June 30, 2012.

[27] Tanielian TL, Jaycox L, Rand C. Invisible wounds of war: psychological and cognitive injuries, their consequences, and services to assist recovery. Santa Monica, CA: RAND;2008.

[28] Leslie DL, Mohamed S, Rosenheck RA . Off-label use of antipsychotic medications in the department of veterans affairs health care system. *Psychiatric Services.* 2009; 60:1175-1181.

[29] Alfonso CA. Dynamic psychopharmacology and treatment adherence. *The Journal of the American Academy of Psychoanalysis and Dynamic Psychiatry.* 2009;37:269-285.

[30] Gabbard GO. *Psychodynamic Psychiatry in Clinical Practice.* Washington, DC: American Psychiatric Pub;2005.

[31] Li TCW. Psychodynamic aspects of psychopharmacology. *Psychiatry Journal of the American Academy of Psychoanalysis and Dynamic Psychiatry*. 2010;38:655-674.

[32] Mintz D. Psychodynamic Trojan horses: using psychopharmacology to teach psychodynamics. *The Journal of the American Academy of Psychoanalysis and Dynamic Psychiatry*. 2006;34:151-161.

[33] Milrod BL, Busch FN. Combining psychodynamic psychotherapy with medication in the treatment of panic disorder: Exploring the dynamic meaning of medication. *Psychoanalytic Inquiry*. 1998;18(5):702.

[34] Löffler W, Kilian R, Toumi M et.al. Schizophrenic patients' subjective reasons for compliance and noncompliance with neuroleptic treatment. *Pharmacopsychiatry*. 2003;36:105-112.

[35] Rettenbacher MA, Hofer A, Eder U et al. Compliance in schizophrenia: psychopathology, side effects, and patients' attitudes toward the illness and medication. *The Journal of Clinical Psychiatry*. 2004;65:1211-1218.

[36] Vlastelica M. Effects of meaning or psychodynamic psycopharmacotherapy. *Psychiatria Danubina*. 2010;22:313-316.

[37] Hogan TP, Awad AG, Eastwood R. A self-report scale predictive of drug compliance in schizophrenics: reliability and discriminative validity. *Psychological Medicine*. 1983;13:177-183.

[38] Margetic B, Aukst-Margetic B. Neuroleptic malignant syndrome and its controversies. *Pharmacoepidemiology and Drug Safety*. 2010;19:429-435.

[39] Merrill DB, Dec GW, Goff DC . Adverse cardiac effects associated with clozapine. *Journal of Clinical Psychopharmacology*.2005;25:32-41.

[40] Griswold KS, Pastore PA, Smith SJ et al. Primary care after psychiatric crisis: A qualitative analysis. *Annals of Family Medicine*. 2008;6:38-43.

[41] Hahm HC, Segal SP. Failure to seek health care among the mentally ill. *The American Journal of Orthopsychiatry* 2006;75:54-62.

[42] Marder SR, Essock SM, Miller AL etal. Physical health monitoring of patients with schizophrenia. *The American Journal of Psychiatry*. 2004;161:1334-1349.

[43] De Hert M, Vancampfort D, MerckenV et al. Guidelines for screening and monitoring of cardiometabolic risk in schizophrenia: Systematic evaluation. *British Journal of Psychiatry*. 2011;199: 99-105.

[44] Farooq S, Taylor M. Clozapine: dangerous orphan or neglected friend? *The British Journal of Psychiatry: the Journal of Mental Science*. 2011198:247-249.

[45] Jindal RD, Keshavan MS. Classifying antipsychotic agents: Need for new terminology. *CNS Drugs*. 2008; 22:1047-1059.

[46] Richelson E. Receptor pharmacology of neuroleptics: relation to clinical effects. *The Journal of Clinical Psychiatry*. 1999;60:5-14.

[47] Shayegan DK, Stahl SM. Atypical antipsychotics: matching receptor profile to individual patient's clinical profile. *CNS Spectrums*. 2004;9:6-14.

[48] Ishibashi T, Horisawa T, Tokuda K et al. Pharmacological profile of lurasidone, a novel antipsychotic agent with potent 5-hydroxytryptamine 7 (5-HT7) and 5-HT1A receptor activity. *Journal of Pharmacology and Experimental Therapeutics*. 2010;334:171-181.

[49] Kroeze WK, Hufeisen SJ, Popadak BA et al. H1-histamine receptor affinity predicts short-term weight gain for typical and atypical antipsychotic drugs. *Neuropsychopharmacology*.2003;28(3):519-526..

[50] Richelson E, Souder T. Binding of antipsychotic drugs to human brain receptors. *Lifescience.* 2000;68:29-39.
[51] Druss BG, Zhao L, Von Esenwein S et al. Understanding excess mortality in persons with mental illness: 17-year follow up of a nationally representative US survey. *Medical Care.* 2011;49:599-604.
[52] Eaton WW, Martins SS, Nestadt G et al. The burden of mental disorders. *Epidemiologic Reviews.* 2008;30:1-14.
[53] Tiihonen J, Lönnqvist J, Wahlbeck K et al. 11-year follow-up of mortality in patients with schizophrenia: a population-based cohort study (FIN11 study). *Lancet.* 374(9690):620-627.
[54] Casey DE, Haupt DW, Newcomer JW et al. Antipsychotic-induced weight gain and metabolic abnormalities: implications for increased mortality in patients with schizophrenia. *The Journal of Clinical Psychiatry.* 2004;65:4-18.
[55] Sacks FM. Metabolic syndrome: epidemiology and consequences. *The Journal of Clinical Psychiatry.* 2004;65:3-12.
[56] Falissard B, Mauri M, Shaw K et al.The METEOR study: frequency of metabolic disorders in patients with schizophrenia. Focus on first and second generation and level of risk of antipsychotic drugs. *International Clinical Psychopharmacology.* 2011;26:291-302.
[57] McEvoy JP, Meyer JM, Goff DC et al. Prevalence of the metabolic syndrome in patients with schizophrenia: baseline results from the Clinical Antipsychotic Trials of Intervention Effectiveness (CATIE) schizophrenia trial and comparison with national estimates from NHANES III. *Schizophrenia Research.* 2005;80:19-32.
[58] Grundy SM, Brewer HB Jr, Cleeman JI et al. Definition of metabolic syndrome: Report of the National Heart, Lung, and Blood Institute/American Heart Association conference on scientific issues related to definition. *Circulation.* 2004;109:433-438.
[59] Allison DB, Mentore JL, Heo M et al. Antipsychotic-induced weight gain: a comprehensive research synthesis. *The American Journal of Psychiatry.* 1999;156:1686-1696.
[60] Newcomer JW. Metabolic considerations in the use of antipsychotic medications: a review of recent evidence. *The Journal of Clinical Psychiatry.* 2007;68:20-27.
[61] Stroup TS, Lieberman JA. Antipsychotic trials in schizophrenia the CATIE project. 2007.http://public.eblib.com/EBLPublic/PublicView.do?ptiID=501322. Accessed June 30, 2012.
[62] Janssen I, Katzmarzyk PT, Ross R. Body mass index, waist circumference, and health risk: evidence in support of current National Institutes of Health guidelines. *Archives of Internal Medicine.* 2002;162:2074-2079.
[63] Gentile S. Contributing factors to weight gain during long-term treatment with second-generation antipsychotics. A systematic appraisal and clinical implications. *Obesity Reviews: An Official Journal of the International Association for the Study of Obesity.* 2009;10:527-542.
[64] Rummel-Kluge C, Komossa K, Schwarz S et al. Head-to-head comparisons of metabolic side effects of second generation antipsychotics in the treatment of schizophrenia: A systematic review and meta-analysis. *Schizophrenia Research.* 2012;123:225-233.

[65] Lieberman JA, Stroup TS, McEvoy JP et al. Effectiveness of antipsychotic drugs in patients with chronic schizophrenia. *The New England Journal of Medicine.* 2005;353:1209-1223.

[66] Wirshing DA. Schizophrenia and obesity: impact of antipsychotic medications. *The Journal of Clinical Psychiatry.* 2004;65:13-26.

[67] Weiden PJ, Mackell JA, McDonnell DD. Obesity as a risk factor for antipsychotic noncompliance. *Schizophrenia Research.* 2004;66:51-57.

[68] Wong MMC, Chen EYH, Lui SSY etal. Medication adherence and subjective weight perception in patients with first-episode psychotic disorders. *Clinical Schizophrenia and Related Psychoses.* 2011;5(3):135-141.

[69] Dasgupta A, Singh OP, Rout JK et al. Insulin resistance and metabolic profile in antipsychotic naive schizophrenia patients. *Progress in Neuropsychopharmacology and Biological Psychiatry.* 2010;34:1202-1207.

[70] Dixon L, Weiden P, Delahanty J et al. Prevalence and correlates of diabetes in national schizophrenia samples. *Schizophrenia Bulletin.* 2000; 26:903-912.

[71] Kohen D. Diabetes mellitus and schizophrenia: historical perspective. *The British Journal of Psychiatry.* 2004;47: 64-66.

[72] Chaggar PS, Shaw SM, Williams SG. Effect of antipsychotic medications on glucose and lipid levels. *Journal of Clinical Pharmacology.* 2011;51:631-638.

[73] Stahl SM, Mignon L, Meyer J M. Clinical overview: Which comes first: atypical antipsychotic treatment or cardiometabolic risk? *Acta Psychiatrica Scandinavica.* 2009;119(3):171-179.

[74] Roerig J, Steffen K, Mitchell J.Atypical antipsychotic-induced weight gain: insights into mechanisms of action. *CNS Drugs.2011*;25:1035-1059.

[75] Lee SY, Park MH, Pae CU. A retrospective comparison of BMI changes and the potential risk factors among schizophrenic inpatients treated with aripiprazole, olanzapine, quetiapine or risperidone. *Progress in Neuro-Psychopharmacology and Biological Psychiatry.* 2011;33:490-6.

[76] McIntyre RS. Asenapine: A review of acute and extension phase data in bipolar disorder. *CNS Neuroscience andTherapeutics.* *2011*;17(6):645-8.

[77] Cutler AJ, Kalali AH, Weiden PJ et al. Four-week, double-blind, placebo- and ziprasidone-controlled trial of iloperidone in patients with acute exacerbations of schizophrenia. *Journal of Clinical Psychopharmacology.* 2008;28:20-28.[78] Ray WA, Chung CP, Murray K et al. Atypical antipsychotic drugs and the risk of sudden cardiac death. *The New England Journal of Medicine.* 2009;360:225-235.

[79] Nielsen J, Graff C, Kanters JK et al. Assessing QT interval prolongation and its associated risks with antipsychotics. *CNS Drugs.* 2011;25:473-490.

[80] Harrigan EP, Miceli JJ, Anziano R et al. A randomized evaluation of the effects of six antipsychotic agents on QTc, in the absence and presence of metabolic inhibition. *Journal of Clinical Psychopharmacology.* 2004;24:62-69.

[81] Pierre JM. Extrapyramidal symptoms with atypical antipsychotics: incidence, prevention and management. *Drug Safety: An International Journal of Medical Toxicology and Drug Experience.* 2005;28:191-208.

[82] Meltzer HY, Matsubara S, Lee JC. Classification of typical and atypical antipsychotic drugs on the basis of dopamine D-1, D-2 and serotonin2 pKi values. *The Journal of Pharmacology and Experimental Therapeutics.* 1989;251: 238-246.

[83] Correll CU, Leucht S, Kane JM. Lower risk for tardive dyskinesia associated with second-generation antipsychotics: a systematic review of 1-year studies. *The American Journal of Psychiatry.* 2004; 161:414-425.

[84] Caroff SN, Hurford I, Lybrand J et al. Movement disorders induced by antipsychotic drugs: implications of the CATIE schizophrenia trial. *Neurologic Clinics.* 201;29:127-148.

[85] Jones PB, Barnes TR, Davies L et al. Randomized controlled trial of the effect on Quality of Life of second- vs first-generation antipsychotic drugs in schizophrenia: Cost Utility of the Latest Antipsychotic Drugs in Schizophrenia Study (CUtLASS 1). *Archives of General Psychiatry.* 2006;63:1079-1087.

[86] Montgomery J, Winterbottom E, Jessani M et al. Prevalence of hyperprolactinemia in schizophrenia: association with typical and atypical antipsychotic treatment. *The Journal of Clinical Psychiatry.* 2004;66:1491-1498.

[87] Milano W, D'Acunto CW, De Rosa M et al. Recent clinical aspects of hyperprolactinemia induced by antipsychotics. *Reviews on Recent Clinical Trials.* 2011;6:52-63.

[88] Cournos F, Guido JR, Coomaraswamy S et al. Sexual activity and risk of HIV infection among patients with schizophrenia.*The American Journal of Psychiatry.*1994;151: 228-232.

[89] Lambert M, Conus P, Naber D. Impact of present and past antipsychotic side-effects on attitude toward typical antipsychotic treatment and compliance. *Schizophrenia Research.* 2003;60(1):360.

[90] Bobes J, Garcia-Portilla MP, Rejas J et al. Frequency of sexual dysfunction and other reproductive side-effects in patients with schizophrenia treated with risperidone, olanzapine, quetiapine, or haloperidol: the results of the EIRE study. *Journal of Sex and Marital Therapy.*2003;29:125-147.

[91] Urichuk L, Dursun S, Prior Ti et al. Metabolism of atypical antipsychotics: Involvement of cytochrome P450 enzymes and relevance for drug-drug interactions. *Current Drug Metabolism.* 2008; 9:410-418.

[92] Essock SM, Schooler NR, Stroup TS et al. Effectiveness of switching from antipsychotic polypharmacy to monotherapy. *The American Journal of Psychiatry.* 2011;168:702-708.

[93] Misawa F, Shimizu K, Fujii Yetal. Is antipsychotic polypharmacy associated with metabolic syndrome even after adjustment for lifestyle effects?: a cross-sectional study. *BMC Psychiatry.* 2011;11:118.

[94] Haro JM, Novick D, Suarez D et al. Antipsychotic treatment discontinuation in previously untreated patients with schizophrenia: 36-month results from the SOHO study.*Journal of Psychiatric Research.* 2009;43:265-273.

[95] Bushe C, Haddad P, Peveler R et al. The role of lifestyle interventions and weight management in schizophrenia. *Journal of Psychopharmacology.* 2005;19:28-35.

[96] Dixon LB, Bellack AS, Bennett M et al. The 2009 schizophrenia PORT psychosocial treatment recommendations and summary statements. *Schizophrenia Bulletin.* 2010;36:48-70.

[97] Pendlebury J, Bushe CJ, Wildgust HJ et al. Long-term maintenance of weight loss in patients with severe mental illness through a behavioural treatment programme in the UK. *Acta psychiatrica Scandinavica. 2007; 115*(4):286-294.

[98] McKibbin CL, Golshan S, Griver K et al. A healthy lifestyle intervention for middle-aged and older schizophrenia patients with diabetes mellitus: A 6-month follow-up analysis. *Schizophrenia Research.* 2010;121:203-206.

[109] Alvarez-Jimenez M, Martinez-Garcia O, Perez-Iglesias R etal. Prevention of antipsychotic-induced weight gain with early behavioural intervention in first-episode psychosis: 2-year results of a randomized controlled trial. *Schizophrenia Research.* 2010;116:16-19.

[100] Littrell KH, Hilligoss NM, Kirshner CD etal. The effects of an educational intervention on antipsychotic-induced weight gain. *Journal of Nursing Scholarship.* 2003;35:237-241.

[101] Warren K, Ball M, Feldman S etal. Exercise program adherence using a 5-kilometer (5K) event as an achievable goal in people with schizophrenia. *Biological Research for Nursing.* 2011;13:383-390.

[102] Forsberg KA, Lindqvist O, Bjorkman TN et al. Meanings of participating in a lifestyle programme for persons with psychiatric disabilities. *Scandinavian Journal of Caring Sciences.* 2011; 25:357-364.

[103] Perlman LM, Cohen JL, Altiere MJ et al. A multidimensional wellness group therapy program for veterans with comorbid psychiatric and medical conditions. *Professional Psychology: Research and Practice.* 2010;41:120-127.

[104] McClave AK, McKnight-Eily LR, Davis SP et al. Smoking characteristics of adults with selected lifetime mental illnesses: results from the 2007 National Health Interview Survey. *American Journal of Public Health.* 2010;100:2464-2472.

[105] Mann-Wrobel MC, Bennett ME, Weiner EE et al. Smoking history and motivation to quit in smokers with schizophrenia in a smoking cessation program. *Schizophrenia Research.* 2010;126(1-3), 277-283

[106] Olincy A, Young DA, Freedman R. Increased levels of the nicotine metabolite cotinine in schizophrenic smokers compared to other smokers. *Biological Psychiatry.* 1997;42:1-5.

[107] Aubin HJ, Rollema H, Svensson TH et al. Smoking, quitting, and psychiatric disease: A review. *Neuroscience and Biobehavioral Reviews.* 2012 ;36:271-284.

[108] Tsoi DT, Porwal M, Webster AC . Interventions for smoking cessation and reduction in individuals with schizophrenia. *Cochrane Database of Systematic Review.* 2010; (6):CD007253.

[109] Ziedonis D, Hitsman B, Beckham JC et al. Tobacco use and cessation in psychiatric disorders: National Institute of Mental Health report. *Nicotine and Tobacco Research : Official Journal of the Society forResearch on Nicotine and Tobacco.* 2008;10:1691-1715.

[110] Tchoukhine E, Takala P, Hakko H etal. Orlistat in clozapine- or olanzapine-treated patients with overweight or obesity: a 16week open-label extension phase and both phases of a randomized controlled trial. *The Journal of Clinical Psychiatry.* 2011;72:326-330.

[111] Ellinger LK, Ipema HJ, Stachnik JM. Efficacy of metformin and topiramate in prevention and treatment of second-generation antipsychotic-induced weight gain. *The Annals of Pharmacotherapy*. 2010;44:668-679.

[112] Ko YH, Joe SH, Jung IK et al. Topiramate as an adjuvant treatment with atypical antipsychotics in schizophrenic patients experiencing weight gain. *ClinicalNeuropharmacology*. 2005;28:169-75.

[113] Mathews M, Gratz S, Adetunji B et al. Antipsychotic-induced movement disorders: evaluation and treatment. *Psychiatry* 2005;2:36-41.

[114] Simpson GM, Angus JW. A rating scale for extrapyramidal side effects. *Acta psychiatrica Scandinavica*. Supplementum 1970;212:11-19.

[115] Barnes TR, McPhillips MA. Critical analysis and comparison of the side-effect and safety profiles of the new antipsychotics. The *British Journal of Psychiatry*. Supplement 1999;38:34-43.

[116] Guy W. Abnormal involuntary movement scales (AIMS). *ECDEU Assessment Manual for Psychopharmacology Revised*. Rockville, MD: Alcohol Drug Abuse and Mental Health Administration, National Institute of Health,1996.

[117] Evans S, Newton R, Higgins S. Nutritional intervention to prevent weight gain in patients commenced on olanzapine: a randomized controlled trial. *Australian and New Zealand Journal of Psychiatry*. 2005,39:479-486.

In: Antipsychotic Drugs
Editors: T.L. Schwartz, J. Megna and M.E. Topel
ISBN: 978-1-62100-071-6

Chapter 9

MODELING THE METABOLIC SIDE EFFECTS OF ANTIPSYCHOTICS IN THE MALE RAT

Hermier Dominique[1,2,*], Minet-Ringuet Julie[1,2], Victoriano Montserrat[1,2] and de Beaurepaire Renaud[3]

[1]UMR914, INRA, Physiologie de la Nutrition et du Comportement Alimentaire, Paris, France

[2]UMR914, AgroParisTech, Physiologie de la Nutrition et du Comportement Alimentaire, Paris, France

[3]Laboratoire de Psychopharmacologie, Groupe Hospitalier Paul-Guiraud, Villejuif, France

ABSTRACT

Introduction: The previous chapter discusses the overall clinical issue regarding weight gain as an adverse effect of psychotropic prescribing. This chapter focuses on the second generation antipsychotics (SGAs) that are known to cause weight gain and metabolic alterations, including hyperlipidemia and glucose regulation dysfunction. Specifically, an animal model was developed to study the metabolic effects of antipsychotics in the male rat.

Conclusion: The authors determined that the most consistent effects of the SGA olanzapine in this model were to produce abnormalities in glucose regulation and an accumulation of adipose tissue. The accumulation of adipose tissue is associated with an inflammatory phenotype. Olanzapine also disrupted feeding pattern sequences. In the present chapter, the authors discuss these specific animal model results in the light of other data and information from other relevant literature, and in the context of the use of SGAs in clinical situations.

[*] dominique;hemier@agroparistech.fr.

A. INTRODUCTION

1. Metabolic Side Effects of Antipsychotics during Clinical Use

SGAs are widely prescribed for the treatment of schizophrenia. However, approximately 50% of antipsychotic-treated patients gain weight, this effect being much greater with certain SGAs than with first-generation antipsychotics (FGAs), with a substantial number of patients developing metabolic abnormalities. [1,2] In 2004, a consensus of the American Diabetes Association and the American Psychiatric Association claimed that treatment with olanzapine or clozapine, two major SGAs, is associated with greater risk of weight gain and associated metabolic disorders (Consensus development conference, 2004). These metabolic disturbances differ among patients, who exhibit generally an increase in serum cholesterol and triglyceride concentration, or an imbalance in glucose homeostasis, leading to insulin resistance. [3,4] The onset of these side effects is characteristic of the metabolic syndrome, which places patients at higher risk of type 2 diabetes and cardiovascular diseases. [5,6] Despite that insulin resistance is thought to be most often secondary to hypertrophy of adipose tissue, it may occur independently of weight gain and obesity, in normal subjects as well as in AAP-treated patients. Similarly, dyslipidemia should not be necessarily considered as associated to weight gain, but sometimes as an independent element of the metabolic syndrome. [7] Besides, the relative increases in plasma concentration of glucose, cholesterol, or triglycerides, depend on the type of SGA. [8,9]

2. Origin of Metabolic Disorders in Antipsychotic-Treated Patients

Weight gain and metabolic abnormalities found in atypical antipsychotic-treated patients likely result from an imbalance in energy metabolism, of which various causes have been noted , such as increased appetite and binge eating, reduced energy expenditure, and alterations in metabolic and endocrine regulations. [10-14] Because these phenomena are often combined and interrelated, they are still matters of controversy, and their precise mechanisms remain largely unknown.

A number of hypotheses has been proposed regarding the mechanisms by which antipsychotics may alter weight and metabolism. Antipsychotics directly act on several brain monoamine receptors, including dopamine, serotonin, norepinephrine, acetylcholine and histamine receptors, and most of these receptors are in one way or another involved in appetite, and weight and metabolism regulation. Increased appetite and weight gain have been associated with dopamine D2 receptor blockade, serotonin 5-HT2A and 5-HT2C blockade and histamine H1 blockade. Furthermore, genetic studies have found evidence of associations between the weight promoting effects of SGAs and genes for 5-HT2A/C and dopamine D2 receptors. Antipsychotics may also indirectly alter food intake, weight and metabolism through interactions between brain neurotransmitter receptors and neuropeptides involved in appetite or incentive drive to eat, such as PYY, NPY, and the melanin-concentrating hormone (MCH) system.[15,16]

However, studies in rodents suggest than SGAs may induce metabolic disorders by directly impacting peripheral tissues, independently of their primary action on the central nervous system. The present review will focus on these peripheral side-effects and their possible mechanisms.

3. Animal Models

Preclinical studies remain difficult especially since, until recently, no reliable animal models of the metabolic effects of antipsychotics were available. In general, antipsychotics induce weight gain in female rats and mice, but not in males. [17-27] In addition, female rats appear to be particularly responsive to antipsychotics, since it has been shown that antipsychotics that do not induce weight gain in humans, such as aripiprazole and ziprasidone, induce weight gain in female rats.[28-30]

These observations do not match the clinical situation in humans in which antipsychotic treatments induce a weight gain and an increase in food intake in both males and females. [1,2,31] However, there have been controversies regarding gender differences in the metabolic effects of antipsychotics in humans. Some studies have shown that body weight increase during SGA-treatment is greater in women than in men [32-34], while other studies found no gender differences. [35,36] According to Coccurello and Moles [7], conclusive data in support of a major liability of women patients to the weight promoting effects of antipsychotics are still lacking. Therefore, the differences observed in animals (almost no weight gain in males, excessive sensitivity in females) are out of proportion with what is observed in humans (nonconsistent differences). Thus, the use of female rats in the study of antipsychotic-induced metabolic effects may not be optimal because of the excessive sensitivity of females to antipsychotics. This is the reason why we decided to use male rats in our experiments.

B. Development of a Male Rat Model

To investigate the metabolic disorders associated with SGAs, we developed a model of antipsychotic-induced metabolic syndrome in the male Sprague-Dawley rat. [37-39] This model is based on self-administration of the drugs in the diet and on the composition of the diet.

1. Drug Administration

Three antipsychotics were tested, two SGAs (olanzapine and ziprasidone) and a first generation antipsychotic antipsychotic (FGA, haloperidol). In our first experiment using male rats, drugs were given orally once a day in a small volume of sweetened solution, and failed to alter body composition. [38] A possible explanation was the short plasma half-life of antipsychotics in the rat (the plasma half-life of haloperidol in humans is 24 h vs 1.5 h in rats, and plasma half-life of olanzapine is 33 h in humans vs 2.5 h in rats). Thus, to favor a more continuous delivery throughout the day-night cycle than by injections or gavages, drugs were given mixed with food in the following experiments. Food was prepared daily. Ziprasidone

(Pfizer Inc., NY, USA) was suspended in10% absolute ethanol solution. Dispersible olanzapine tablets (Lilly, France), which have been designed to be dissolved in water, were so solubilized (1mg active susbtance/1ml) and blended in the plain diet. Haloperidol (Janssen, France) was used as a FGA without pronounced metabolic side-effects in humans. It was provided in aqueous solution and was directly blended in the plain diet (in experiments involving ziprasidone, haloperidol and olanzapine were solubilized in 10% ethanol). The control group continued receiving the plain diet. Food intake was measured twice a week, so that the amounts of drugs to be added were adjusted every week according to the mean food intake of the previous week.

2. Drug Dosage

As noted above, in our model as well as in other studies, hyperphagia and weight gain resulting from chronic SGA treatment were inconsistently reported in the male rat. [16,37-41] Even olanzapine doses up to 8 mg/kg failed to induce weight gain in males when given once a day in a cookie dough for 2 weeks, whereas it was effective in females. [17] In Sprague-Dawley male rats, self-administration of 5 mg/kg olanzapine enhanced food intake, and body weight gain after 13 and 17 days of treatment, but not over a longer period of time, whereas higher doses (7.5 and 10 mg/kg) were less effective. [42] In the same study, no significant effect was reported in response to ziprasidone. In our own studies with Sprague-Dawley male rats, we used 1-2 mg/kg olanzapine and 1 mg/kg haloperidol, which corresponds to 3 to 6-fold the human doses. Despite these doses usually not enhancing weight gain, a higher adiposity was consistently reported in response to 2 mg/kg olanzapine for several weeks, whereas 1 mg/kg haloperidol had no effect. [16,37,39,41] This appears to be independent of the manner of drug administration and of the breed of rats, since *i.p.* injections of olanzapine (1-4 mg/kg) to male Wistar rats resulted in increased adiposity without hyperphagia or increased body weight. [40]

3. Diet Composition and Acceptance

In order to approach the human western diet, the rat diet was moderately high in lipid, providing (in % energy) 14% protein, 31% lipid, and 54% carbohydrate. Thus, this regimen greatly differs from the usual rodent regimen (approximately 20% protein, 10% lipid and 70% carbohydrate). Before establishing this model, we performed preliminary food-selection experiments, in which rats were fed with three separate sources of pure macronutrients (protein, lipid, carbohydrate). [37,38] Under these conditions, quantitative food intake, but also self-selection, and, thus, food preferences, were not altered by olanzapine, ziprasidone, or haloperidol. In all groups, lipids accounted for a major energy source, showing that drug administration, given orally in solution [38] or mixed with food (39)would not alter the high acceptance of a moderately lipid-rich diet.

A possible inconvenience of this administration is a taste aversion due to the presence of drugs in the food. Thus, a preference test was performed in male rats, and allowed to conclude that no significant difference was observed in food intake between supplemented or non-supplemented diets, which indicates the absence of taste aversion relative to the drug used. [16] Besides, daily food intake or repartition of meals throughout the 24-hr cycle were not affected by either olanzapine or haloperidol. [16]

4. Advantages of the Model

Our animal model of antipsychotic-induced weight gain in the rat is the result of a process of progressive establishment of the best (according to us) experimental procedures to mimic the side-effects of SGAs in humans. The first step was to choose male rats instead of females, the major reason being the excessive sensitivity of females to antipsychotics (see above). A second step was reached when we observed that, when olanzapine was mixed with food, it produced a significant increase in fat accumulation, whereas the accumulation of fat was not significant when it was given by gavage. Drug administration in food has several advantages. First of all, it ensures a more continuous delivery than when given once a day orally or by injection. This is of major interest due to the very short half-life of antipsychotics in the rat. Besides, in animal studies investigating chronic pharmacological treatment, it reduces animal stress and the possible adverse events associated with repeated injections or oral gavages. Also, it does not induce food aversion nor alter food preferences. Very recently, another research group used our original mixing procedure, slightly modified by using grounded olanzapine crystals directly in the food, rather than dissolving olanzapine in water then mixing the solution with food. [43] Alternately, olanzapine was provided in cookie dough every 8 hours. [44] Taken together, our studies and others suggest that oral self-administration is the best method for antipsychotic delivery resembling therapeutic administration in human patients.

Most importantly, even though hyperphagia and body weight gain were not consistently reproducible across the experiments, the accumulation of adipose fat tissue during olanzapine treatment was very consistent. Thus, our findings demonstrate that, in the male rat, SGAs, and especially olanzapine, can enhance fat deposition independently of hyperphagia and increased body weight. Thus, and despite the fact that male are less responsive than females, this model appears to be relevant to investigate the undesirable metabolic side effects of SGAs, in a situation where these side effects cannot be accounted for by an increase in energy intake.

C. Metabolic Side Effects of Second Generation Antipsychotics in the Male Rat

1. Adiposity

As noted above, olanzapine treatment generally does not increase significantly body weight in male rats, but results in a change in body composition, which manifests as a significant increase in adiposity. In contrast, haloperidol and the SGAs ziprasidone and risperidone do not consistently affect body composition. This was the case in our male rat model, but also in other studies. [16,18,40,42,43,46]. In this respect, investigations using female rodents do not provide appropriate models, given that females gain weight and/or accumulate adipose tissue when treated with SGAs that do not produce weight gain in humans, such as aripiprazole and ziprasidone. [28-30]

2. Dyslipidemia and Hepatosteatosis

Plasma

To our knowledge, there is no evidence of any consistent dyslipidemia in SGA-treated rats, whether male or female. In our model of chronic olanzapine administration in food, a rise in plasma cholesterol concentration was found in response to chronic treatment by 1 mg/kg olanzapine [37], but further studies failed to reproduce this finding, even at higher doses.[16,39] In female rats, plasma triglyceride concentration increased transiently 1 hour after an acute clozapine (25 mg/kg) or olanzapine injection (5 mg/kg). [47]

Studies in the mouse reported various lipid abnormalities. In male mice, a high clozapine dose (10 mg/kg) increased plasma triglycerides. [48] In female mice, triglyceride plasma concentration increased in response to risperidone and olanzapine. [49-51] Plasma cholesterol concentration increased in response to olanzapine [49], but decreased in response to risperidone and quetiapine. [51] As in healthy subjects or patients treated acutely or chronically with SGAs [45,52,53] the rise in free fatty acid (FFA) plasma concentration was attenuated in male Sprague-Dawley rats treated acutely (two doses) or chronically (28 days) by olanzapine. [18,55] In summary, the literature dealing with the effects of antipsychotics on lipids in the animal is still elusive on many aspects, and a consistent model of the effects of antipsychotics on lipid metabolism remains to be established; however, it should be noted that the effects of antipsychotics on lipid metabolism in the clinic differ from one antipsychotic to the other, that they are generally mild, and that there is important interindividual variability.

Liver

Acutely SGA-treated female rats exhibit triglyceride accumulation in the liver, i.e. hepatosteatosis. Indeed, lipids (triglycerides, cholesterol, and phospholipids) accumulated in the liver of female rats 48 hours after a single injection of high-dose clozapine (40 mg/kg). [56] In response to 25 mg/kg clozapine, triglyceride accumulation was transient, being maximal at 12 hours after injection, and disappearing after 24 hours. [56] Similarly, an acute dose of olanzapine (5 mg/kg) induced lipid accumulation in the liver of females rats, most pronounced for triglycerides after 12 hours. [47] To our knowledge, the steatohepatosis in male rats under SGA treatment has not been investigated so far. However, in response to haloperidol, olanzapine, or ziprasidone, the liver weight of treated rats did not differ from the control group, which indicates the absence of a marked hepatosteatosis. [37,39]

In summary, animal studies dedicated to antipsychotic-induced dyslipidemia and hepatosteatosis are largely inconsistent and deserve further investigations.

3. Dysregulation of Glucose Homeostasis

Our male rat model allows investigating the effects of antipsychotics after either acute or chronic administration.

Acute Treatment

When a glucose tolerance test (GTT) was performed in drug-naive male Sprague-Dawley rats fed a standard rodent chow diet, both fasting blood glucose and plasma insulin levels were significantly increased after haloperidol (0.25 mg/kg), quetiapine (10 mg/kg) or clozapine (10 mg/kg) injections [57]. These drugs also induced significant impairments in the ability to clear a glucose load. The effect was greatest for the SGA drugs, and especially clozapine, with haloperidol having only a minor effect. Similarly, in the same male rat model, both blood glucose and plasma insulin levels were significantly increased by 1 h after olanzapine injection (10 mg/kg) [46]. Despite this impairment in glucose tolerance, insulin sensitivity was not altered by a single olanzapine treatment [46]. Rather, the raise in plasma glucose after acute SGA injection would have resulted from a primary and direct effect of the drugs on pancreatic glucagon secretion (see below Section D for the possible mechanisms).

In healthy volunteers receiving three days of oral placebo or olanzapine (10 mg/day), an oral GTT showed that the area under curve for glucose, but not for insulin, was higher in the olanzapine-treated group [18]. According to the authors, this suggested alterations in pancreatic insulin secretion and/or in insulin sensitivity. In view of the studies in the rat, it may be hypothesized that hyperglycaemia may also result from a stimulation by acute olanzapine treatment of glucagon secretion, which was not assessed in the human volunteers study. In this respect, the relevance of the rat model to the early effects of SGAs in human patients remains to be clarified.

Chronic Treatment

The response to chronic treatment depends on the dietary conditions. In the chow-fed rat, the absence of an increase in plasma glucose after 2 to 4 weeks of olanzapine treatment was consistently reported when olanzapine was given orally, in females as well as in males. [17,21,40] The only report of an early occurrence of hyperglycaemia (2-week treatment) was in chow-fed female rats treated by subcutaneous infusion of olanzapine (1.75 mg/day). In male rats fed a standard rodent chow diet and injected daily with SGAs for 7 or 28 days, administration of both quetiapine and clozapine did not induced hyperglycemia or hyperinsulinemia. However, it significantly impaired glucose disposal and increased plasma insulin levels during a GTT. [57] In contrast, haloperidol was no longer able to have a significant effect on glucose metabolism. A small but significant defect in glucose tolerance remained 48 h after the final injection of quetiapine or clozapine. However, this difference was normalized by 7 days following drug removal. Thus, the impairment in glucose tolerance following chronic injections of SGAs appears to be transient and reversible.

The situation may be different in our male rat model, which were fed diets rich in fat and/or saccharose, resembling the human western diets. Male Srague-Dawley rats were treated with either vehicle, olanzapine (2 mg/kg) or haloperidol (1 mg/kg) mixed with food.[16] In a first experiment, fasting concentrations of blood glucose and plasma insulin did not differ between groups after 26 days of treatment. In a second experiment, rats were treated for 46 days. During an oral GTT performed after 31 days of treatment, fasting blood glucose concentration was higher in the olanzapine-treated rats than in the control ones and remained higher 10 min after the glucose load. This corresponded to a more rapid increase in glycaemia after the glucose load since the difference in glucose concentrations between T0 and T+10 min was significantly higher in the olanzapine-treated group than in the control one. Haloperidol-treated rats did not differ from either control or olanzapine-treated rats at any time. In contrast, insulin response was similar in control and both treated groups at all times, as well as the difference between T0 and T+10 min. For both glucose and insulin, areas under the curve (AUC) did not show any significant difference. Similarly, the fasting HOMA index of insulin resistance did not differ between treatments. After 46 days of treatment, fasting plasma glucose (measured in samples taken from the heart) was still significantly higher in olanzapine-treated rats than in control rats. Besides, the relative hyperglycaemia in olanzapine-treated rats was more pronounced than after 31 days. In haloperidol-treated rats, fasting plasma glucose was intermediary between those of control and olanzapine-treated rats. Plasma insulin concentration and HOMA were the highest in the olanzapine-treated group; however, the difference between the control and haloperidol-treated groups was not statistically significant. Interestingly, body weight and total food intake did not differ with treatment at any time. In contrast, adiposity, as assessed by the proportion of the epididymal adipose tissue, was the same in all groups after 26 days of treatment, but was significantly higher in olanzapine-treated rats after 46 days treatment, suggesting that dysregulation of glucose homeostasis precedes the changes in body composition, and cannot be accounted for by obesity-induced insulin resistance.

Another approach reported in the literature has been to test the effects of repeated daily injections of SGAs in male Sprague-Dawley rats fed a diet rich in fat and saccharose.[46,58] After 42 days under these dietary conditions, control rats (injected with the vehicle) became obese and insulin resistant, and exhibited a lower glucose tolerance than rats on the chow diet. Daily injections of clozapine, quetiapine, or olanzapine (10 mg/kg of each drug) did not aggravate the body fat content. In response to an oral GTT, glycaemic and insulinemic curves were above chow-fed controls in rats fed the obesogenic diet; besides, both curves were higher in SGA-treated rats than in vehicle-treated controls, whatever the drug. Thus, chronic injections of quetiapine, clozapine and olanzapine induced impairments in glucose tolerance in chow-fed rats, but also over and above those induced by obesity in high fat/high saccharose-fed rats. In contrast, in response to an insulin injection (insulin tolerance test), glucose concentration decreased less in rats fed the obesogenic diet than in those fed the chow diet, indicating a decrease in insulin sensitivity; however, none of the three drugs had additional effects over those resulting from obesity alone.

Interestingly, these observations in the rat are consistent with the situation in treated schizophrenic patients. [59] In response to an oral GTT, the glycemic curve did not differ from controls in FGA-treated patients. In contrast, it was significantly higher at all time points in olanzapine-treated patients, and less pronounced in clozapine- and risperidone-treated patients. Whatever the drug, the insulin curve did not significantly differ from controls. These effects of glucose homeostasis were independent of the severity of adiposity.

Taken together, these findings strongly suggest that, in the male rat model, dysregulations of glucose homeostasis occur early in response to SGAs. The main effects of SGA treatment are a hyperglycemia and a decrease in glucose tolerance, which could not be accounted for by obesity-induced insulin resistance. Possible mechanisms are described below.

D. POSSIBLE MECHANISMS

1. Dysregulation of Energy Homeostasis

Increase in body weight and/or adiposity results from an imbalance in energy homeostasis, due to either an increased energy intake and/or a decreased energy expenditure.

Decreased Energy Expenditure

In olanzapine- or clozapine-treated patients, it has been hypothesized that body weight gain and obesity may result from a decreased energy expenditure, not only accounted for by an impaired physical activity, but also by a decrease in substrate oxidation or in thermogenesis. [60, 61] *In vivo* resting energy expenditure has been shown to decrease in mice after chronic treatment with olanzapine, [62] which also reduced thermogenesis and UCP-1 expression in brown adipose tissue of the female rat.[63] Until now, there has been few investigation of *in vivo* energy metabolism in the male rat. In male Sprague-Dawley rats acutely treated with olanzapine (10 mg/kg by oral gavage), locomotor activity was lowered in all dimensions during the night and day phases, whereas body temperature did not differ from control.[18] Surprisingly, despite the decrease in locomotor activity, overall energy expenditure was not modified by olanzapine treatment. In the same study, when rats were chronically treated with olanzapine (increased dosing from 4 to 12 mg/kg in 2 weeks, then 12 mg/kg, in cookie dough), locomotor activity did not differ from controls after 3 weeks treatment (Albaugh et al., 2011). In male Wistar rats, olanzapine treatment (1, 2.5 of 7.5 mg/kg for 9 days, or 6.5 mg/kg for 4 weeks), locomotor activity was decreased under all conditions, whereas body temperature decreased only after a 3-week treatment.[64] However, in our chronic male rat model, *ex vivo* mitochondrial thermogenesis of brown adipose tissue was not altered by a 6-week treatment with either olanzapine, ziprasidone, or haloperidol.[37] These findings remain fragmentary and have to be confirmed by a more global approach of energy homeostasis in chronically-treated rats.

Disruption of Energy Intake

As noted above, in the rat model, males differ from females with respect to the effect of SGAs on energy intake. Indeed, in the male, chronic SGA treatment, whatever the administration mode, generally does not induce hyperphagia, and resulting weight gain, even though hyperphagia and weight gain sometimes occur.[37,42,43] As also noted, total food intake and body weight gain in the male rat are usually not affected in response to up to 2 mg/kg olanzapine. Besides, repartition of meals throughout the 24-hr cycle were not affected by either treatment.[16] According to this model, the absence of hyperphagia and associated weight gain does not preclude a consistent increase in adiposity.

Beyond these quantitative data on energy intake, detailed studies of feeding behavior are also essential for understanding how SGAs alter food intake, by providing information on potential specific alterations of appetite or satiety systems mechanisms. Furthermore, although there is no clearly established relationship between obesity and meal patterns [65], it may be hypothesized that abnormal feeding patterns participate in the development of obesity and metabolic disorders. In this respect, using our male rat model, a more detailed recording of the feeding pattern for 23 hours showed significant modifications in response to olanzapine. Indeed, chronic olanzapine treatment (2 mg/kg in food for 3 weeks) resulted in an increase in the number of meals, together with a decrease in meal size and inter-meal interval, without a change in meal duration.[16] In contrast, haloperidol did not alter the feeding pattern.

This differs from the changes in meal pattern that were observed in female rats, which exhibit an increase in meal size and meal duration, without a change in meal frequency. In females treated with olazapine for 7 days, these alterations typically result in an increase in energy intake, and consequently in body weight [66], which are both absent in the males.[16]

Our results may also have some theoretical implications regarding the effects of olanzapine on satiety systems. First it should be emphasized that olanzapine-induced alterations in feeding patterns are not related to potential sedative effects of the drug, for at least two reasons. The first is that in our study the latency before the first meal was the same in all groups (antipsychotics and control), and the second is that haloperidol treatment, which is known to be as sedative as olanzapine, did not modify the feeding patterns. Concerning the interactions between antipsychotics and neurotransmitter receptors, it has been suggested that olanzapine may alter feeding patterns through a dopamine D2 blockage. However, according to these authors, a dopamine D2 blockage may increase meal size and reduce meal frequency, while the opposite was observed in our study. Therefore, the results of our study cannot be explained by the D2 blockade potency of olanzapine. Serotonin agonists and antagonists, as well as histamine antagonists, alter food intake in complex ways, but the particular feeding pattern profile observed with olanzapine in our experiments (reduced meal size and increased meal frequency) has never been reported in relation to manipulations of the serotonergic or histaminergic systems. Therefore, the effects on feeding patterns observed with olanzapine in our experiments are unlikely related to its serotonin 5HT2, or histamine H1, blockade, and, more generally, to a direct effect of blockade of classical neurotransmitter receptors.

The control of feeding behavior is also known to depend on two major peptidergic systems, a satiation system, represented by the melanocortin system (alpha-MSH, agouti and agouti-related peptides, MC receptors and mahogany protein), and a feeding-initiation system, represented by the melanin-concentrating hormone (MCH) system (pro-MCH-derived peptides and MCH receptors). Abnormalities in the melanocortin system have never been associated with antipsychotic treatment, while a linkage study has associated the MCH gene with antipsychotic-induced weight gain [67], and a prepro-MCH gene polymorphism has been specifically associated with olanzapine-induced weight gain [68] Olanzapine, like other antipsychotics, is known to act in the nucleus accumbens, and it has been shown that MCH peptide neurons are located in the lateral hypothalamus [69] and project to the nucleus accumbens to modulate the incentive drive for food. [70] It has also been shown that olanzapine simultaneously activates c-Fos in the nucleus accumbens and orexin neurons in the lateral hypothalamus . This set of elements leads us to propose the hypothesis that an interaction between olanzapine and MCH peptide in the nucleus accumbens and/or lateral hypothalamus drives the brain feed-initiation system. This could explain the increased number of meals observed in chronically olanzapine-treated rats in our experiments, and this would be in accordance with the observation that olanzapine increases binge eating in treated patients. [11,71] The normal functioning of the satiation system in the male rat may explain why chronic olanzapine treatment in male rats generally does not produce weight gain [26,39] or increases weight very moderately.[37] It is also consistent with data showing that total food intake is not increased in olanzapine-treated rats. [16] We think that a decrease in meal size along with no difference in meal duration, associated with an increase in meal number and a decrease in the inter-meal interval, more likely indicates that the satiation systems are preserved during chronic olanzapine treatment. However, because olanzapine reinforces the incentive drive for food, rats compensate for decreased ingestion rate and meal size by increasing meal number and thus maintained the same 24-h food intake as controls. Further specific investigations of the feed-initiation and satiety/satiation systems underlying the resilience of feeding behavior in response to olanzapine are needed in animal models, as well as investigations in the clinic.

There is increasing evidence that certain metabolic side effects of SGAs are due, at least in part, to direct effects on peripheral tissues, and especially on insulin targets, such as liver, muscle, and adipose tissue. Indeed, it has been repetitively hypothesised that insulin resistance could occur very early in SGA-treated patients. The following section will thus focus on the potential mechanisms involved in the action of SGAs in the peripheral tissues.

2. Pancreas

Insulin

In naive male Srague-Dawley rats treated acutely with a single injection of either haloperidol (0.25 mg/kg), quetiapine (10 mg/kg), or clozapine (10 mg/kg), and then challenged with a glucose load (oral GTT), plasma glucose and insulin concentrations increased, with clozapine>quetiapine>haloperidol in response. [57] Similarly, plasma glucose and insulin concentrations increased in rats after an acute injection of olanzapine (10 mg/kg).[46] However, in both studies, insulin sensitivity and insulin signaling remained the same as in control rats suggesting that, under these experimental conditions, acute rises in plasma concentration of glucose and insulin were not associated with insulin resistance. Rather, hyperglycemia resulted from an enhanced hepatic glucose production under an increased glucagon secretion by the pancreas (see below). Thus, the increase in insulin concentration was interpreted by the authors as a secondary secretory response of the pancreas to compensate for glucagon-induced hyperglycaemia. In parallel, other studies focused on insulin secretion by using the hyperglycaemic clamp procedure, which is the gold standard for addressing this issue. This approach was used in naive male Srague-Dawley rats treated acutely with a single injection of either haloperidol (0.25 mg/kg), olanzapine (3.0 mg/kg), clozapine (10 mg/kg), risperidone (1 mg/kg) or ziprasidone (3 mg/kg). [72] In response to the hyperglycaemic clamp, clozapine and olanzapine decreased insulin secretion, which is indicative of an impaired beta cell function. Other drugs had no effects. These findings are consistent with an *in vitro* study, in which pancreatic islets isolated from male Srague-Dawley rats were incubated with clozapine. [73] After 7 days of treatment with 1.0 μmol/l (therapeutic concentration), insulin secretion was significantly impaired via multiple mechanisms involving pancreatic glucose metabolism and the distal step of insulin exocytosis. In another study, using pancreatic islets from male Sprague-Dawley rats, perfusion with 10 nM or 100 nM of atropine, clozapine or olanzapine decreased carbachol-potentiated insulin secretion, whereas 100 nM of haloperidol, ziprasidone, or risperidone had no effects. [74] In the same study, olanzapine and clozapine, but not the three other drugs, were shown to be potent muscarinic M_3 antagonists, which led the authors concluding that therapeutic concentrations of olanzapine and clozapine can markedly and selectively impair cholinergic-stimulated insulin secretion by blocking M3 receptors. Indeed, M3 and H1 binding of antipsychotics has been linked to their diabetogenic potential. [75,76] In an elegant attempt to investigate the acute mechanisms underlying clozapine and olanzapine effects on insulin secretion in relation to receptor binding, hyperglycaemic clamps were performed in male Sprague-Dawley rats after injection of various specific antagonists. [77] Interestingly, darifenacin, a muscarinic M_3 antagonist, decreased insulin and C-peptide secretion, whereas ketanserin, a $5HT_{2A}$ antagonist, decreased insulin secretion only. Raclopride, a D_2/D_3 antagonist, increased insulin secretion, whereas terfenadine, a H_1 antagonist, had no effects. The effect of darifenacin on insulin and C-peptide response is consistent with the fact that, among SGAs, olanzapine and clozapine exhibit the highest M_3 binding capacity. The absence of effect of the H1 antagonist terfenadine remains to be clarified. Regarding the effects of raclopride-induced D2 blockade, they are in line with recent data supporting D2-mediated inhibition of glucose-stimulated insulin secretion, suggesting that permanent blockage of D2 receptors may results in glucose intolerance. [78] According to Hahn et al., a prolonged D2 blockade with antipsychotics may lead to a depletion of insulin stores, eventually compromising pancreatic compensation. [77]

Unfortunately, to our knowledge, studies on the effects of chronic SGA treatment on insulin secretion in the male rat under a hyperglycaemic clamp are lacking. In female Sprague-Dawley rats, treated for 4 weeks with olanzapine (2.0 or 7.5 mg/kg), there was no depression of insulin and C-peptide secretion under a hyperglycaemic clamp. [79] Consistently, in our own male rat model, insulin response to a GTT was not altered by 31 days of treatment by olanzapine (2.0 mg/kg). [16] This suggests that the lack of olanzapine effects on insulin secretion in rats under chronic treatment may reflect their adaptation to the drug over a several week period. This is consistent with human studies suggesting a complex effect of SGAs on insulin secretion. Most recently, a time-study of insulin secretion in schizophrenic olanzapine-treated patients clearly demonstrated that, in response to intravenous GTT, insulin secretion was impaired at 2 weeks, returned to baseline, at 4 weeks, then increased at 8 weeks. [80] However, in long-term treated patients (3 months to >21 months), there was no evidence that SGA medication by itself (olanzapine, risperidone, ziprasidone, or FGAs) altered insulin secretion, which was rather significantly correlated with adiposity in healthy controls as well as in treated patients. [81] Thus, in the former study, one cannot exclude the possibility that the impaired β-cell dysfunction observed after 8 weeks of olanzapine treatment may be secondary to the observed increase in adiposity found in these patients.[80] In our male rat model, in which animals do not gain weight, the possibility that insulin secretion increases after prolonged treatment, in relation with the appearance of insulin resistance remains to be assessed via hyperglycaemic clamp.

Glucagon

Besides insulin and C-peptide, glucagon secretion may also be altered by SGA treatment. Indeed, studies from the group of Shepherd and colleagues strongly suggest, that, in response to acute treatment of naïve male Srague-Dawley rats with either quetiapine (10 mg/kg), olanzapine (10 mg/kg) or clozapine (10 mg/kg), glucagon secretion is enhanced. (46,57,58) In parallel, GLP-1 plasma concentration was decreased. [46,58] According to the authors' hypothesis, this dysregulation of glucagon during the acute phase of SGA treatment would be the primary and direct effect of SGAs on the pancreas, with increases in plasma insulin and glucose concentrations being only secondary (see above and below). However, the reasons for this dysregulation remain unclear. This could be a direct effect via antagonism of alpha-2 adrenergic receptors as these are important for controlling glucagon secretion, but may also arise from the decreased plasma concentration of GLP-1, which is a brake of glucagon secretion. Interestingly, most SGAs are muscarinergic receptor antagonists, and GLP-1 secretion is known to be blocked by muscarinergic receptor antagonists in human and rat L-cells. [82,83] The persistence of these abnormalities after long-term treatment, in parallel with insulin resistance, remains to be investigated in the rat, as well as the relevance of these observations for the human patient.

In human patients, increases in plasma glucagon concentration have been reported after treatment by olanzapine, clozapine, and risperidone. [84] In this respect, animal models should help to determine whether the reported increase in glucagon results from a primary, direct effect of SGAs on the pancreatic α-cell or is secondary to the defects in the synthesis and secretion of gut hormones, and especially GLP-1, that normally inhibits glucagon secretion. [59]

3. Adipose Tissue

Adipose tissue in not a passive compartment destined for triglyceride storage in adipocytes. It is an active endocrine tissue involved in the control of energy homeostasis. Besides, cells other than adipocytes also play a major role in the synthesis of adipokines, involved in various physiological pathways, such as immunity and inflammation.

Thus, adipose tissue is likely to be a very complex target of SGAs.

Cellularity

In a first study using our male rat model, haloperidol (1 mg/kg body weight), olanzapine (1 mg/kg body weight), or ziprasidone (10 mg/kg) were given in food for 5 weeks, then rats were killed and adipose pads were dissected for *ex vivo* studies.[26] Mean adipocyte size and diameter distribution did not differ from controls in haloperidol- and ziprasidone-treated rats, whereas adipocytes isolated from the olanzapine-treated group were larger and heavier than in controls.

In Wistar rats treated with the equivalent of 6 mg/kg olanzapine in drinking water, adipocyte hyperplasia was already detectable after 3 days treatment (*ie* before rats started to gain weight) in females in the subcutaneous adipose tissues, but not in the visceral ones. [85] The authors indicate that the same effect was visible in males after a prolonged period of treatment, and without significant weight gain. Hyperplasia was also detected in visceral adipose tissue of female Wistar rats treated for 12 days by *sc* injections of risperidone (0.5 mg/kg) or sulpiride (20 mg/kg) [10] and in our male rat model receiving olanzapine (2 mg/kg) in food for 5 weeks. [41] In human adipose-derived stem cells, clozapine, olazapine and haloperidol slightly stimulated the transcriptional program of adipogenesis, without significant effect on subsequent differentiation. [86]

Lipid Metabolism

In our male rat model, changes in adipose tissue cellularity were accompanied by alterations in lipid metabolism. [26] In response to stimulation by the β-adrenergic agonist isoprenaline, intra-abdominal adipocytes from chronic olanzapine-treated rats exhibited decreased lipolytic activity. In parallel, adipose mRNA levels of hormone sensitive lipase (HSL, a key element in lipolysis) and fatty acid synthase (FAS, involved in lipogenesis) were significantly modified by olanzapine treatment, with HSL being less expressed and FAS being overexpressed. The observed mRNA changes were therefore in agreement with the diminished lipolytic capacity, the increased adipocyte size and the extended fat depots reported above for olanzapine-treated rats.

The other antipsychotics (haloperidol and ziprasidone) did not significantly alter adipocyte lipolytic capacity. The intimate mechanisms of olanzapine action remained unclear, since our results showed that a decrease activation of α1-, α2-, and β-adrenergic receptors was not responsible for the decreased lipolysis. Thus, this study showed for the first time that cell functions of a peripheral organ actively participating in energy homeostasis, namely the adipose tissue, are clearly disturbed after olanzapine treatment, which may contribute to fat deposition. Impaired lipolysis was confirmed by showing that, in fasted Sprague-Dawley rats, acute (2 doses) or chronic (28 days) treatment with olanzapine (10 mg/kg, given orally), plasma concentration of both free fatty acids and glycerol (which originates from the adipose tissue in the fasted state) was lower than in controls. [18, 55] Consistently with our *in vitro* study [26], *in vivo* rise in plasma glycerol and free fatty acid following an isoproterenol challenge was blunted in acutely olanzapine-treated male Srague-Dawley rats.[18]

As concerns lipogenesis, our finding of FAS overexpression [26] is consistent with an increased adipose lipogenesis in male Sprague-Dawley rats acutely treated with olanzapine. [18] Taken together, these studies clearly showed that, in the male rat model, impaired adipose tissue lipolysis and enhanced liopgenesis are early and persistent events that largely contribute to the increase in fat mass induced by SGA treatment.

Hexose Metabolism

In male Wistar Han rats acutely treated with 10 mg/kg of olanzapine (single injection), clozapine (single or 5 daily injections) or ziprasidone (single injection), insulin-stimulated glucose uptake by isolated adipocytes decreased in respone to clozapine, but not in response to olanzapine or ziprasidone. [87]

In our model of chronically treated male rats, basal or insulin-stimulated glucose uptake into adipocytes was not modified in the antipsychotic-treated groups. [26] Accordingly, mRNAs levels of the key elements of glucose utilization, namely the glucose transporters GLUT1 and GLUT4, did not show notable changes.

This is consistent with a recent *in vivo* study using the hyperinsulinemic-euglycemic clamp in male Sprague-Dawley rats acutely treated with olanzapine, and showing that glucose (deoxyglucose) uptake was higher than in controls in subcutaneous adipose tissue, but remained unchanged in visceral adipose tissues. [18]

When assessed on cultured 3T3 adipocytes, insulin-stimulated deoxyglucose uptake was not affected after incubation with therapeutically relevant concentrations (1 μmol/l) of clozapine, quetiapine, or haloperidol, and marginally decreased when concentrations were tenfold higher (10 μmol/l). [57] Consistently, in the same study, insulin signaling in the adipose tissue, as assessed in acutely treated male Sprague-Dawley rats by the phosphorylation of serine 473 on Akt/PKB, was not decreased in response to haloperidol (0.25 mg/kg), quetiapine (10 mg/kg), or clozapine (10 mg/kg).

Taken together, these data suggest that acute or chronic treatment with SGAs affects only marginally hexose uptake by adipose tissue, which does not appear to be the main tissue responsible for the observed insulin resistance in the rat model.

Inflammation and Related Cytokines

When using our male rat model in which rats were treated with haloperidol (1 mg/kg body weight) or olanzapine (2 mg/kg body weight) for 46 days, epididymal adipose tissue from olanzapine-treated rats showed a shift towards an inflammatory phenotype, with extensive macrophage infiltration and a two-fold increase in TNFα expression. [41] In plasma, TNFα and IL-1β concentrations were slightly elevated, which is consistent with a low-grade inflammation. Because the low-grade inflammation initiated in the adipose tissue and the subsequent increase in cytokines have been repeatedly associated with an increased risk of insulin resistance and cardiovascular diseases, these alterations in adipose phenotype may contribute to the impairment of glucose homeostasis observed in our rat model, as well as in human patients, in response to olanzapine.

This low-grade inflammation of the adipose tissue in our male rat model is relevant to the clinical situation. In the general population, obesity is associated with an inflammatory state. [88] Consistently, antipsychotics that induce weight gain have been shown to increase circulating TNFα. [89, 90] or other markers of inflammation [91], whereas antipsychotics that do not increase weight, such as haloperidol, produced no increase in circulating proinflammatory cytokines, including TNFα. [91] Another study showed that TNFα levels increased with body mass index in olanzapine-treated patients, while IL-6 levels were not affected. There have also been controversies as to whether low-grade inflammation has a primary or a secondary role in the development of weight gain in antipsychotic-treated patients. [13] Our results would favor the hypothesis that the presence of macrophages in the adipose tissue is an early event that precedes the overexpression of TNFα, since, in our model, overexpression of TNFα is likely secondary to the accumulation of macrophages in the adipose tissue, even in the absence of pronounced adiposity.

Leptin and Adiponectin

Finally, adipose tissue plays an endocrine role, since it is the major site of leptin and adiponectin synthesis and secretion. In our male rat model, after 6 weeks of SGA treatment, plasma leptin concentration was increased (vs control) in response to olanzapine (1 mg/kg) and haloperidol (1 mg/kg), but not to ziprasidone (10 mg/kg). [37] This was consistent with the higher adiposity in olanzapine- and haloperidol-treated rats. In further studies, under the same experimental conditions, only olanzapine (1 or 2 mg/kg), but not haloperidol increased adiposity; however, leptin plasma concentration and mRNA level did not differ from control rats. [26, 41] Leptin concentration also increased in female Sprague-Dawley rats after 20 treatment days with olanzapine (4 then 8 mg/kg given once a day in cookie dough). [17] Other studies reported no significant increase in leptin concentration in response to various doses of olanzapine, clozapine or ziprasidone, in male or female rats, despite consistent increases in body weight and/or adiposity. [20,40,58,92, 93] Taken together, these findings suggest that olanzapine treatment does not consistently result in an increase in leptin synthesis. This is consistent with data in human SGA-treated patients, showing that plasma leptin increase results primarily from the weight gain and resulting obesity, rather than from a direct impact on leptin physiology. [94]

Compared to leptin, there are fewer studies on adiponectin. In female Sprague-Dawley rats treated for 20 days with olanzapine (4 then 8 mg/kg given once a day in cookie dough), adiponectin plasma concentration was not altered. [17] In female Wistar Han rats treated with clozapine for 20 days, adiponectin plasma concentration significantly increased in response to 4 mg/kg (two daily injections), whereas a trend was observed in response to 1 and 2 mg/kg. [92] The same increase, but only in response to intermediary doses, was observed in male Wistar Han rats under the same experimental conditions. [40] In both studies, the increase in adiponectin was associated with a higher adiposity. Studies in humans led to conflicting results. Most recently, a 3-month prospective study in drug-naive schizophrenics showed that adiponectin plasma concentration slightly increased in response to risperidone, but decreased in response to olanzapine, and did so independently of adiposity or the presence/absence of metabolic syndrome. [95] The differential effect of risperidone *vs* olanzapine suggested a direct and specific effect of SGAs on adipose tissue. This hypothesis could be validly tested by comparing rodent models with or without SGA-induced adiposity.

In conclusion, our results and others indicate that the adipose tissue may be a key target of SGAs, not only through the previously known increase in adiposity, but also through the occurrence of low-grade inflammation. Both of these phenomena contribute to the etiology of metabolic syndrome that is frequently observed in SGA-treated patients.

4. Liver

Liver metabolism is impacted by SGA treatment, as concerns both glucose and lipids.

Glucose

As noted above, in male Sprague-Dawley rats, acute treatment with clozapine (10 mg/kg) enhances hepatic gluconeogenesis and glucose output following glycerol or pyruvate challenge . Besides, these effects are transient, and disappeared by 48 hours after drug injection . This increase in hepatic glucose production was confirmed by means of hyperinsulinic-euglycaemic clamps in male Sprague-Dawley rats treated with acute injections of clozapine (1 mg/kg) or olanzapine (3 mg/kg). [72] In contrast, ziprasidone (3 mg/kg) decreased hepatic glucose output, whereas haloperidol (0.25 mg/kg) and risperidone (1 mg/kg) had no effects. [72] Similarly, hyperinsulinic-euglycaemic clamps were used in male Wistar rats, showing that single doses of clozapine (10 mg/kg) or olanzapine (10 mg/kg) increased hepatic glucose output. [87]

In the same study, ziprasidone (10 mg/kg) had no effects. Consistently, even in females, mRNA level of phosphoenoylpryruvate carboxykinase (*Pepck*) was transiently (up to 3 hours post-injection) increased in the liver of rats after a single injection of olanzapine (5 mg/kg) and, to a lesser extent, clozapine (25 mg/kg).

The reasons for these enhanced gluconeogenesis and glucose outputs remain unclear. According to the group of Shepherd and colleagues, they would not result from a direct effect of clozapine on the liver, but would rather be secondary to the enhanced glucagon secretion. [46,57] However, the possibility of direct effects of SGAs on the liver cannot be excluded, since they interact with a number of cell receptors. [96] As concerns glucose metabolism, acetylcholine enhances hepatic glucose uptake, whereas adrenergic activation stimulates gluconeogenesis and glucose output. Thus, strong M_3 antagonists, such as olanzapine and clozapine, could block the parasympathic pathway, leading to a shift towards adrenergic-stimulated glucose production.

Finally, these early effects remain to be investigated in response to long-term treatment, to assess if increased hepatic glucose production is accounted for by a persistence of glucagon hypersecretion, or results rather from a hepatic insulin resistance failing to regulate gluconeogenesis.

Lipids

To our knowledge, mechanistic effects of chronic treatments with SGAs on hepatic lipid metabolism have not been investigated *in vivo* in the male rat, with the exception of one study using our own model and of a study using risperidone. [97] After 46 days of olanzapine (2 mg /kg) or haloperidol (1 mg/kg) in food, there was no significant effect of either drug on the expression of the two major transcription factors involved in hepatic lipid homeostasis (PPARα and SREBP-1c), or in the expression of target enzymes that control fatty acid synthesis (AcetylCoA carboxylase, fatty acid synthase) or β-oxidation (AcylCoA oxidase, carnitine palmitoyl transferase 1). This was consistent with the absence of changes in the plasma lipid profile, especially in triglyceride concentration, that we reported in a previous study [16], but not with the study by Lauressergues et al. [97], where SREBP-1c was elevated in the liver. This contrasts with acute studies in the female rat reporting an immediate up-regulation (up to 3 hours after injection) of some SREBP-controlled lipogenic enzymes after a single injection of olanzapine (5 mg/kg) or clozapine (25 mg/kg), whereas other lipogenic genes were down-regulated later on (3-24 hours post-injection). [47,56]

Consistently, plasma triglyceride concentration was transiently increased (1 hour after both drug injections) [56]. Hepatic lipid content was also altered by a single clozapine injection [47]. After 25 or 50 mg/mg, triglycerides and phospholipids increased between 6-48 hours after injection, whereas cholesterol content was increased only 48 hours after injection. Surprisingly, this accumulation corresponded to the time when lipogenic enzymes were down-regulated, suggesting that clozapine altered the hepatic balance in lipid synthesis, secretion (as lipoproteins) and storage.

Short-term effects of SGAs on hepatic lipogenesis were confirmed by *in vitro* studies. [98] Hepatocytes isolated from male Sprague-Dawley rats were incubated for 24 hours with clozapine (25 μM), olanzapine (25 μM), haloperidol (25 μM), quetiapine (25 μM), and aripiprazole (10 μM).Triglyceride synthesis was increased by olanzapine, and phospholipid synthesis by clozapine olanzapine, and haloperidol. Cholesterol synthesis increased in response to clozapine, and, to a lesser extent, to olanzapine, whereas it was decreased by haloperidol (for cholesteryl esters only). Quetiapine and aripiprazole had no effect. Consistently, mRNA levels of SREBP-1 and of major lipogenic enzymes FAS and stearoylCoA desaturase 1 (*SCD1*), as well as the protein content of the mature form of SREBP-1, were all increased in response to clozapine and, to a lesser extent, to olanzapine and haloperidol. In contrast, they were down-regulated by quetiapine, whereas aripiprazole had no effect. As concerns hepatic cholesterol metabolism, clozapine up-regulated HMGCoA reductase (key-enzyme of cholesterol synthesis) and LDL receptors (cholesterol uptake), and increased the protein level of SREBP-2, which control most of the genes involved in cholesterol metabolism. The same genes were also up-regulated, but to a lesser extent, by olanzapine and quetiapine. Unfortunately, lipids secretion in the culture medium was not assayed, and the balance among lipid synthesis, storage, and exportation could not be quantified. When hepatocytes isolated from male Srague-Dawley rats were incubated with risperidone (25 μM for 24 hours), FAS and, to a lesser extent, SREBP-1c mRNA levels were increased, as well as triglyceride, phospholipids, and free cholesterol synthesis and hepatic content [97] Expression level of genes involved in cholesterol metabolism was unchanged [97].

Other aspects of lipid metabolism have been investigated in Sprague-Dawley rats acutely treated with olanzapine (2 oral administration of 10 mg/kg over 48 hours). [55] Free fatty acid uptake was two-fold higher than in controls, whereas VLDL secretion was unchanged, suggesting that olanzapine enhanced hepatic fatty acid oxidation to the detriment of their release.[55]

Taken together, *in vivo* and *in vitro* studies suggest that hepatic lipid synthesis is transiently enhanced by various SGAs, the major effects being observed with clozapine and, to a lesser extent, with olanzapine. SREBP activation appears to be a key-player in these alterations. However, long-term studies are now needed to follow the effects of chronic SGA treatments on hepatic lipid metabolism, in relation to the lack of alterations in the plasma lipid profile which is generally observed in the rat models.

In the female mouse, 11-week treatment with weekly injections of long-lasting risperidone (12.5 mg/kg) failed to alter the hepatic content of triglycerides, phospholipids, and cholesterol, as well as the plasma lipid profile. [98] In the same mice, risperidone up-regulated the expression of hepatic genes involved in both fatty acid synthesis (SREPB-1c, FAS) and oxidation, (acylCoA oxidase), whereas the mRNA level of SREPB-2, which controls cholesterogenesis, was depressed. Thus, at least in this mouse model, despite some variations in gene expression, the hepatic balance of lipid synthesis, secretion, and storage, remains unchanged.

Finally, how SGAs activate SREPB-1 and 2, and other transcription factors (PPARs, LXR), remains also to be investigated.

Inflammation and Related Cytokines

In our rat model, and in contrast with adipose tissue, a 6 week treatment by olanzapine failed to enhance expression of TNFα in the liver. [41] This suggests that, at this early stage, the liver does not contribute to the low-grade inflammation found in our model. [41]

5. Muscle

Acute or chronic action of SGAs on skeletal muscle remains poorly investigated. $_{14}$C-deoxyglucose (2DG) is a glucose analog which is normally up-taken by tissues, but is not further metabolized, which allows to assess *in vivo* insulin sensitivity in terms of glucose uptake.

In male Srague-Dawley rats acutely treated with 10 mg/kg of clozapine, olanzapine, or ziprasidone, glucose uptake by the *soleus* and the *quadriceps* muscles was impaired in response to clozapine, but not to olanzapine or ziprasidone.[87] This suggests that clozapine induces a very early insulin resistance in skeletal muscle. However, this effect was transient as it disappeared after a 5-day treatment.

The use of a hyperinsulinmic-euglycemic clamp in acutely treated male Sprague-Dawley rats also revealed that olanzpine (10 mg/kg) impaired glucose uptake by muscle as a result of early insulin resistance.[18] A couple of *ex vivo* and *in vitro* studies also addressed this question. In *soleus* muscle isolated from naïve male Srague-Dawley rats, incubation for 30 min with 1 μM or 10 μM clozapine, quetiapine, or haloperidol, and in presence of insulin, did not alter glucose uptake, showing that, under these conditions, insulin sensitivity was not altered by the three tested SGAs. [57] In *epitrochlearis* muscle isolated from female Sprague-Dawley rats, incubations with either olanzapine or clozapine (0.1-10 mM), and in presence of insulin, failed to alter 2DG uptake. [87] Thus, in contrast with *in vivo* studies, these *ex vivo* and *in vitro* studies do not support the hypothesis of a short-term insulin resistance in skeletal muscle, as far as it is assessed *via* glucose uptake.

In Srague-Dawley rats treated acutely with olanzapine (two oral administrations over 48 hours, 10 mg/kg), free fatty acid uptake was enhanced in skeletal muscle, which also showed an increased content of carnitine derivatives of β-oxidation, suggesting that olanzapine simulates fatty acid disposal by skeletal muscle. [55] According to the authors' hypothesis, acute SGA treatment results in a rapid shift in the oxidation of metabolic fuels from mostly carbohydrates to mostly lipids, which precedes the development of insulin resistance. Thus, the contribution of the skeletal muscles to whole body insulin resistance resulting from SGA treatment, in relation to the complex interactions between carbohydrate and lipid metabolism, remains to be further investigated, especially under chronic treatment.

6. Gastrointestinal System

Gastrointestinal peptides such as cholecystokinin (CCK), peptide YY (PYY) and ghrelin are known regulators of appetite and, thus, influence energy intake. This is quite important as a number of monoamine neurotransmitter receptors, the SGA target, have been identified in the enteric nervous system, in parallel with their well-known localization in the central nervous system. However, to date, only a few studies of SGA effects on ghrelin concentrations in schizophrenic patients are available. A recent review concluded that there is a decrease in serum-active ghrelin levels compared with baseline in response to short-term treatment and an increase during longer periods.(99 In healthy volunteers, short-term treatment with olanzapine (10 mg/day for 8 days) did not modify the plasma concentration of any gut peptides. [53] Long-term studies are still lacking.

In male rats acutely treated with a single clozapine injection, plasma ghrelin concentration was significantly higher than in control rats. [100, 101] In response to an acute olanzapine injection in male rats, meal-related ghrelin concentration, but not baseline concentration, was significantly higher than in the control group. [101] In female rats sub-chronically treated for 14 days with olanzapine (0.25, 0.5, 1.0 and 2.0 mg/kg) in food, the plasma levels of ghrelin, and, to a lesser extent, CCK, increased, whereas that of PYY was unchanged. 44) Ghrelin concentration was positively and significantly correlated with food intake, body weight, and total white adipose tissue mass whereas CCK concentration tended to be positively correlated with total white adipose tissue mass. In this female rat model, increased weight gain and adiposity result largely from drug-induced hyperphagia. The findings of these studies are thus consistent with the known role of ghrelin in the stimulation of food intake. Moreover, the acute studies in the male rat [100,101] clearly showed that the increase in plasma ghrelin is a very early event.

In female rats treated sub-chronically with olanzapine, CCK plasma concentration was higher than in control rats. [44] Since CCK is an anorectic hormone, the increase in plasma CCK is rather surprising, but may be interpreted as a compensatory mechanism in response to ghrelin-induced hyperphagia [44]. This is consistent with the finding that, contrary to ghrelin, CCK concentration was not affected in male rats acutely treated with a single olanzapine injection. [101]

In response to olanzapine, PYY concentration did not differ from control rats in acutely treated male rats [101], or in sub-chronically treated female rats [44]

GLP-1 counteracts hyperglycemia by inducing glucose-dependent stimulation of insulin secretion while suppressing glucagon secretion, and has thus been involved in the dysregulation of pancreas metabolism by SGAs (see above). In the male rat, GLP-1 plasma concentration was not affected by acute olanzapine injection. [101] In chronically-treated male rats, after 42 days on a low- or a high-fat diet, olanzapine (10 mg/kg), clozapine (10 mg/kg), or quetiapine (10 mg/kg), decreased GLP-1 plasma concentration. [46] Interestingly, under these experimental conditions, this effect of SGAs on GLP-1 is independent of hyperphagia, weight gain, and obesity.

Taken together, these findings strongly suggest that, among gastrointestinal hormones, ghrelin and GLP-1 are the most responsive to SGAs. Increase in plasma ghrelin is a very early event, whereas decrease in plasma GLP-1 occurs later. The molecular mechanisms by which SGAs may enhance ghrelin synthesis and/or secretion in the intestine, and in particular the identification of the involved receptors, remain to be investigated.

CONCLUSION

In conclusion, there is increasing evidence that SGAs exert peripheral actions, independently of their well-known effects on the central nervous system. The use of rodent models allows characterizing the metabolic alterations resulting from either acute or chronic SGA administration. However, in response to chronic SGA administration, it may remain unclear whether metabolic disturbances result from a direct effect of the drug on peripheral tissues, or are secondary to the increased food intake and consequent adiposity that are usually found in human patients, but also in some rodent models. For these reasons, we developed a male rat model in which SGAs are chronically administered in food. Under these conditions, there is no increase in food intake and weight gain, whereas adiposity increases significantly, but moderately, after a 6 week-treatment. Longitudinal studies using this model gave insights into the temporal pattern of the alterations of energy homeostasis in response to SGA treatment. Our results show that chronic olanzapine treatment alters meal patterns in a way that suggests it activates brain feeding-initiation systems, whereas satiation systems are preserved. The fact that, in this study, metabolic abnormalities (glucose elevation and fat accumulation) occurred after the alterations in feeding behaviour, and seemed to progressively worsen along with the duration of treatment, raises the hypothesis of a temporal relationship between meal pattern abnormalities and the development of metabolic abnormalities. Metabolic abnormalities are accompanied with a low-grade inflammation, which originates from the accumulation of macrophages in the visceral adipose tissue. Interestingly, infiltration of adipose tissue by macrophages is an early event, occurring in the absence of pronounced adiposity.

As concerns the underlying mechanisms of the alterations of glucose and lipid metabolism by SGAs, several target tissues have been identified: pancreas, adipose tissue, liver, muscle, and gastrointestinal tract. All these tissues display a number of SGA target receptors. Studies in our male rat model focused primarily on adipose tissue. The impact of SGAs on other peripheral tissues remains to be investigated. There is also a need for longitudinal studies of the occurrence of metabolic disturbances in relation to what is observed in patients. Indeed, the identification of early events occurring together with, but probably independently of weight gain, such as low-grade inflammation, would be of great help in the prevention and/or care of SGA side-effects.

ACKNOWLEDGMENTS

Julie Minet-Ringuet was financially supported by Pfizer Laboratories, and Montserrat Victoriano by Servier Laboratories.

REFERENCES

[1] Allison, D.B., Mentore, J.L., Heo, M., Chandler, L.P., Cappelleri, J.C., Infante, M.C., and Weiden, P.J. Antipsychotic-induced weight gain: a comprehensive research synthesis. *Am. J. Psychiatry*. 1999;156:1686-1696.

[2] Baptista, T. Body weight gain induced by antipsychotic drugs: mechanisms and management. *Acta Psychiatr. Scand*. 1999;100:3-16.

[3] Kelly, D.L., Conley, R.R., Love, R.C., Morrison, J.A., and McMahon, R.P. Metabolic risk with second-generation antipsychotic treatment: a double-blind randomized 8-week trial of risperidone and olanzapine. *Ann. Clin. Psychiatry*. 2008;20:71-78.

[4] Wirshing, D.A., Boyd, J.A., Meng, L.R., Ballon, J.S., Marder, S.R., and Wirshing, W.C. The effects of novel antipsychotics on glucose and lipid levels. *J. Clin. Psychiatry*. 2002;63:856-865.

[5] Henderson, D.C., and Doraiswamy, P.M. Prolactin-related and metabolic adverse effects of atypical antipsychotic agents. *J. Clin. Psychiatry*. 2008;69 Suppl 1:32-44.

[6] Newcomer, J.W. Antipsychotic medications: metabolic and cardiovascular risk. *J. Clin. Psychiatry*. 2007;68 Suppl 4:8-13.

[7] Coccurello, R., and Moles, A. Potential mechanisms of atypical antipsychotic-induced metabolic derangement: clues for understanding obesity and novel drug design. *Pharmacol. Ther*. 2010;127:210-251.

[8] Casey, D.E. Dyslipidemia and atypical antipsychotic drugs. *J. Clin. Psychiatry*. 2004;65 Suppl 18:27-35.

[9] Rummel-Kluge, C., Komossa, K., Schwarz, S., Hunger, H., Schmid, F., Lobos, C.A., Kissling, W., Davis, J.M., and Leucht, S. Head-to-head comparisons of metabolic side effects of second generation antipsychotics in the treatment of schizophrenia: a systematic review and meta-analysis. *Schizophr. Res.* 2010;123:225-233.

[10] Baptista, T., de Baptista, E.A., Lalonde, J., Plamondon, J., Kin, N.M., Beaulieu, S., Joober, R., and Richard, D. Comparative effects of the antipsychotics sulpiride and risperidone in female rats on energy balance, body composition, fat morphology and macronutrient selection. *Prog. Neuropsychopharmacol. Biol. Psychiatry.* 2004;28:1305-1311.

[11] Gebhardt, S., Haberhausen, M., Krieg, J.C., Remschmidt, H., Heinzel-Gutenbrunner, M., Hebebrand, J., and Theisen, F.M. Clozapine/olanzapine-induced recurrence or deterioration of binge eating-related eating disorders. *J. Neural. Transm.* 2007;114:1091-1095.

[12] Gothelf, D., Falk, B., Singer, P., Kairi, M., Phillip, M., Zigel, L., Poraz, I., Frishman, S., Constantini, N., Zalsman, G., Weizman, A., and Apter, A. Weight gain associated with increased food intake and low habitual activity levels in male adolescent schizophrenic inpatients treated with olanzapine. *Am. J. Psychiatry.* 2002;159:1055-1057.

[13] Kluge, M., Schuld, A., Schacht, A., Himmerich, H., Dalal, M.A., Wehmeier, P.M., Hinze-Selch, D., Kraus, T., Dittmann, R.W., and Pollmacher, T. Effects of clozapine and olanzapine on cytokine systems are closely linked to weight gain and drug-induced fever. *Psychoneuroendocrinology* 2009;34:118-128.

[14] Roerig, J.L., Mitchell, J.E., de Zwaan, M., Crosby, R.D., Gosnell, B.A., Steffen, K.J., and Wonderlich, S.A. A comparison of the effects of olanzapine and risperidone versus placebo on eating behaviors. *J. Clin. Psychopharmacol.* 2005;25:413-418.

[15] Guesdon, B., Denis, R.G., and Richard, D. Additive effects of olanzapine and melanin-concentrating hormone agonism on energy balance. *Behav. Brain Res.* 2010;207:14-20.

[16] Victoriano, M., Hermier, D., Even, P.C., Fromentin, G., Huneau, J.F., Tome, D., and de Beaurepaire, R. Early perturbation in feeding behaviour and energy homeostasy in olanzapine-treated rats. *Psychopharmacology* (Berl) 2009;206:167-176.

[17] Albaugh, V.L., Henry, C.R., Bello, N.T., Hajnal, A., Lynch, S.L., Halle, B., and Lynch, C.J. Hormonal and metabolic effects of olanzapine and clozapine related to body weight in rodents. *Obesity* (Silver Spring) 2006;14:36-51.

[18] Albaugh, V.L., Judson, J.G., She, P., Lang, C.H., Maresca, K.P., Joyal, J.L., and Lynch, C.J. Olanzapine promotes fat accumulation in male rats by decreasing physical activity, repartitioning energy and increasing adipose tissue lipogenesis while impairing lipolysis. *Mol. Psychiatry.* 2011;16:569-581.

[19] Arjona, A.A., Zhang, S.X., Adamson, B., and Wurtman, R.J. An animal model of antipsychotic-induced weight gain. *Behav. Brain Res.* 2004;152:121-127.

[20] Cooper, G.D., Pickavance, L.C., Wilding, J.P., Halford, J.C., and Goudie, A.J. A parametric analysis of olanzapine-induced weight gain in female rats. *Psychopharmacology* (Berl) 2005;181:80-89.

[21] Fell, M.J., Marshall, K.M., Williams, J., and Neill, J.C. Effects of the atypical antipsychotic olanzapine on reproductive function and weight gain in female rats. *J. Psychopharmacol.* 2004;18:149-155.

[22] Fell, M.J., Neill, J.C., and Marshall, K.M. Effects of the classical antipsychotic haloperidol and atypical antipsychotic risperidone on weight gain, the oestrous cycle and uterine weight in female rats. *Eur. Neuropsychopharmacol.* 2004;14:385-392.

[23] Goudie, A.J., Cooper, G.D., and Halford, J.C. Antipsychotic-induced weight gain. *Diabetes Obes. Metab.* 2005;7:478-487.

[24] Goudie, A.J., Smith, J.A., and Halford, J.C. Characterization of olanzapine-induced weight gain in rats. *J. Psychopharmacol.* 2002;16:291-296.

[25] Kaur, G., and Kulkarni, S.K. Studies on modulation of feeding behavior by atypical antipsychotics in female mice. *Prog. Neuropsychopharmacol. Biol. Psychiatry.* 2002;26:277-285.

[26] Minet-Ringuet, J., Even, P.C., Valet, P., Carpene, C., Visentin, V., Prevot, D., Daviaud, D., Quignard-Boulange, A., Tome, D., and de Beaurepaire, R. Alterations of lipid metabolism and gene expression in rat adipocytes during chronic olanzapine treatment. *Mol. Psychiatry.* 2007;12:562-571.

[27] Pouzet, B., Mow, T., Kreilgaard, M., and Velschow, S. Chronic treatment with antipsychotics in rats as a model for antipsychotic-induced weight gain in human. *Pharmacol. Biochem. Behav.* 2003;75:133-140.

[28] Cope, M.B., Nagy, T.R., Fernandez, J.R., Geary, N., Casey, D.E., and Allison, D.B. Antipsychotic drug-induced weight gain: development of an animal model. *Int. J. Obes.* (Lond) 2005;29:607-614.

[29] Kalinichev, M., Rourke, C., Daniels, A.J., Grizzle, M.K., Britt, C.S., Ignar, D.M., and Jones, D.N. Characterisation of olanzapine-induced weight gain and effect of aripiprazole vs olanzapine on body weight and prolactin secretion in female rats. *Psychopharmacology* (Berl) 2005;182:220-231.

[30] Kalinichev, M., Rourke, C., and Jones, D.N. Body weights and plasma prolactin levels in female rats treated subchronically with ziprasidone versus olanzapine. *Behav. Pharmacol.* 2006;17:289-292.

[31] Ganguli, R., Brar, J.S., and Ayrton, Z. Weight gain over 4 months in schizophrenia patients: a comparison of olanzapine and risperidone. *Schizophr. Res.* 2001;49:261-267.

[32] Hakko, H., Komulainen, M.T., Koponen, H., Saari, K., Laitinen, J., Jarvelin, M.R., and Lindeman, S. Are females at special risk of obesity if they become psychotic? The longitudinal Northern Finland 1966 Birth Cohort Study. *Schizophr. Res.* 2006;84:15-19.

[33] Russell, J.M., and Mackell, J.A. Bodyweight gain associated with atypical antipsychotics: epidemiology and therapeutic implications. *CNS Drugs* 2001;15:537-551.

[34] Taylor, D.M., and McAskill, R. Atypical antipsychotics and weight gain--a systematic review. *Acta Psychiatr. Scand.* 2000;101:416-432.

[35] Ascher-Svanum, H., Stensland, M.D., Kinon, B.J., and Tollefson, G.D. Weight gain as a prognostic indicator of therapeutic improvement during acute treatment of schizophrenia with placebo or active antipsychotic. *J. Psychopharmacol.* 2005;19:110-117.

[36] Meltzer, H.Y., Perry, E., and Jayathilake, K. Clozapine-induced weight gain predicts improvement in psychopathology. *Schizophr. Res.* 2003;59:19-27.

[37] Minet-Ringuet, J., Even, P.C., Lacroix, M., Tome, D., and de Beaurepaire, R. A model for antipsychotic-induced obesity in the male rat. *Psychopharmacology* (Berl) 2006;187:447-454.

[38] Minet-Ringuet, J., Even, P.C., Guesdon, B., Tome, D., and de Beaurepaire, R. Effects of chronic neuroleptic treatments on nutrient selection, body weight, and body composition in the male rat under dietary self-selection. *Behav. Brain Res.* 2005;163:204-211.

[39] Minet-Ringuet, J., Even, P.C., Goubern, M., Tome, D., and de Beaurepaire, R.. Long term treatment with olanzapine mixed with the food in male rats induces body fat deposition with no increase in body weight and no thermogenic alteration. *Appetite* 2006;46:254-262.

[40] Cooper, G.D., Pickavance, L.C., Wilding, J.P., Harrold, J.A., Halford, J.C., and Goudie, A.J. Effects of olanzapine in male rats: enhanced adiposity in the absence of hyperphagia, weight gain or metabolic abnormalities. *J. Psychopharmacol.* 2007;21:405-413.

[41] Victoriano, M., de Beaurepaire, R., Naour, N., Guerre-Millo, M., Quignard-Boulange, A., Huneau, J.F., Mathe, V., Tome, D., and Hermier, D. Olanzapine-induced accumulation of adipose tissue is associated with an inflammatory state. *Brain Res.* 2010;1350:167-175.

[42] Shobo, M., Yamada, H., Koakutsu, A., Hamada, N., Fujii, M., Harada, K., Ni, K., and Matsuoka, N. Chronic treatment with olanzapine via a novel infusion pump induces adiposity in male rats. *Life Sci.* 2011;88:761-765.

[43] Shobo, M., Yamada, H., Mihara, T., Kondo, Y., Irie, M., Harada, K., Ni, K., Matsuoka, N., and Kayama, Y. Two models for weight gain and hyperphagia as side effects of atypical antipsychotics in male rats: validation with olanzapine and ziprasidone. *Behav. Brain Res.* 2011;216:561-568.

[44] Weston-Green, K., Huang, X.F., and Deng, C. Olanzapine treatment and metabolic dysfunction: a dose response study in female Sprague Dawley rats. *Behav. Brain Res.* 2011;217:337-346.

[45] Albaugh, V.L., Singareddy, R., Mauger, D., and Lynch, C.J. A double blind, placebo-controlled, randomized crossover study of the acute metabolic effects of olanzapine in healthy volunteers. *PLoS ONE 2011* 62001;e22662.

[46] Smith, G.C., Vickers, M.H., and Shepherd, P.R. Olanzapine effects on body composition, food preference, glucose metabolism and insulin sensitivity in the rat. *Arch Physiol. Biochem.*2011;117(4):241-9.

[47] Jassim, G., Skrede, S., Vazquez, M.J., Wergedal, H., Vik-Mo, A.O., Lunder, N., Dieguez, C., Vidal-Puig, A., Berge, R.K., Lopez, M., Steen, V.M., and Ferno, J. Acute effects of orexigenic antipsychotic drugs on lipid and carbohydrate metabolism in rat. *Psychopharmacology* (Berl) 2012; 219:783-94.

[48] Cheng, C.Y., Hong, C.J., and Tsai, S.J. Effects of subchronic clozapine administration on serum glucose, cholesterol and triglyceride levels, and body weight in male BALB/c mice. *Life Sci.* 2005;76:2269-2273.

[49] Coccurello, R., Caprioli, A., Conti, R., Ghirardi, O., Borsini, F., Carminati, P., and Moles, A. Olanzapine (LY170053, 2-methyl-4-(4-methyl-1-piperazinyl)-10H-thieno[2,3-b][1,5] benzodiazepine), but not the novel atypical antipsychotic ST2472 (9-piperazin-1-ylpyrrolo[2,1-b][1,3]benzothiazepine), chronic administration induces weight gain, hyperphagia, and metabolic dysregulation in mice. *J. Pharmacol. Exp. Ther.* 2008;326:905-911.

[50] Coccurello, R., Caprioli, A., Ghirardi, O., Conti, R., Ciani, B., Daniele, S., Bartolomucci, A., and Moles, A. Chronic administration of olanzapine induces metabolic and food intake alterations: a mouse model of the atypical antipsychotic-associated adverse effects. *Psychopharmacology* (Berl) 2006;186:561-571.

[51] Cope, M.B., Jumbo-Lucioni, P., Walton, R.G., Kesterson, R.A., Allison, D.B., and Nagy, T.R.. No effect of dietary fat on short-term weight gain in mice treated with atypical antipsychotic drugs. *Int. J. Obes.* (Lond) 2007;31:1014-1022.

[52] Kaddurah-Daouk, R., McEvoy, J., Baillie, R.A., Lee, D., Yao, J.K., Doraiswamy, P.M., and Krishnan, K.R. Metabolomic mapping of atypical antipsychotic effects in schizophrenia. *Mol. Psychiatry*. 2007;12:934-945.

[53] Vidarsdottir, S., de Leeuw van Weenen, J.E., Frolich, M., Roelfsema, F., Romijn, J.A., and Pijl, H. Effects of olanzapine and haloperidol on the metabolic status of healthy men. *J. Clin. Endocrinol. Metab.* 2010;95:118-125.

[54] Vidarsdottir, S., Roelfsema, F., Streefland, T., Holst, J.J., Rehfeld, J.F., and Pijl, H. Short-term treatment with olanzapine does not modulate gut hormone secretion: olanzapine disintegrating versus standard tablets. *Eur. J. Endocrinol.* 2010;162:75-83.

[55] Albaugh, V.L., Vary, T.C., Ilkayeva, O., Wenner, B.R., Maresca, K.P., Joyal, J.L., Breazeale, S., Elich, T.D., Lang, C.H., and Lynch, C.J. Atypical Antipsychotics Rapidly and Inappropriately Switch Peripheral Fuel Utilization to Lipids, Impairing Metabolic Flexibility in Rodents. *Schizophr. Bull.*2010; 38(1):153-66.

[56] Fernø, J., Vik-Mo, A., Jassim, G., Håvik, B., Berge, K., Skrede, S., Gudbrandsen, O., Waage, J., Lunder, N., Mørk, S., Berge, R., Jørgensen, H., and Steen, V. Acute clozapine exposure in vivo induces lipid accumulation and marked sequential changes in the expression of SREBP, PPAR, and LXR target genes in rat liver. *Psychopharmacology* 2009;203:73-84.

[57] Smith, G.C., Chaussade, C., Vickers, M., Jensen, J., and Shepherd, P.R. Atypical antipsychotic drugs induce derangements in glucose homeostasis by acutely increasing glucagon secretion and hepatic glucose output in the rat. *Diabetologia* 2008;51:2309-2317.

[58] Smith, G.C., Vickers, M.H., Cognard, E., and Shepherd, P.R. Clozapine and quetiapine acutely reduce glucagon-like peptide-1 production and increase glucagon release in obese rats: implications for glucose metabolism and food choice behaviour. *Schizophr. Res.* 2009;115:30-40.

[59] Newcomer, J.W., Haupt, D.W., Fucetola, R., Melson, A.K., Schweiger, J.A., Cooper, B.P., and Selke, G. Abnormalities in glucose regulation during antipsychotic treatment of schizophrenia. *Arch. Gen. Psychiatry*. 2002;59:337-345.

[60] Procyshyn, R.M., Chau, A., and Tse, G. Clozapine's effects on body weight and resting metabolic rate: a case series. *Schizophr. Res.* 2004;66:159-162.

[61] Virkkunen, M., Wahlbeck, K., Rissanen, A., Naukkarinen, H., and Franssila-Kallunki, A. Decrease of energy expenditure causes weight increase in olanzapine treatment - a case study. *Pharmacopsychiatry* 2002;35:124-126.

[62] Coccurello, R., Brina, D., Caprioli, A., Conti, R., Ghirardi, O., Schepis, F., and Moles, A. 2009. 30 days of continuous olanzapine infusion determines energy imbalance, glucose intolerance, insulin resistance, and dyslipidemia in mice. *J. Clin. Psychopharmacol.* 2009;29:576-583.

[63] Stefanidis, A., Verty, A.N., Allen, A.M., Owens, N.C., Cowley, M.A., and Oldfield, B.J. The role of thermogenesis in antipsychotic drug-induced weight gain. *Obesity* (Silver Spring) 2009;17:16-24.

[64] van der Zwaal, E.M., Luijendijk, M.C., Evers, S.S., la Fleur, S.E., and Adan, R.A. Olanzapine affects locomotor activity and meal size in male rats. *Pharmacol. Biochem. Behav*. 2010;97 :130-137.

[65] Bellisle, F., McDevitt, R., and Prentice, A.M. Meal frequency and energy balance. *Br. J. Nutr*. 1997;77 Suppl 1:S57-70.

[66] Davoodi, N., Kalinichev, M., Korneev, S.A., and Clifton, P.G. Hyperphagia and increased meal size are responsible for weight gain in rats treated sub-chronically with olanzapine. *Psychopharmacology* (Berl) 2009;203:693-702.

[67] Chagnon, Y. C., C. Merette, et al. A genome wide linkage study of obesity as secondary effect of antipsychotics in multigenerational families of eastern Quebec affected by psychoses. *Mol. Psychiatry*. 2004;9(12): 1067-1074.

[68] Chagnon, Y. C., A. Bureau, et al. Possible association of the pro-melanin-concentrating hormone gene with a greater body mass index as a side effect of the antipsychotic olanzapine. *Am. J. Med. Genet. B Neuropsychiatr. Genet.* 2007;144B: 1063-1069.

[69] Bittencourt JC, Presse F, Arias C, Peto C, Vaughan J, Nahon JL, Vale W, Sawchenko PE. The melanin-concentrating hormone system of the rat brain: an immuno- and hybridization histochemical characterization. *J. Comp. Neurol. 1992;*319*:* 218–245.

[70] The Hypothalamic Neuropeptide Melanin-Concentrating Hormone Acts in the Nucleus Accumbens to Modulate Feeding Behavior and Forced-Swim Performance Dan Georgescu, Robert M. Sears Jonathan D. Hommel *The Journal of Neuroscience* 2005;25: 2933-2940.

[71] Kluge, M., Schuld, A., Himmerich, H., Dalal, M., Schacht, A., Wehmeier, P.M., Hinze-Selch, D., Kraus, T., Dittmann, R.W., and Pollmacher, T. Clozapine and olanzapine are associated with food craving and binge eating: results from a randomized double-blind study. *J. Clin. Psychopharmacol*. 2007;27:662-666.

[72] Chintoh, A.F., Mann, S.W., Lam, L., Giacca, A., Fletcher, P., Nobrega, J., and Remington, G. Insulin resistance and secretion in vivo: effects of different antipsychotics in an animal model. *Schizophr. Res*. 2009;108:127-133.

[73] 73.Sasaki, N., Iwase, M., Uchizono, Y., Nakamura, U., Imoto, H., Abe, S., and Iida, M. The atypical antipsychotic clozapine impairs insulin secretion by inhibiting glucose metabolism and distal steps in rat pancreatic islets. *Diabetologia* 2006;49:2930-2938.

[74] Johnson, D.E., Yamazaki, H., Ward, K.M., Schmidt, A.W., Lebel, W.S., Treadway, J.L., Gibbs, E.M., Zawalich, W.S., and Rollema, H. Inhibitory effects of antipsychotics on carbachol-enhanced insulin secretion from perifused rat islets: role of muscarinic antagonism in antipsychotic-induced diabetes and hyperglycemia. *Diabetes* 2005;54:1552-1558.

[75] Matsui-Sakata, A., Ohtani, H., and Sawada, Y. Receptor occupancy-based analysis of the contributions of various receptors to antipsychotics-induced weight gain and diabetes mellitus. *Drug Metab. Pharmacokinet.* 2005;20:368-378.

[76] Silvestre, J.S., and Prous, J. Research on adverse drug events. I. Muscarinic M3 receptor binding affinity could predict the risk of antipsychotics to induce type 2 diabetes. *Methods. Find. Exp. Clin. Pharmacol.* 2005;27:289-304.

[77] Hahn, M., Chintoh, A., Giacca, A., Xu, L., Lam, L., Mann, S., Fletcher, P., Guenette, M., Cohn, T., Wolever, T., Arenovich, T., and Remington, G. Atypical antipsychotics and effects of muscarinic, serotonergic, dopaminergic and histaminergic receptor binding on insulin secretion in vivo: An animal model. *Schizophr. Res.* 2011; 131:90-95.

[78] Garcia-Tornadu, I., Ornstein, A.M., Chamson-Reig, A., Wheeler, M.B., Hill, D.J., Arany, E., Rubinstein, M., and Becu-Villalobos, D. Disruption of the dopamine d2 receptor impairs insulin secretion and causes glucose intolerance. *Endocrinology* 2010;151:1441-1450.

[79] Chintoh, A.F., Mann, S.W., Lam, L., Lam, C., Cohn, T.A., Fletcher, P.J., Nobrega, J.N., Giacca, A., and Remington, G. Insulin resistance and decreased glucose-stimulated insulin secretion after acute olanzapine administration. *J. Clin. Psychopharmacol.* 2008;28:494-499.

[80] Chiu, C.C., Chen, C.H., Chen, B.Y., Yu, S.H., and Lu, M.L. The time-dependent change of insulin secretion in schizophrenic patients treated with olanzapine. *Prog. Neuropsychopharmacol. Biol. Psychiatry.* 2010;34:866-870.

[81] Haupt, D.W., Fahnestock, P.A., Flavin, K.A., Schweiger, J.A., Stevens, A., Hessler, M.J., Maeda, J., Yingling, M., and Newcomer, J.W. Adiposity and insulin sensitivity derived from intravenous glucose tolerance tests in antipsychotic-treated patients. *Neuropsychopharmacology* 2007;32:2561-2569.

[82] Anini, Y., and Brubaker, P.L. Muscarinic receptors control glucagon-like peptide 1 secretion by human endocrine L cells. *Endocrinology* 2003;144:3244-3250.

[83] Anini, Y., Hansotia, T., and Brubaker, P.L. Muscarinic receptors control postprandial release of glucagon-like peptide-1: in vivo and in vitro studies in rats. *Endocrinology* 2002;143:2420-2426.

[84] Elias, A.N., and Hofflich, H. Abnormalities in glucose metabolism in patients with schizophrenia treated with atypical antipsychotic medications. *Am. J. Med.* 2008;121:98-104.

[85] Tan, W., Fan, H., and Yu, P.H. Induction of subcutaneous adipose proliferation by olanzapine in rodents. *Prog. Neuropsychopharmacol. Biol. Psychiatry.* 2010;34:1098-1103.

[86] Sertie, A.L., Suzuki, A.M., Sertie, R.A., Andreotti, S., Lima, F.B., Passos-Bueno, M.R., and Gattaz, W.F. Effects of antipsychotics with different weight gain liabilities on human in vitro models of adipose tissue differentiation and metabolism. *Prog. Neuropsychopharmacol. Biol. Psychiatry.* 2011; 35:1884-90.

[87] Houseknecht, K.L., Robertson, A.S., Zavadoski, W., Gibbs, E.M., Johnson, D.E., and Rollema, H. Acute effects of atypical antipsychotics on whole-body insulin resistance in rats: implications for adverse metabolic effects. *Neuropsychopharmacology* 2007;32:289-297.

[88] Weisberg, S.P., McCann, D., Desai, M., Rosenbaum, M., Leibel, R.L., and Ferrante, A.W., Jr. Obesity is associated with macrophage accumulation in adipose tissue. *J. Clin. Invest.* 2003;112:1796-1808.

[89] Birkas Kovats, D., Palik, E., Faludi, G., and Cseh, K. [Possible connection between ghrelin, resistin and TNF-alpha levels and the metabolic syndrome caused by atypical antipsychotics]. *Neuropsychopharmacol. Hung.* 2005;7:132-139.

[90] Pollmacher, T., Hinze-Selch, D., Fenzel, T., Kraus, T., Schuld, A., and Mullington, J. Plasma levels of cytokines and soluble cytokine receptors during treatment with haloperidol. *Am. J. Psychiatry*. 1997;154:1763-1765.

[91] Meyer, J.M., McEvoy, J.P., Davis, V.G., Goff, D.C., Nasrallah, H.A., Davis, S.M., Hsiao, J.K., Swartz, M.S., Stroup, T.S., and Lieberman, J.A. Inflammatory markers in schizophrenia: comparing antipsychotic effects in phase 1 of the clinical antipsychotic trials of intervention effectiveness study. *Biol. Psychiatry*. 2009;66:1013-1022.

[92] Cooper, G.D., Harrold, J.A., Halford, J.C., and Goudie, A.J. Chronic clozapine treatment in female rats does not induce weight gain or metabolic abnormalities but enhances adiposity: implications for animal models of antipsychotic-induced weight gain. *Prog. Neuropsychopharmacol. Biol. Psychiatry*. 2008;32:428-436.

[93] von Wilmsdorff, M., Bouvier, M.L., Henning, U., Schmitt, A., and Gaebel, W. The impact of antipsychotic drugs on food intake and body weight and on leptin levels in blood and hypothalamic ob-r leptin receptor expression in wistar rats. *Clinics* (Sao Paulo) 2010;65:885-894.

[94] Jin, H., Meyer, J.M., Mudaliar, S., and Jeste, D.V. Impact of atypical antipsychotic therapy on leptin, ghrelin, and adiponectin. *Schizophr. Res*. 2008;100:70-85.

[95] Wampers, M., Hanssens, L., van Winkel, R., Heald, A., Collette, J., Peuskens, J., Reginster, J.Y., Scheen, A., and De Hert, M. Differential effects of olanzapine and risperidone on plasma adiponectin levels over time: Results from a 3-month prospective open-label study. *Eur. Neuropsychopharmacol.* 2011; 22:17-26.

[96] Reynolds, G.P., and Kirk, S.L. Metabolic side effects of antipsychotic drug treatment--pharmacological mechanisms. *Pharmacol. Ther.* 2010;125:169-179.

[97] Lauressergues, E., Martin, F., Helleboid, A., Bouchaert, E., Cussac, D., Bordet, R., Hum, D., Luc, G., Majd, Z., Staels, B., and Duriez, P. Overweight induced by chronic risperidone exposure is correlated with overexpression of the SREBP-1c and FAS genes in mouse liver. *Naunyn. Schmiedebergs. Arch. Pharmacol*. 2011;383:423-436.

[98] Lauressergues, E., Staels, B., Valeille, K., Majd, Z., Hum, D.W., Duriez, P., and Cussac, D. Antipsychotic drug action on SREBPs-related lipogenesis and cholesterogenesis in primary rat hepatocytes. *Naunyn. Schmiedebergs. Arch. Pharmacol.* 2010;81:427-439.

[99] Sentissi, O., Epelbaum, J., Olie, J.P., and Poirier, M.F. Leptin and ghrelin levels in patients with schizophrenia during different antipsychotics treatment: a review. *Schizophr. Bull.* 2008;34:1189-1199.

[100] Murashita, M., Kusumi, I., Hosoda, H., Kangawa, K., and Koyama, T. Acute administration of clozapine concurrently increases blood glucose and circulating plasma ghrelin levels in rats. *Psychoneuroendocrinology* 2007;32:777-784.

[101] van der Zwaal, E.M., Merkestein, M., Lam, Y.K., Brans, M.A., Luijendijk, M.C., Bok, L.I., Verheij, E.R., la Fleur, S.E., and Adan, R.A. The acute effects of olanzapine on ghrelin secretion, CCK sensitivity, meal size, locomotor activity and body temperature. *Int. J. Obes.* (Lond) 2011; 36:254-61.

In: Antipsychotic Drugs
Editors: T.L. Schwartz, J. Megna and M.E. Topel

ISBN: 978-1-62100-071-6

Chapter 10

PHARMACOGENETICS AND GENOMICS OF ANTIPSYCHOTIC-INDUCED WEIGHT GAIN AND OBESITY: AN INTEGRATED REVIEW

Yvon C. Chagnon*

Centre de Recherche de l'Institut Universitaire en Santé Mentale de Québec, Québec, Canada

ABSTRACT

Introduction: Excess body weight gain induced by antipsychotics (APS) is a major concern since the increasing use of these medications in multiple mental disorders including schizophrenia, bipolar disorder, autism, Tourette's syndrome, Attention-Deficit/Hyperactivity Disorder, Parkinson and Alzheimer diseases. Dramatically, the use of APS is also growing in children and adolescents where this side-effect could be devastating. The percentage of patients gaining excess weight following APS medication can reach up to 80% according to the APS used, with around 30% developing obesity that could contribute to medical morbidity. Multiple factors, genetic and environmental, play a role in individual susceptibility to gain excess weight with APS medication. The genetic analysis of adverse effects of APS on weight highlighted single nucleotide polymorphisms (SNP) within 32 associated genes, while 44 additional genes showed negative results. The most studied genes include the serotonin receptor 2C (HTR2C; 30 studies), leptin receptor (9 studies) and leptin (13 studies), the serotonin 2A receptor (7 studies), and the guanine nucleotide binding protein (G protein), beta polypeptide 3 (6 studies) and insulin induced gene 2 (5 studies). The adrenergic B3 and adrenergic alpha-2A receptors had 4 studies each.

Conclusion: Except for HTR2C, results are generally not well reproduced among studies, one or the other of the two alternative alleles being at risk across studies, and negative results being commonly observed. We can speculate that different genomic contexts and environmental conditions modulate the phenotype expression and produce these discrepancies. For instance, until recently rarely conducted, studies using genomic

*Tel: 418-663-5747 ext. 4717, Fax : 418-663-8756, E-Mail yvon.chagnon@crulrg.ulaval.ca

approaches such as genome-wide linkage and association studies have identified new candidate genes for APS-induced obesity such as the pro-melanin concentrating hormone. Genome-wide studies of RNA expression and DNA methylation, that are environmentally, epigenetic-induced DNA modifications affecting gene expression, are even more scarce, none reporting on APS side-effects. The simultaneous study of gene RNA expression and DNA methylation in response to APS, together with the analysis of structural variations such as SNPs, should integrate the genomic information needed to provide biomarkers of drug side-effect on body weight.

1. INTRODUCTION

1.1. Biological and Clinical Aspects of the Antipsychotics

In depression and schizophrenia, effective drug therapy is available, but 30% to 50% of all patients do not respond sufficiently to the initial treatment [1], with the identification of nonresponders taking 3 to 6 weeks. Moreover, severe side effects from correctly applied drug therapy have been repeatedly shown to be a major problem with considerable health burden and cost. [2-6] A new generation of antipsychotics (APS) allowed mitigation against major neuromotor abnormalities induced by first generation APS but substituted metabolic side effects such as excessive weight gain that contributes to non-compliance with treatment and may lead to medical morbidity when obesity is reached. [7] Mitigation of APS excess weight gain could be effected via the use of an alternative APS, which may be problematic for the therapy, and/or by dieting and physical activity programs that could, however, be difficult to initiate and maintain, or inefficient in some cases.

The use of APS concentrations below those used for acute treatment could also be a strategy for minimizing side effects [8] but should also be monitored closely for therapeutic efficiency. In any case, there is a need for an efficient way to predict the individual response of a patient to the prescribed APS at the initiation of treatment. A pharmacogenetics approach is expected to provide such a predictive tool [9, 10], particularly if based on genomic parameters integrating genetic and environmental information.

Demographic factors, diet, substance abuse, smoking, concomitant treatments, and comorbidities may all affect the actions of APS. [10] The relative importance of these factors in body weight gain following APS medication is controversial.

Gender, age, therapeutic response and clinical outcome, lower or higher baseline body mass index (BMI; kg/m2), paternal BMI, children or adolescent states, race and ethnicities could be involved, but not apparently APS history and doses nor illness duration. [11-20] Variable magnitude of weight gain is observed according to the APS used [11], the greatest gain being observed with olanzapine, which could also exceptionally induce a weight loss as reported in an adolescent [21], and with clozapine that is associated with a percentage of weight gain ranging between 13% to 85%. [22] In comparison, fluphenazine showed a range between 25% to 50% after one month to one year of treatment. [23] Ziprasidone induces the lowest weight gain, and molindone is associated with a reduction of weight. [11] The APS-induced weight gain could also reach a plateau as with olanzapine at approximately 36 weeks of up to three years of medication. [24] From these highly variable and controversial observations, it could be hypothesized that for patients biologically similar in age, gender, race and ethnicity, living within a particular environment and following similar eating and exercise practices, there are intrinsic characteristics that can explain the variable effects of any given APS, namely genetic factors.

1.2. Pharmacogenetics

Pharmacogenetics deals with the influence of genetic variation on drug response in patients by correlating DNA single-nucleotide polymorphisms (SNPs) and/or gene expression changes with a drug's efficacy or toxicity. There are many intricacies in the design and analysis of pharmacogenetic association studies, including having adequate power, selecting proper endpoints, detecting and correcting the effects of population stratification (races and ethnicities within races), modeling genetic and nongenetic covariates accurately, and validating the results. [25] Properly designed and analyzed pharmacogenetic association studies have the potential to improve the discovery, the development and, ultimately, the prescription and clinical usage of drugs by identifying DNA sequence variations that are associated with safety and efficacy of drugs.

However, at this point there are no formal guidelines on the design and analysis of pharmacogenetic studies. Usually, pharmacogenetic studies are case–control association studies looking at patients with and without a certain clinical response that are selected from a cohort being studied for clinical efficacy. They then usually correspond to hypothesis-testing studies assessing the potential of one or more genetic variants contributing to either drug response or another predefined endpoint. On the other hand, hypothesis generating studies focusing on discovery of genes and variations that impact a clinical endpoint are becoming more used. In a blind approach, these studies often test large numbers of genes and genetic variants covering the entire genome to investigate potential genetic effects, and this analysis of all the genome simultaneously is then called a pharmacogenomics study (see 3.0 below).

The intended use of the marker and regulatory implications often guide the design of the prospective test of the hypothesis. [26] Hence, biomarkers used for patient selection may be based on 1) better response observed among the biomarker positive group in pre-clinical or early phase trials, or 2) retrospective analysis of existing clinical trial data.

For the first category, common issues may include results extrapolation from pre-clinical data, using convenient, small sample size and non-representative patient samples, or questionable/incomplete clinical information. For the second category, common issues may include retrospective analysis without an *a priori* hypothesis, and "false positive" results from multiple comparisons.

Pharmacogenetics has been developed mostly based on a candidate gene approach. In these studies, genes showing affinity for the tested drugs or genes known to be involved in drug metabolism, such as the CYP450 genes family, or those genes suspected to be candidates for the disease were prime candidates for drug effects. This approach is theoretically valuable but suffers from many flaws as highlighted by the mitigated results observed where sensitivity and specificity of response prediction are generally low. Some factors could explain these poor results.

First, it could be that wrong candidate genes and/or not all genes involved in the drug response were identified and consequently included in the predictive model. Second, since drug response is a complex trait involving multiple genes and environmental factors such as diet and way of life, analyses integrating gene-gene and gene-environment interactions should be done systematically, and/or alternatively, the analysis of variables integrating these interactions such as RNA gene expression should be explored. Third, SNP markers used for association studies are genomic static markers that are not altered by environmental or biological changes such as aging, pathological states or medication. Therefore, if the effect of the drug is effected through an epigenetic modification of the DNA such as a methylation, it will 'not' be detected by a SNP analysis alone. [27]

2. RESULTS

2.1. Candidate Gene for the Antipsychotic-Induced Weight Gain

Table 1. presents the genes that have showed positive associations with APS-induced weight gain or other variables related to obesity, while Table 2 presents those genes giving negative association results. It has to be emphasized that the results included in these Tables are not necessarily exhaustive, and some studies and genes could be missing. However, they should be sufficient to provide a good overview of where we are and what is needed to progress in our comprehension of APS-induced excess weight gain.

All studies, except one in autistic children, were made on schizophrenic patients (SZ), some studies analyzing APS drug-naive SZ while others studied SZ that were switched to a different APS, or a group of patients taking various APS. Also, samples were generally comprised of a variable proportion of the two genders, and of single or multiple races and ethnicities. However, there is no clear evidence that these variable characteristics change the association results since positive and negative associations were observed for almost all situations (Table 1).

First, candidate genes analyzed were selected according to the putative mechanisms of action of APS (i.e.,genes originally candidates for SZ and the effect of APS), and according to those genes related to the APS kinetics such as their metabolizing enzymes. Genes involved in energy and food intake controls, in energy storage and in obesity in the general population were next selected.

2.1.1. Genes Related to the Mechanism of Action and the Kinetics of Antipsychotics

The mechanism of the effects of APS is probably multifactorial [28], and focused on serotonergic, dopaminergic, alpha adrenergic, muscarinic, histaminergic, and cholinergic neurotransmitter systems. [29, 30] Some 13 APS belonging to typical or atypical classes showed binding affinity for almost all the ten serotonergic receptors among which the 5-hydroxytryptamine (serotonin) receptors 1A (HTR1A), 2A (HTR2A), 2C (HTR2C) and 6 (HTR6), the five dopaminergic receptors DRD1 to DRD5, the five alpha-adrenergic receptors including ADRA1A, ADRA2A and ADRA2C, and the histamine receptor 1 (HRH1). However, they showed low affinity for other histaminic receptors including HRH2 and HRH3, the six nicotinic receptors, the two beta-adrenergic receptors including ADRB3, the cannabinoid receptor CNR1, and for the dopamine and serotonin (SLC6A4) transporters. [31]

Table 1. Candidate genes showing significant effect at p≤ 0.05 for the antipsychotic (APS) side effect on weight. Mixed gender samples of schizophrenic patients have been studied except when indicated. Number of different APS used among the patients are indicated between parentheses

Gene	Variant	Patients	APS	Effect	Risk allele	Ref
5-hydroxytryptamine (serotonin) receptor 2C (HTR2C)	rs3813928 (alias -997G/A)	128 Caucasian (German)	various (5)	No difference in weight change	na	(Opgen-Rhein et al. 2010)
		427 Caucasian	various (4+)	No difference in BMI	na	(Al-Janabi et al. 2009)
	rs3813929 (alias -759C/T)	96 Asian (Chinese)	various (5)	Smaller gain in BMI in T/TC than C/CC Greater frequency of C in 7% BMI gainers	C	(Reynolds et al. 2002)
		80 Caucasian / African-American	Clozapine	Greater weight gain in T than C for males	T	(Basile et al. 2002a)
		32 Asian (Chinese)	Clozapine	Smaller gain in BMI in T than C for males	C	(Reynolds et al.)
		42 Caucasian	Olanzapine	Greater frequency of C in 10% BMI gainers No difference in 5% and 7% BMI gainers	C	(Ellingrod et al. 2005)
		73 Caucasian	various (7)	Smaller gain in BMI in T/TC than C/CC Greater frequency of C in 7% BMI gainers	C	(Templeman et al. 2005)
		107 Caucasian	Olanzapine	Smaller frequency of T in 10% BMI gainers	C	(Godlewska et al. 2009)
		40 Caucasian / African-American / Hispanic	Clozapine	Smaller gain in percent BMI in T/TC than C/CC Smaller frequency of T in 7% BMI gainers	C	(Miller et al. 2005)
		123 Asian (Chinese)	Risperidone	Smaller gain in weight in T/TC	C	(Lane et al. 2006)

Table 1. (Continued)

Gene	Variant	Patients	APS	Effect	Risk allele	Ref
5-hydroxytryptamine (serotonin) receptor 2C (HTR2C)	rs3813929 (alias -759C/T)	588 Caucasian / African-American / Asian	various	Smaller gain in weight in T	C	(De Luca et al. 2007a)
		84 Asian (Korean)	various (5)	Smaller BMI in T than C Smaller frequency of T in 7% weight gainers	C	(Ryu et al. 2007)
		170 Asian (Chinese)	various	Greater frequency of C/CC in 7% weight gainers	C	(Shao et al. 2008)
		85 Asian (Chinese)	various	Greater frequency of C in 7% weight gainers	C	(Wu et al. 2011)
		32 Caucasian (autistic children)	Risperidone	Smaller gain in BMI for T carriers	C	(Hoekstra et al. 2010)
		392 Caucasian/Asian/African-American	Iloperidone	No difference in weight change	na	(Thompson et al. 2010)
		80 Asian (Chinese)	Clozapine	No difference in BMI change	na	(Tsai et al. 2002)
		97 Causasian	Clozapine	No difference in allele frequency for 7% BMI gainers	na	(Theisen et al. 2004)
		108 Caucasian (females only)	various (2)	No difference in allele frequency for 7% weight gainers	na	(Kuzman et al. 2008)
		79 Asian (Korean)	Olanzapine	No difference in 7% weight gainers	na	(Park et al. 2008)
		276 Caucasian / mixed	various (3+)	No difference with the presence of the metabolic syndrome	na	(Mulder et al. 2007)
		427 Caucasian	various (4+)	No difference in BMI	na	(Al-Janabi et al. 2009)
		128 Caucasian (German)	various (5)	No difference in weight gain	na	(Opgen-Rhein et al. 2010)
		146 Asian (Korean)	Clozapine	No difference in weight or waist	na	(Kang et al. 2011)

Gene	Variant	Patients	APS	Effect	Risk allele	Ref
5-hydroxytryptamine (serotonin) receptor 2C (HTR2C)	rs518147 (alias -697G/C)	170 Asian (Chinese)	various	Greater frequency of G/CG-GG in 7% weight gainers	G	(Shao et al. 2008)
		85 Asian (Chinese)	various	Greater frequency of G in 7% weight gainers	G	(Wu et al. 2011)
		107 Caucasian	Olanzapine	Smaller frequency of C in 10% BMI gainers	G	(Godlewska et al. 2009)
		276 Caucasian / mixed	various (3+)	No difference in the metabolic syndrome	na	(Mulder et al. 2007)
		146 Asian (Korean)	Clozapine	No difference in weight or waist	na	(Kang et al. 2011)
	rs6318 (Cys23Ser)	152 Caucasian	Clozapine	No difference in 7% and 10% BMI gainers	na	(Rietschel et al. 1997)
		80 Caucasian / African-American	Clozapine	No difference in weight change	na	(Basile et al. 2001a)
		93 Asian (Chinese)	Clozapine	No difference in percent weight change	na	(Hong et al. 2001)
		102 Caucasian (German)	various (17)	No difference in BMI change	na	(Popp et al. 2009)
		128 Caucasian (German)	various (5)	No difference in weight gain	na	(Opgen-Rhein et al. 2010)
		427 Caucasian	various (4+)	No difference in BMI	na	(Al-Janabi et al. 2009)
	rs1414334	276 Caucasian / mixed	various (3+)	Greater frequency of C with the presence of the metabolic syndrome	C	(Mulder et al. 2007)
	rs498177	456 Asian (Chinese)	various (3)	Greater percentage of CC in the presence of the metabolic syndrome	C	(Bai et al. 2011)
	rs498207	128 Caucasian (German)	various (5)	Greater weight gain in AA/A than GG/G	A	(Opgen-Rhein et al. 2010)

Table 1. (Continued)

Gene	Variant	Patients	APS	Effect	Risk allele	Ref
5-hydroxytryptamine (serotonin) receptor 2C (HTR2C)	rs543229	39 Caucasian	Clozapine	Greater waist circumference in: CC than TA/AA	C	(Chagnon 2009)
	rs5988087			TT than CT/CC	T	
	rs11167436			AA than CA/CC	A	
	Haplotype rs3813929 rs518147 rs1414334 142948 (GT)n	138 Caucasian / other	various (12)	Increased risk for the metabolic syndrome with the haplotype C/C/C/n13	C/C/C/n13	(Mulder et al. 2007)
	Haplotype rs3813929 rs518147 rs6318	46 Caucasian	various (2)	Greater frequency of the haplotype C/G /G in obese	C/G/G	(Gunes et al. 2008)
	Haplotype rs3813929 GT12-18/CT4-5	139 Caucasian / African-American	various (?)	No difference in weight gain	na	(De Luca et al. 2007b)
5-hydroxytryptamine (serotonin) receptor 2A (HTR2A)	rs6311 (alias -1438G/A)	84 Asian (Chinese)	Risperidone Chlorpromazine	No difference in weight gain	na	(Mou et al. 2005)
	rs6313 (alias 102T/C)	164 Asian (Japanese)	Olanzapine	Smaller percent BMI gain in CC	T	(Ujike et al. 2008)
		123 Asian (Chinese)	Risperidone	Smaller weight gain in CC than TT	T	(Lane et al. 2006)
		93 Asian	Clozapine	No difference in percent weight gain	na	(Hong et al. 2001)
		427 Caucasian	various (4+)	No difference in BMI	na	(Al-Janabi et al. 2009)
		80 Caucasian / African-American	Clozapine	No difference in weight gain	na	(Basile et al. 2001a)

Gene	Variant	Patients	APS	Effect	Risk allele	Ref
5-hydroxytryptamine (serotonin) receptor 2A (HTR2A)	rs2770296	34 Caucasian	Risperidone	Smaller BMI and waist circumference with T	C	(Chagnon 2009)
	rs6314 (His452Tyr)	80 Caucasian / African-American	Clozapine	No difference in weight gain	na	(Basile et al. 2001a)
5-hydroxytryptamine (serotonin) receptor 6 (HTR6)	267C/T	123 Asian (Chinese)	Risperidone	Weight gain greater in CC/CT than TT	C	(Lane et al. 2006)
		164 Asian (Japanese)	Olanzapine	No difference in percent BMI change	na	(Ujike et al. 2008)
		93 Asian	Clozapine	No difference in percent weight change	na	(Hong et al. 2001)
Serotonin transporter (SLC6A4)	rs4795541 (alias 5-HTT L/S)	94 Caucasian (females only)	Olanzapine	Greater gain in BMI for SS/S	S	(Bozina et al. 2007)
		427 Caucasian	various (4+)	Greater frequency of SS in BMI greater than 30 kg/m^2	S	(Al-Janabi et al. 2009)
		93 Asian	Clozapine	No difference in percent weight change	na	(Hong et al. 2001)
	rs8071667	235 Caucasian	various (4)	Greater BMI in TT than CT/CC	T	(Chagnon 2009)
	rs140700	56 Caucasian	Olanzapine	Greater BMI in GG than AG	G	
Histamine receptor H1 (HRH1)	rs346074 rs346070	430 Caucasian	various (5+)	Greater frequency of GG/CC than GA/CT than AA/TT with obesity	G/C	(Vehof et al. 2011)
	rs2067467 (Glu349Asp)	88 Asian	Clozapine	No difference in weight and BMI change, percent weight change	na	(Hong et al. 2002)
		85 Asian (Chinese)	various	No difference in 7% weight gainers	na	(Wu et al. 2011)
	rs2067470 (Leu449Ser)	164 Asian (Japanese)	Olanzapine	No difference in percent BMI change	na	(Ujike et al. 2008)

Table 1. (Continued)

Gene	Variant	Patients	APS	Effect	Risk allele	Ref
Leptin (LEP)	rs7799039 (alias – 2548A/G)	577 Asian (Taiwan)	Various (3+)	Greater BMI and waist circumference in AA than AG/GG	A	(Kuo et al. 2011)
		85 Asian (Chinese)	various	Greater frequency of A in 7% weight gainers	A	(Wu et al. 2011)
		128 Caucasian (German)	various (5)	Greater weight gain in AA/A than GG/G	A	(Opgen-Rhein et al. 2010)
		128 Asian (Chinese)	various (2)	Greater gain in BMI in AA than AG/GG	A	(Zhang et al. 2003a)
		102 Asian (Chinese)	Clozapine	Smaller gain in BMI in AA than AG/GG in males	G	(Zhang et al. 2007)
		74 Asian (Korean)	Olanzapine	Greater weight gain in AG than AA	G	(Kang et al. 2008)
		73 Caucasian	various (7)	Greater gain in BMI in GG than AG/AA	G	(Templeman et al. 2005)
		37 Caucasian	Olanzapine	Greater gain in BMI for G in LEPR rs113701 G carriers with a concentration of olanzapine greater than 20.6 ng/ml	G	(Ellingrod et al. 2007)
		134 Caucasian (Irish)	various (3)	Smaller BMI in AA than AG/GG in those also carrying CC at HTR2C rs3813929 C/T	G	(Yevtushenko et al. 2008)
		200 Caucasian (Dutch)	various (3)	No difference in weight	na	(Gregoor et al. 2011)
		205 Hispanic (Spanish)	various (6)	No difference in weight gain	na	(Perez-Iglesias et al. 2010)
		56 Hispanic (Venezualian)	Clozapine	No difference in weight, BMI, waist changes	na	(Fernandez et al. 2010)
	rs4731426	130 Asian (Indian)	Olanzapine	Weight gain	C	(Srivastava et al. 2008)

Gene	Variant	Patients	APS	Effect	Risk allele	Ref
Leptin receptor (LEPR)	rs1137101 (Gln223R)	101 Caucasian / African-American	Risperidone	Lower frequency of G in subjects weighting more than100 kg	A	(Ruano et al. 2007)
		200 Caucasian (Dutch)	various (3)	Greater weight in females carrying AA than GG	A	(Gregoor et al. 2011)
		37 Caucasian	Olanzapine	Greater gain in BMI for G in LEP rs7799039 G carriers with a concentration of olanzapine greater than 20.6 ng/ml	G	(Ellingrod et al. 2007)
		205 Hispanic (Spanish)	various (6)	No difference in weight gain	na	(Perez-Iglesias et al. 2010)
		577 Asian (Taiwan)	Various (3+)	No difference in BMI, waist circumference	na	(Kuo et al. 2011)
		56 Hispanic (Venezualian)	Clozapine	No difference in weight, BMI, waist change	na	(Fernandez et al. 2010)
	rs8179183 (Lys656Asn)	101 Caucasian / African-American	Risperidone	Lower frequency of G in subjects weighting more than100 kg	C	(Ruano et al. 2007)
		261 Caucasian (Belgium)	various (6+)	No difference in BMI, weight, waist changes	na	(Moons et al. 2011)
	rs7602, rs1171276	168 Caucasian / African-American / Hispanic / Others	various (2)	No difference in weight gainers	na	(Ruano et al. 2007)
Insulin induced gene 2 (INSIG2)	rs17587100	160 Caucasian (German)	Clozapine	Greater gain in BMI in CC than CA than AA	C	(Le Hellard et al. 2009)
		154 Caucasian / African-American	various (4)	No difference in weight change, percent of change and 7% change	na	(Tiwari et al. 2010)
		577 Asian (Taiwan)	Various (3+)	No difference in BMI or waist circumference	na	(Kuo et al. 2011)

Table 1. (Continued)

Gene	Variant	Patients	APS	Effect	Risk allele	Ref
Insulin induced gene 2 (INSIG2)	rs10490624	160 Caucasian (German)	Clozapine	No difference in BMI gain	na	{Le Hellard, 2009
		128 Caucasian (German)	various (5)	No difference in weight change	na	(Opgen-Rhein et al. 2010)
		154 Caucasian / African-American	various (4)	No difference in weight change, percent of change and 7% change	na	(Tiwari et al. 2010)
	rs17047764	160 Caucasian (German)	Clozapine	No difference in BMI gain	na	{Le Hellard, 2009
		128 Caucasian (German)	various (5)	No difference in weight change	na	(Opgen-Rhein et al. 2010)
		154 Caucasian / African-American	various (4)	No difference in weight change, percent of change and 7% change	na	(Tiwari et al. 2010)
	rs7566605	154 Caucasian / African-American	various (4)	No difference in weight change, percent of change and 7% change	na	(Tiwari et al. 2010)
		128 Caucasian (German)	various (5)	No difference in weight change	na	(Opgen-Rhein et al. 2010)
		756 European / African	various (?)	No difference in BMI change	na	(Skelly et al. 2007)
		577 Asian (Taiwan)	Various (3+)	No difference in BMI or waist circumference	na	(Kuo et al. 2011)
	rs889904	577 Asian (Taiwan)	Various (3+)	No difference in BMI or waist circumference	na	(Kuo et al. 2011)
Guanine binding protein 3 (GNB3)	rs5443 (alias 825C/T)	164 Asian (Japanese)	Olanzapine	Greater percentage of BMI gain in TT/TC	T	(Ujike et al. 2008)
		134 Asian (Chinese)	Clozapine	Greater weight gain in TT than TC/CC	T	(Wang et al. 2005b)
		402 Asian / Caucasian / African-American	various (2+)	Smaller BMI and weight gain in CC	T	(Souza et al. 2008)

Gene	Variant	Patients	APS	Effect	Risk allele	Ref
Guanine binding protein 3 (GNB3)	rs5443 (alias 825C/T)	104 Asian (Korean)	Olanzapine	No difference in weight and BMI	na	(Park et al. 2009)
		42 Caucasian	Olanzapine	No change in weight	na	(Bishop et al. 2006)
		87 Asian	Clozapine	No difference in weight and percent gain	na	(Tsai et al. 2004)
Cytochrome P450, family 2, subfamily D, polypeptide 6 (CYP2D6)	*1/*1, *1/*3, *4	11 Caucasian (males only)	Olanzapine	Greater gain in percent BMI in *1*3 and *4 than *1*1	*3, *4	(Ellingrod et al. 2002)
	188C/T	123 Asian (Chinese)	Risperidone	Lower weight gain in CC than CT than TT	T	(Lane et al. 2006)
	rs764481	56 Caucasian	Olanzapine	Greater BMI and waist circumference in GG than GA/AA	G	(Chagnon 2009)
Multidrug resistance p-glycoprotein (MDR1; alias ABCB1)	2677G/T 3435C/T	108 Caucasian	various (2)	Smaller frequency of G2677/C3435 in those with a percent gain in weight greater than 7%	T/T	(Kuzman et al. 2008)
Adiponectin, C1Q (ADIPOQ)	rs17300539	160 Caucasian (German)	Clozapine	Greater gain in BMI	A	(Jassim et al. 2011)
	276G/T	85 Asian (Chinese)	various	Greater frequency of G in 7% weight gainers	G	(Wu et al. 2011)
		164 Asian (Japanese)	Olanzapine	No difference in percent BMI change	na	(Ujike et al. 2008)
	45T/G	85 Asian (Chinese)	various	No difference in 7% weight gainers	na	(Wu et al. 2011)
Fat mass and obesity associated (FTO)	rs9922047	732 Caucasian / African-American / Other	various (5)	Greater gain in percent weight change in CG than CC/GG	CG	(Tiwari et al. 2011a)
	rs9939609	160 Caucasian (German)	Clozapine	No difference in BMI change	na	(Jassim et al. 2011)
		205 Hispanic (Spanish)	various (6)	No difference in weight change	na	(Perez-Iglesias et al. 2010)

Table 1. (Continued)

Gene	Variant	Patients	APS	Effect	Risk allele	Ref
Melanocortin receptor 4 (MC4R)	rs2229616	577 Asian (Taiwan)	Various (3+)	Greater waist circumference in CC/CT than TT	C	(Kuo et al. 2011)
	rs17782313			No difference in BMI, waist circumference	na	
Pro-melanin concentrating hormone (PMCH)	rs7973796	72 Caucasian (males only)	Olanzapine	Greater BMI in GG than AA	G	(Chagnon et al. 2007a)
Apolipoprotein A-IV (APOA4)	rs5092	67 Caucasian / African-American / Hispanic / Others	Olanzapine	Greater weight gain with G	G	(Ruano et al. 2007)
	rs675	168 Caucasian / African-American / Hispanic / Others	various (2)	No difference in weight gain	na	
Apolipoprotein E (APOE)	rs7412 (Arg176Cys)	67 Caucasian / African-American / Hispanic / Others	Olanzapine	Greater frequency of C in those ≥100 kg	C	(Ruano et al. 2007)
	rs405509 rs439401 rs446037 rs429358	168 Caucasian / African-American / Hispanic / Others	various (2)	No difference in weight gain	na	
Fatty acid amide hydrolase (FAAH)	rs324420 (Pro129Tyr) (alias 385C/A)	83 Caucasian	various (5)	Greater frequency of A in 7% weight gainers	A	(Monteleone et al. 2010)
		164 Asian (Japanese)	Olanzapine	No difference in percent BMI change	na	(Ujike et al. 2008)
Scavenger receptor class B, member 1 (SCARB1)	rs4765623	67 Caucasian / African-American / Hispanic / Others	Olanzapine	Greater weight gain with T	T	(Ruano et al. 2007)
	rs11057830	39 Caucasian	Clozapine	Greater waist circumference in AA than AG/GG	A	(Chagnon 2009)
	rs10846744	168 Caucasian / African-American / Hispanic / Others	various (2)	No difference in weight gain	na	(Ruano et al. 2007)

Gene	Variant	Patients	APS	Effect	Risk allele	Ref
Paraoxonase 1 (PON1)	rs705381	101 Caucasian / African-American	Risperidone	Greater frequency of G in those of ≥100 kg	G	(Ruano et al. 2007)
	rs662, rs854572, rs3917550	168 Caucasian / African-American / Hispanic / Others	various (2)	Weight gain	na	
Adrenergic alpha-2A receptor (ADRA2A)	rs1800544 (alias -1291C/G)	93 Asian (Chinese)	Clozapine	Greater weight gain in GG than CC Greater frequency of G in 7% weight gainer	G	(Wang et al. 2005a)
		62 Asian (Chinese)	Olanzapine	Greater weight gain in GG than GC/CC Greater frequency of G in 10% weight gainer	G	(Park et al. 2006)
		139 Caucasian / African-American / Hispanic / Others	various (4)	No difference in weight gain	na	(De Luca et al. 2011)
	rs7096359	35 Caucasian	Risperidone	Smaller BMI in TT than TC/CC	C	(Chagnon 2009)
Adrenergic B3 receptor (ADRB3)	rs4994 (Trp64Arg)	164 Asian (Japanese)	Olanzapine	Greater percent BMI change in ArgArg	CC	(Ujike et al. 2008)
		87 Asian	Clozapine	No difference in weight and percent change	na	(Tsai et al. 2004)
		80 African-American / Caucasian	Clozapine	No difference in weight change	na	(Basile et al. 2001a)
		139 Caucasian / African-American / Hispanic / Others	various (4)	No difference in weight gain	na	(De Luca et al. 2011)

Table 1. (Continued)

Gene	Variant	Patients	APS	Effect	Risk allele	Ref
Dopamine receptor D2 (DRD2)	rs4436578 12 SNPs	479 Asian (Chinese)	various (3)	Greater risk of weight gain in CC then TC/TT	C	(Hong et al. 2010)
	rs1799732 (alias −141C Ins/Del)	58 Caucasian/African-American/ Asian/Hispanic/Other	various (2)	Greater weight gain in carriers of -141C Del	-141C Del	(Lencz et al. 2010)
	rs1079598	206 Caucasian/African-American	various (4)	Greater frequency of C in 7% weight gainer	C	(Muller et al. 2010)
	Ser311Cys	164 Asian (Japanese)	Olanzapine	No difference in percent BMI change	na	(Ujike et al. 2008)
		123 Asian (Chinese)	Risperidone	No difference in weight change	na	(Lane et al. 2006)
Dopamine receptor D4 (DRD4)	48bp VNTR E3	102 Caucasian (German)	various (17)	Smaller frequency of 7-fold repeat in smaller BMI change for males	not 7-fold repeat	(Popp et al. 2009)
	3 SNPs	58 Caucasian/African-American/ Asian/Hispanic/Other	various (2)	No difference in weight change	na	(Muller et al. 2010)
	48 bp VNTR E3 12 bp E1 13 bp Del E1 Gly11Arg E	149 Caucasian	Clozapine	No difference in weight change	na	(Rietschel et al. 1996)
Neuropeptide Y receptor Y5 (NPY5R)	rs6837793	101 Caucasian / African-American	Risperidone	Greater frequency of G in those of ≥100 kg	G	(Ruano et al. 2007)
	rs11100494	168 Caucasian / African-American / Hispanic / Others	various (2)	Weight gain	na	
Brain derived neurotrophic factor (BDNF)	rs6265 (Val66Met)	196 Asian (Chinese)	various (7)	Greater BMI gain in AA for males	A	(Zhang et al. 2008)
		123 Asian (Chinese)	Risperidone	Smaller weight gain in AA than GG	G	(Lane et al. 2006)
Solute carrier family 30 member 8 (SLC30A8)	rs13269119	732 Caucasian / African-American / Other	various (5)	Greater gain in percent weight change in GG the CG than CC	G	(Tiwari et al. 2011a)

Gene / Chr	Variant	Patients	APS	Effect	Risk allele	Ref
Potassium Channel Inwardly Rectifying Subfamily J Member11 (KCNJ11)	rs2237988			Greater gain in percent weight change in TT than CT/CC	T	
Glucocorticoid receptor (NR3C1)	rs6196	261 Caucasian (Belgium)	various (6+)	Greater BMI and waist in G	G	(Moons et al. 2011)
	rs6190, rs6195, rs258751			No difference in BMI, weight, waist changes	na	
Synaptosomal-associated protein, 25kDa (SNAP25)	DdeI T/C MnlI T/G TaiI T/C	162 Caucasian	various (5)	Greater weight gain in DdeI CC/TC than TT	C	(Musil et al. 2008)
	rs6077693	35 Caucasian	Risperidone	Smaller waist circumference in AA than AG/GG	G	(Chagnon 2009)
	rs363040			Smaller waist circumference in TT than GT/GG	G	
	DdeI T/C MnlI T/G TaiI T/C	59 Caucasian	various (4)	No difference in weight change	na	(Muller et al. 2005b)
	401C/T 1065T/G 1069T/C	164 Asian (Japanese)	Olanzapine	No difference in percent BMI change	na	(Ujike et al. 2008)

Table 1. (Continued)

Gene / Chr	Variant	Patients	APS	Effect	Risk allele	Ref
GWA	492K SNPs	738 Caucasian / African-American / others	various (6)			(Adkins et al. 2011)
Meis homeobox 2 (MEIS2)	rs1568679		Risperidone	C greater gain in BMI	C	
Protein kinase cAMP-dependent regulatory type II beta (PRKAR2B)	rs13224682		Clozapine	G greater gain in BMI	G	

Table 2. Non-significant effect at p≤ 0.05 of different candidate genes for antipsychotics (APS) side effect on weight

Gene	Name	Variant	Patients	APS	Phenotype	Ref
TNFA	Tumor necrosis factor, alpha	-308G/A	80 Caucasian / African-American	Clozapine	Weight change	(Basile et al. 2001a)
			247Caucasian / African-American / others	mixed	Weight change	(Zai et al. 2006)
		-308G/A, -857C/T	164 Asian (Japanese)	Olanzapine	Percent BMI change	(Ujike et al. 2008)
TNFRSF1A	Tumor necrosis factor receptor superfamily, member 1A	38A/G	164 Asian (Japanese)	Olanzapine	Percent BMI change	(Ujike et al. 2008)
TNFRSF1B	Tumor necrosis factor receptor superfamily, member 1B	Met196Arg				
GHRL	Ghrelin/obestatin prepropeptide	Leu72Met				
		rs26312	168 Caucasian / African-American / Hispanic / Others	various (2)	Weight gain	(Ruano et al. 2007)
PPARG	Peroxisome proliferator-activated receptor gamma	rs1805192 (Pro12Ala)	164 Asian (Japanese)	Olanzapine	Percent BMI change	(Ujike et al. 2008)
		161C/T	146 Asian (Korean)	Clozapine	Weight, waist	(Kang et al. 2011)
PPARA	Peroxisome proliferator-activated receptor alpha	V227A				

Table 2. (Continued)

Gene	Name	Variant	Patients	APS	Phenotype	Ref
FABP3	Fatty acid-binding protein 3	7 SNPs	160 Caucasian (German)	Clozapine	BMI change	(Jassim et al. 2011)
PRKAA1	Protein kinase, AMP-activated, alpha 1 catalytic subunit	5 SNPs				
PRKAA2	Protein kinase, AMP-activated, alpha 2 catalytic subunit	9 SNPs				
PRKAB1	Protein kinase, AMP-activated, beta 1 non-catalytic subunit	3 SNPs				
PRKAG1	Protein kinase, AMP-activated, gamma 1 non-catalytic subunit	4 SNPs				
PRKAG2	Protein kinase, AMP-activated, gamma 2 non-catalytic subunit	33 SNPs				
PRKAG3	protein kinase, AMP-activated, gamma 3 non-catalytic subunit	2 SNPs				
CCK	Cholecystokinin	2 SNPs	215 Caucasian	various (2)	Percent weight change	(Tiwari et al. 2011b)
CCKA	Cholecystokinin A receptor	4 SNPs				
CCKB	Cholecystokinin B receptor	4SNPs, CTn				

Gene	Name	Variant	Patients	APS	Phenotype	Ref
CHRM3	Muscarinic acetylcholine receptor M3	rs3738435	430 Caucasian	various (5+)	BMI, obesity	(Vehof et al. 2011)
SH2B1	Src homology 2	rs7498665	205 Hispanic (Spanish)	various (6)	Weight gain	(Perez-Iglesias et al. 2010)
PNLIP (alias Tag Lipase)	Pancreatic lipase	rs2915748, rs2234972	130 Asian (Indian)	Olanzapine	Weight gain	(Srivastava et al. 2008)
CL	Citrate lyase	rs2304497				
LPL	Lipoprotein lipase	rs320, rs285, rs4922115, rs328, rs326				
APOA1	Apolipoprotein A1	rs5070, rs4225	168 Caucasian / African-American / Hispanic / Others	various (2)	Weight gain	(Ruano et al. 2007)
APOA2	Apolipoprotein A2	rs5085				
APOB	apolipoprotein B	rs3791981, rs1801701, rs676210				
NPY	neuropeptide Y	rs1468271				
SCARB2	Scavenger receptor class B, member 2	rs3853188, rs894251				
GAL	Galanin	rs694066				
MC3R	Melanocortin receptor-3	rs3746619	261 Caucasian (Belgium)	various (6+)	BMI, weight, waist changes	(Moons et al. 2011)
PER2	Period 2	rs934945				
SDC3	Syndecan 3	rs4949184, rs2282440				

Table 2. (Continued)

Gene	Name	Variant	Patients	APS	Phenotype	Ref
CNR1	Cannabinoid receptor 1	1359G/A	83 Caucasian	various (5)	Weight change	(Monteleone et al. 2010)
HTR1A	5-hydroxytryptamine (serotonin) receptor 1A	CA	80 Caucasian / African-American	Clozapine	Weight change	(Basile et al. 2001a)
CYP1A2	Cytochrome P450, subfamily I, polypeptide 2	IVS1 CA				
HRH2	Histamine receptor H2	-1018G/A	80 Caucasian / African-American	Clozapine	Weight change	(Basile et al. 2001a)
			164 Asian (Japanese)	Olanzapine	Percent BMI change	(Ujike et al. 2008)
HRH3	Histamine receptor H3	Ser332Ser	164 Asian (Japanese)	Olanzapine	Percent BMI change	(Ujike et al. 2008)
DRD1, 3, 5	Dopamine receptor D1, D3, D5	3, 14, 3 SNPs	58 Caucasian/African-American/ Asian/Hispanic/Other	various (2)	Weight gain	(Muller et al. 2010)
TPH2	Tryptophan hydroxylase subtype 2	-366T/C, -8933A/G	427 Caucasian	various (4+)	BMI	(Al-Janabi et al. 2009)
ADRA1A	Adrenergic, alpha-1A-receptor	rs1048101 (Arg347Cys)	80 Caucasian / African-American	Clozapine	Weight change	(Basile et al. 2001a)
			139 Caucasian / African-American / Hispanic / Others	various (4)	Weight gain	(De Luca et al. 2011)
		-563C/T, -4155G/C, -4884A/G	427Caucasian	mixed	BMI	(Saiz et al. 2008)
ADRA2C	Adrenergic, alpha-2C-receptor	rs11269124	139 Caucasian / African-American / Hispanic / Others	various (4)	Weight gain	(De Luca et al. 2011)
MAOA	monoamine oxidase A	u-VNTR, rs6323				
COMT	catechol-O-methyl transferase	rs4680 (Val108/158Met)				
DBH	dopamine b-hydroxylase	rs251915 (alias TaqIB), (GT)n, 19bp Ins/Del				

Table 3. Expression for several genes and variants related to APS-induced weight

Gene	Variants	Samples	Effects	Ref
Serotonin receptor 2C	−759C/T −697G/C	SH-SY5Y neuroblastoma cell lines	Lower expressions for -759T and -697C	(Hill and Reynolds 2007)
	6 haplotypes −1165A/G −1028GT −997G/A −759C/T	Cell lines : -HEK293t (human embryo kidney) -TE671 (medulloblastoma/rhabdomyosarcoma	Lower expression for haplotypes containing the -759C than T allele, and for −997A allele	(Buckland et al. 2005)
Serotonin receptor 2A	−1438A/G	SH-SY5Y neuroblastoma and HeLa cell lines	-1438G lower level	(Parsons et al. 2004)
		human fibroblast cell lines	-1438G lower level	(Myers et al. 2007)
	rs6313 (102T/C)	-Prefrontal cortex of post-mortem brain from SZ -Peripheral blood lymphocytes controls	-102C lower level than 102T -monoallelic expression : 102T (19% of subjects), 102C (29%) -unequal biallelic expression in 52% of subjects (102C 10%-81% of HTR2A expression level)	(Fukuda et al. 2006)
		Temporal cortex of post-mortem brain from SZ or controls	102C lower level than 102T (ratio 0.8)	(Polesskaya and Sokolov 2002)
		Temporal cortex of post-mortem brain (American) Peripheral leukocytes (Russian)	2 CpG sites specific to 102C methylated in proportion of level of expression	(Polesskaya et al. 2006)
		Postmortem brain from suicidals and controls	102C lower level	(Turecki et al. 1999)
	His452Tyr	blood platelets	lower level 452Tyr	(Ozaki et al. 1997)

Table 3. (Continued)

Gene	Variants	Samples	Effects	Ref
Serotonin transporter	5HTTLPR S/L	control lymphoblast cell lines	-S had a lower amounts of mRNA transcription than L -CpG methylation higher and mRNA production lower in females than males	(Philibert et al. 2008)
Dopamine receptor 3, 5	na	-Blood lymphocytes from SZ receiving APS for 3 years, free for 3 months, naive or from controls	Lower expression of DRD3 and DRD5 in those free for 3 months but higher in those of 3 years of medication. No effect in drug-naive subjects.	(Kwak et al. 2001)
Histamine H1 receptor	na	Cell lines : -human airway smooth muscle_HASM -bronchial epithelial cell line [BEAS2B) Others : -primary cultured bronchial epithelial cells -placenta -brain	Variable and specific expression of different H1R1 isoforms according to tissues	(Swan et al. 2006)
Genes associated with weight gain (Table 1)	na	Immortalized lymphocyte cell lines from SZ being obese or not while taking APS and stimulated with a clinical dose of olanzapine	Lower expression in obese: -Paraoxonase 1 -Potassium Channel Inwardly Rectifying Subfamily J Member11 -Protein kinase cAMP-dependent regulatory type II beta Higher expression in obese: -Adrenergic alpha-2A receptor	(Chagnon 2007b)

Tables 1. and 2. reported association results including some of the previous genes for which the abbreviations are given, that were investigated for APS-induced weight gain. Among these genes, the three serotonergic genes showing affinity for APS (HTR2A, HTR2C and HTR6) also showed positive association with APS-induced weight gain (Table 1), while HTR1A showed no association (Table 2). Even if showing low affinity for APS, the serotonin transporter SLC6A4 was positively associated (Table 1). Similarly, among the five dopaminergic receptors, the three alpha-adrenergic receptors and the histaminic receptor showing good affinity for APS, only DRD2, DRD4, ADRA2A and HRH1 have some association with APS-induced weight gain (Table 1), but not DRD1, 3, 5, ADRA1A and ADRA2C (Table 2). As expected, because of their low affinity for APS, HRH2 and HRH3, ADRB3 and CNR1 showed no association with APS-induced weight gain (Table 2). From these results it can be seen that the level of affinity of a receptor for APS will not necessarily be predictive of its association with APS effect, and conversely, its low affinity, as with the serotonin transporter SLC6A4, of its absence of association. However, as illustrated below, the interpretation of these negative and positive results could change if more studies are conducted which reveal the complexity of the factors involved.

2.1.2. Serotonin Receptors

2.1.2.1. Serotonin HTR2C Receptor

Of all the genes studied in relation to APS-induced weight gain, HTR2C, located on human chromosome Xq24, is the most studied, mostly the –759C/T variant, now named rs3813929 and located in the promoter region of HTR2C. HTR2C has been evaluated in 30 different studies, including 24 positive associations and 20 negative ones, with more than one marker being evaluated in several studies (see Table 1). HTR2C was the first gene, together with CYP2P6 [32], to be reported associated with APS-induced weight gain by Reynolds et al [33]. In their study of a mixed gender sample of Asian Chinese SZ patients, they reported a lower susceptibility to gain weight while taking APS in those SZ carrying the T allele at the variant -759C/T. They reported an APS–induced weight gain three times lower (ΔBMI 0.41±1.02) in those carrying the -759T variant allele than in those not-carrying the T allele (ΔBMI 1.38±1.21; p=0.0003). Later, they confirmed their result, but in males only, in first-episode Chinese patients (ΔBMI=0.03±0.72 vs 1.26±0.90; p=0.008). [34] In contrast, Basile et al. [35] reported an opposite borderline significant result (p=0.05) where carriers of the –759T allele showed a higher weight gain than non-carriers (ΔBW=7.2±3.9 and 3.6±4.9). However, in the following years, ten additional studies confirmed that carriers of the -759T allele gain less weight while taking APS medication than non-carriers in various races and ethnies, and for different APS (Table 1). On the other hand, eight other studies reported no effect at all of the -759T/C variant on APS-induced weight gain (Table 1). Despite these contradictory results, it is highly probable that the HTR2C -759C/T polymorphism is involved in the control of weight gain in the presence of APS, but additional unknown factors modulating its effect in the different samples studied should also be present.

This conclusion is supported by the fact that the -759T/C variant is a functional variant with haplotypes containing the -759C allele showing *in vitro* less transcriptional activity than the -759T allele [36], but the inverse was also reported with the -759T allele showing a lower activity, the discrepancies between the two results being explained by the different cell type used for the test. [37, 38] The HTR2C KO mice, that have no HTR2C activity at all, overeat and become obese [39] while stimulating HTR2C with an agonist decreases food intake [40]. From these findings, it could be hypothesized that the known antagonistic effect of APS on HTR2C receptors lowers even more their activity in the -759C allele carriers reaching a level sufficiently low to produce an effect similar to that which is observed in the HTR2C KO mice, i.e., excess weight gain, while carriers of the -759T, allele showing a higher intrinsic activity, are more resistant to their APS antagonistic effect. However, decreased HTR2C RNA expression and altered RNA editing observed in SZ was not related to genetic variations at HTR2C, as evaluated in post-mortem brain, and the authors concluded that independent factors may contribute to the altered HTR2C expression in SZ brains. [41] RNA editing alter DNA splicing and produce different HTR2C isoforms [42] that could have very different properties in their expression over time and in different tissues potentially generating significant functional variation. [43, 44] Alternative splicing is not unusual since the majority of the known genes show it. [45] A mechanism that could alter gene splicing is the environmentally or epigenetic-induced DNA methylation as observed for HTR2A (see below), which is believed to contribute to drug tolerance in some cases. [46]

For its part, the Cys23Ser substitution (rs6318) is encoded in exon 4 and its product is located in the extracellular N-terminus of the protein. The variant Ser23 allele showed reduced affinity binding to serotonin and required higher 5-HT concentrations to induce the same intracellular Ca2+ peak as the Cys23 allele. [47] The Ser23 allele is also constitutively more active than Cys23 [47] and displays a faster and stronger ACTH response to m-chlorophenylpiparezine (mCPP) challenge, an agonist of the HTR2C receptor (48). A reduced hypophagic response to mCPP has been observed in a group of normal female subjects who are carriers of the Ser23 allele. [49] Accordingly, an effect of the Cys23Ser variant on APS-induced weight gain was expected but this was not the case in the six different studies reported (Table 1). Similarly, the polymorphism -997G/A (rs3813928) shows a reduced expression in carriers of the A allele (36) but was not associated with APS-induced change in body weight in two studies (Table 1). The results from these two variants highlight that the analysis of a functional variant does not presage positive association results.

Finally, nine other SNPs or markers, all of them except one (rs498207) being located in introns of HTR2C, were studied individually or combined in haplotypes including the variant –759C/T. Eleven studies reported positive associations with APS-induced weight gain with four negative results (Table 1). These data strengthen previous conclusions that HTR2C is involved in APS-induced weight gain.

2.1.2.2. Serotonin HTR2A Receptor

HTR2A is very central to APS action showing affinities for most of them. (31) Four non-synonymous HTR2A SNPs (Thr25Asn, Ile197Val, Ala447Val, and His452Tyr) were evaluated for APS affinity and potency changes and Ile197Val and His452Tyr exhibited changes for both while Thr25Asn was associated with affinity and Ala447Val for potency only [6]. Interestingly, His452Tyr showed no association with APS-induced weight gain (Table 1) despite its effect on APS affinity and potency, while the other three SNPs are yet to be evaluated.

Two studies reported that the CC genotype of the 102T/C variant, now named rs6313, located in an intron of HTR2A, was associated with a smaller weight gain compared to TT, while three other studies showed no association for this variant (Table 1). Unexpectedly, the

CC genotype of this intronic variant showed lower levels of expression than the TT genotype in SZ and normal individuals, either as monoallelic or unequal biallelic expression [50, 51] (Table 3). This is a consequence of a specific methylation of the C allele. [52] In HTR2A KO mice, with no expression of HTR2A, a higher locomotor activity is observed [53]. It can then be hypothesized that individuals with two C alleles, because of a lower HTR2A expression, are more active which induces a lower weight gain with APS. In contrast, it also has been reported that TT subjects showed a lower BMI than those with CT and CC genotypes because of a differential eating behavior of increasing protein intake that favors a lower body weight. [54] In APS-induced weight gain, we can speculate that this effect on eating behavior could be counterbalanced by APS that are known to stimulate appetite. [55] Again, opposing results observed for the same variant of a gene indicates that additional unknown factors are involved. Two other SNPs give either a positive or a negative association (Table 1).

2.1.2.3. Serotonin HTR6 Receptor and Serotonin Transporter SLC6A4

HTR6 has excitatory effects on cortical neurons and appears to be expressed to a greater degree in inhibitory interneuron's of the cerebral cortex. [56] Few studies have investigated HTR6 variants in relation to APS response [57-60] and even fewer in relation to APS-induced weight gain. One of three studies in Asian populations, analyzing the same 267C/T variant for three different APS, reported a greater weight gain in CC carriers for those taking risperidone in contrast to olanzapine or clozapine (Table 1). However, it is clear from results of previous genes that a greater number of studies is needed to be able to conclude there is a sustained HTR6 effect on APS-induced weight.

For its part, the serotonin transporter SLC6A4 and more particularly its variant characterized by a short and a long repeat allele, has showed a greater weight gain for its short allele variant. (Table 1). For instance, in control lymphoblast cell lines the short allele had a lower amount of mRNA transcription than the long one (Table 3) that could be reinforced by an antagonistic effect of APS. SLC6A4 also showed a higher CpG methylation and a lower mRNA production in females than in males [61] that could eventually be important for APS-induced weight gain.

2.1.3. Other Receptors

Histaminergic neurotransmission is crucial in conveying the effect of leptin since inhibition of histamine antagonizes leptin-induced reduction of food intake in mice. [62] The analysis of the histamine receptor H1 (HRH1) was of particular interest because of its relatively high affinity for almost all APS [31] and its possible direct involvement in body weight gain with APS. [63] However, very few studies have analyzed HRH1 in relation to APS-induced weight gain. From four studies, only one presents a positive association (Table 1) while the two other histaminic receptor studies on HRH2 and HRH3 are negative (Table 2). Additional association studies are needed, particularly for HRH1.

2.2. Metabolizing Enzymes CYP450

Genetic variations in drug metabolizing enzymes modify their activity and the corresponding drugs' therapeutic outcome and/or side effects. Among genes involved in the pharmacokinetics of APS are the cytochrome P450 CYP2D6, CYP1A2 and CYP3A4. [64] The therapeutic level of clozapine is determined in part by the activities of liver isozymes CYP1A2 and CYP3A4, while haloperidol and the risperidone clearances are determined by the number of active CYP2D6 genes [65, 66]. Significant differences have been reported in plasma concentrations of haloperidol at low dosages (<20 mg daily) among CYP2D6 genotypes in Korean SZ [67], and one study showed that CYP2D6 genotypes could be a good predictor of adverse events following haloperidol administration. [65] Only CYP2D6 and CYP1A2 have been studied for APS-induced weight gain, with CYP2D6 providing positive associations in the three studies reported (Table 1) but with three different markers excluding a direct reciprocal confirmation of the associations observed. For its part, CYP1A2 showed negative results (Table 2). CYP7A1 and CYP19 have been associated with BMI [68,69] and CYP19 with abdominal obesity [70], and fat loss following exercise [71], but have not been studied yet for APS-induced weight gain. Once again, in spite of the central role of this category of enzymes in drug metabolism, very few results have been reported.

2.3. Genes Related to Obesity

Theisen et al. [72] have tested affinity for the three APS: clozapine, olanzapine and haloperidol at 14 selected receptors involved in body weight regulation, including the anorexigenic cholecystokinin (CCK) and melanocortin-4 (MC4R) receptors, the orexigenic cannabinoid receptor 1 (CNR1), as well as receptors involved in physiological actions related to digestion and fluid, but not the leptin receptor LEPR. The only tested receptor that showed some APS affinity was the melanin-concentrating hormone receptor for haloperidol. [72] This supports our reported association of the gene encoding the pro-melanin concentrating hormone that is an agonist of this receptor with obesity even if our result was observed for olanzapine. [73] In contrast, these results do not support the hypothesis of a possible effect of APS on weight via these metabolic receptors. For instance, only very recently MC4R showed a positive association with waist circumference in APS medicated SZ in one study (74) (Table 1), while CCK receptors A and B and CNR1 showed no association (Table 2). Other genes have not been tested yet to our knowledge, but without further evidences the aforementioned do not represent, at this time, strong candidate genes for APS-induced weight gain and obesity.

2.3.1. The Leptin (LEP) Gene and Its Receptor (LEPR)

In body weight control, leptin is a central hormone secreted by adipose tissue which transmits to the brain the level of stored fat. Leptin levels were shown to be varied in the presence of APS [75-79] equalizing the natural level difference observed between genders. [80] However, it has to be elucidated if it is a direct effect of APS or in response to the weight gain per se. Almost all, except one of the 13 studies reporting on the leptin gene, analyzed the −2548A/G variant, now named rs7799039, that is located proximal to a binding site for the Sp1 transcription factor in the promoter region. rs7799039 is associated with the transcriptional activity showing a higher expression in the presence of the GG genotype. [81, 82] In contrast to HTR2C, the two alleles of this SNP showed about the same number of positive associations with APS-induced weight gain i.e. four studies with the A allele originally found to be associated [83], five studies with the G allele, and three negative results

(Table 1). Again, no apparent effect of race, ethnicity, nor of the APS used was detected. These opposing results of APS-induced weight gain with respect to one or the other of the A or G alleles of -2548A/G have to be put into their genomic context, meaning that the association of LEP with this phenotype is probably real but requires the expression of some specific interactions with other genes or environmental factors. Then, it will be of great interest to evaluate other genes, and the expression of individual allelic and isoforms in relation to the possible methylation of LEP and other genes in these patients.

For the leptin receptor, the non-synonymous SNP rs1137101 (changing the encoded amino acid glutamine at position 223 for an arginine) showed association either with its A or G allele, while the SNP rs8179183 (changing the lysine 656 for an asparagine) showed one positive and one negative association (Table 1). Carriers of the Arg223 or G allele showed a lower level of leptin [84] that is consistent with the association of this allele with APS-induced weight gain. However, the two other positive studies showed associations with the A allele (Table 1) while exhibiting normal leptin levels. Also, it is not clear at this point how APS could alter LEP and LEPR expression and functions since associations with both alleles are observed for both gene variants.

2.3.2. The Insulin Induced Gene 2 (INSIG2)

Insulin induced gene 2 (INSIG2) is present in the endoplasmic reticulum and mediates feedback control of cholesterol synthesis. [85] One of the SNP analyzed, rs7566605, is located 10 kb upstream of INSIG2 and has been associated in a whole genome association study with BMI in the general population. [86] Over the fourteen analyses using five different SNPs in five studies, only the original study of Le Hellard [87] yielded a positive association with APS-induced greater BMI (Table 1). It could be hypothesized that these overall negative results come from the analysis of morphometric variables such as weight, BMI or waist circumference while INSIG2 is more related to cholesterol level control. From these results, it is likely that INSIG2 is not or is weakly related to APS-induced weight gain.

2.3.3. The Guanine Binding Protein 3 (GNB3)

G proteins are important regulators of the specificity and temporal characteristics of cellular signaling. The 825C/T variant, located in exon 10 of GNB3 (rs5443), does not change the amino acid serine at position 275 but is associated with the occurrence of a splice variant of exon 9 lacking nucleotides 498–620 that is translated into a truncated beta3 subunit [88]. This 825T variant allele was associated with increased signal transduction, ion transport into the cell and enhanced G-protein signaling. [89, 90] The 825T allele was also associated with pathophysiological conditions such as obesity. [91, 92] In APS-induced obesity, three studies showed a consistent association of the same 825T allele with a greater weight or BMI while three others did not (Table 1). These results support that GNB3 could be related to greater APS-induced weight, particularly in Asian populations. However, more studies are needed in Asians and other races to confirm this possible racial effect.

2.3.4. The Dopaminergic Genes

Despite that almost all antipsychotics bind to the dopamine D2 receptor (DRD2), it is noteworthy that this receptor, until recently, was poorly investigated for APS-induced weight gain. The 5′ promoter region contains the variant −141C Ins/Del, now named rs1799732, which alters gene expression *in vitro* and striatal receptor density *in vivo.* [93 , 94] This, and two other variants of DRD2, have shown only recently an association with APS-induced weight gain (Table 1), as well as DRD4 that showed one positive and one negative result (Table 1). A second DRD2 non-synonymous variant Ser311Cys was not associated with APS weight gain in two studies (Table 1). DRD1, DRD3 and DRD5 showed negative results in a single study (Table 2). DRD3 was for a long time considered as central to APS effect, and it is surprising that no additional studies of its possible relation to induced weight gain were done.

Two positive results have been reported for the adrenergic, alpha-2A-, receptor (ADRA2A), both for the -1291C/G polymorphism (Table 1). These two studies showed remarkably similar results and indicated a G at risk allele effect of the ADRA2A –1291C/G variant for APS-induced weight gain, at least in Asian, Chinese, and Korean samples.

3. OMICs

3.1. Pharmacogenomics of Antipsychotics

Analysis of candidate genes selected from biological and biochemical pathways potentially relevant to APS effects could be a tedious task. For instance, the number of APS receptors are relatively large with APS showing few specificities (see 31). Moreover, necessary candidate genes could include a gene, or more probably a combination of genes, from the perturbed metabolic pathway such as weight control where more then 600 genes and loci have been identified. [95] It can be hypothesized that some variant forms of genes not normally sensitive to APS could become responsive and induce abnormal biochemical cascade reactions. More global approaches to study genetic causes of the APS effect on body weight are needed to identify additional candidate genes in the context of the entire genome. For diseases and complex phenotypes, such as response to drugs, integration of multiple Omics sources promises an improved description of the pathophysiology of the disease and of the response to drug, thereby forming the basis for novel diagnostics and therapy but equally important personalized interventions. Thanks to new techniques such as high density microchips and new generation sequencing which allow the analyze at an affordable price of all the coding regions (exon DNA) or of all the functional parts (RNA transcripts of the genome), researchers can now identify the genetic differences involved in drug response thus leading to the development of more effective, safer and better tolerated drugs. This field has the aim to use genomic data to optimize drug therapy, with respect to the patients' genotype, and to ensure maximum drug efficacy with minimal side effects. These approaches are also known as "personalized medicine" or "individualized medicine" – where drugs and drug combinations are optimized for the individual's genetic characteristics. Pharmacogenomics is the whole genome application of pharmacogenetics, which examines the interaction of drugs with single genes. Pharmacogenomics uses mainly whole-genome association and whole-genome expression studies, to which could be added whole-genome methylation and whole-genome metabolome analyses, as new generation sequencing.

3.2. Genome-Wide Linkage Studies (GWL)

To overcome the problem of unknown involved genes, studies without specific hypotheses requiring candidate genes were initiated, such as genome-wide linkage (GWL) analysis in which all chromosomes are tested in family-related affected and unaffected subjects for regions linked to the response or side-effects of the drug. These linked regions generally contain hundreds of genes that have to be evaluated by individual association studies.

We have published the first genome-wide linkage scan on the side-effect of APS on obesity. [96] From a sample of twenty-one large multigenerational pedigrees, including SZ and BP patients taking various APS for several years, we have identified nine informative pedigrees that we probed with 470 microsatellite markers covering all the 22 autosomal and 2 sexual chromosomes. In a non-parametric linkage analysis, we observed one suggestive linkage result at 12q24 (Lod score of 2.8) with no linkage to a phenotype of common obesity, not taking into account the use of APS, and with SZ or bipolar disorder. Close to the linkage signal at 12q24, the pro-melanin concentrating hormone (PMCH) gene is found. In rats, PMCH encodes a neuropeptide involved in the control of food intake and energy expenditure. [97] PMCH KO mice showed reduced body weight and leanness following hypophagia and an increase metabolic rate. [98]

We analyzed the SNP rs7973796 G/A located 5' of PMCH in a sample of 300 unrelated SZ taking APS and 150 controls, and observed an association of the G allele with a higher BMI ($p=0.025$), but only for those SZ taking olanzapine and of less then 50 years of age [73]. Odds ratios for SZ carrying the GA and the GG genotype were 4.4 and 10.2, respectively. On the other hand, we also analyzed three cohorts of healthy Caucasians of the surroundings of Quebec and from France and observed an association of the same PMCH SNP with the common form of obesity, which was modulated, again, according to age, but also gender and ethnicity (unpublished results). This let us conclude that the APS effect on weight in SZ could come from APS acting on a natural genetic susceptibility to gain weight in subjects carrying the GG at risk genotypes.

We also analyzed a second cohort of subjects from new multigenerational pedigrees characterized this time for BMI. [99] To determine chromosomal regions possibly linked to APS-related greater BMI, we used a non-parametric analysis relaying on identity-by-descent associations between sib-pairs (SIBPAL, LODPAL; SAGE 5.1).

We observed four significant ($p\leq0.0001$) and four suggestive ($0.0001<p\leq0.001$) linkages, some of which were located close to already identify candidate genes for APS-induced weight, such as the serotonin receptor 2A at 13q14-q21 and the gamma-aminobutyric acid A receptor beta 3 at 15q12. An association study using 20 SNPs located near and within HTR2A in unrelated SZ taking APS, and in controls, gave a positive association with rs2770296 only.

However, SNPs rs6313 and rs6314 from previous studies yielding positive associations (see Table 1) were not analyzed in our sample. Therefore, association study of these SNPs should also be made in pedigrees from where our linkage was observed [99] because of a possible strong familial component in our linkage results.

3.3. Genome-Wide Association Study (GWA)

A second more recent approach is the genome-wide association (GWA) study in which the entire genome, including all the known genes, is tested simultaneously. This approach has been used for the response and the neuronal and metabolic side-effects of drugs with some success [100-103] including our own GWA [104] study on the obesity side-effect of antipsychotics.

However, the possibilities of these studies are relatively limited since large cohorts of several thousand subjects are needed to overcome multiple testing statistical bias. These large cohorts are difficult to gather since the need to select a sample as homogeneous as possible in regard to the drug used by the patients, the dose and the period time of use, and other factors such as race and population of origin, age, gender and other diseases carried by the subjects, all of which can modulate drug response.

Results from a genome-wide association study of olanzapine-treated SZ patients in relation to weight gain have been reported [105] but not formally published. Patients had taken olanzapine for a minimum of six months, and the 20% extreme weight gainers (N=255) were compared to the 20% extreme non-gainers (N=258).

In this study, from about 1.6 million SNPs compared on pooled DNAs of each group, some 30,000 SNPs showed sufficient differences between the two groups of patients to be genotyped individually. Using Fisher's exact test three hundred eleven (311) SNPs were identified as significantly different ($p<0.001$) between weight gainers and non-gainers. These SNPs need now to be analyzed in independent samples to validate their association with weight gain while receiving olanzapine.

More recently, Adkins et al [102] published results from a GWA based on 738 SZ patients genotyped for ~492,000 SNPs and analyzed in relation to metabolic syndrome variables including weight and waist circumference. They found that the SNP rs1568679, located in an intron of Meis homeobox 2 gene located on chromosome 15q14, mediated the effects of risperidone on hip and waist circumferences. MEIS2 has a transcriptional regulatory function in adults [106] and is a highly complex locus showing at least 27 distinct splice variants. It could be speculate that the transcriptional activity of variants of MEIS2 may be differentially influenced by APS, particularly risperidone, causing changes in downstream metabolic pathways including weight control. Our own GWA [104] including some 250 SZ taking various APS and 150 controls did not reach genome–wide significant results, but provided confirmation of APS-induced higher BMI or waist circumference for several known candidate genes when statistically adjusted for the number of SNPs analyzed by gene. These included SLC6A4 over all the APS used and SLC6A4, SCARB1, HTR2A, HTR2C, ADRA2A, CYP2D6 and SNAP25 when considering specific APS (see Table 1).

3.4. Genome-Wide Expression Studies (GWE)

Few studies have used gene RNA expression to identify biomarkers related to diseases and even fewer for drug response and side-effects. Among these studies, different tissues were used including post-mortem brain or liver, fresh muscle biopsies, blood, mononuclear cells or lymphocytes, primary human neurons, and cultured neuroblastoma, astrocyte or immortalized lymphocyte cells. The best example of the use of gene expression to identify biomarkers comes from the cancer field. Diffuse large B-cell lymphoma (DLBCL), the most common subtype of non-Hodgkin's lymphoma, is clinically heterogeneous: 40% of patients respond well to current therapy and have prolonged survival, whereas the remainder succumb to the disease. In 2000, Stanford researchers published results [107] utilizing expression profiling techniques to stratify DLBCL to two subtypes: germinal center B-like DLBCL and activated B-like DLBCL. The authors studied the expression of 17,856 genes preferentially expressed in lymphoid cells and those with roles in cancer or immunology for 96 normal and malignant lymphocytes. The hierarchical clustering algorithm identified a subset of tumors that would have been labeled DLBCLs by traditional histological methods; however, the expression profiles of these tumors were heterogeneous. When the tumors were re-clustered based on expression of germinal center B-cell genes, a second group of genes characteristic of activated B-cells emerged and were oppositely regulated compared to the first set of genes. Based on these expression patterns, the heterogeneous DLBCL cluster was sub classified to the germinal center B-like DLBCL and activated B-like DLBCL. The distinction of these groups is significant in terms of overall patient survival: the probability of survival for patients with germinal center B-like DLBCLs over 10 years was about 80% while those with activated B-like DLBCLs was lowered to about 40% over a shorter eight-year period. The authors concluded that the new methods of gene expression profiling call for a revised definition of what is deemed a `disease' [107], and we proposed that will be the same for drug treatment response.

In the characterization of drug response using gene expression, one of the most exhaustive studies was made on neuronal cultured cells [108, 109]. Three classes of drugs, including 8 antipsychotics, 20 antidepressants and 8 opioids, were used to stimulate, at pharmaceutically relevant doses neuronal cells for 24 hours followed by a GWE on RNA levels. The approach was successful in reclassifying tested drugs to their respective classes showing that each class has a specific pattern of expression. However, in this study the individual drug signature across different genomes was not investigated. Also, only one drug dose for one period of stimulation was tried precluding the ability to differentiate effects of drug dose, and of short versus long term drug use. Similarly, Sun et al [110] reported in immortalized lymphocytes (IML) of bipolar patients, in contrast to unrelated controls, a lower expression of five genes after lithium stimulation. These studies demonstrated the possibilities of using stimulated cultured cells to identify genes involved in the response and side-effects of drugs. In our preliminary study, we observed differences in the RNA expression of several genes in IML between SZ and controls that were changed for some of them after stimulation of the cells in culture with an antipsychotic. [111, 112] More particularly, the RNA expression of PMCH in pooled RNA from two groups of three obese SZ and two groups of three non obese SZ were analyzed on an Agilent 18K microchips. We observed a possible genotype-dependent higher expression of PMCH in obese in contrast to non-obese patients (+45%; p=0.07) in those carrying the PMCH GG risk genotype associated with APS-induced obesity [111].

In contrast to fresh blood, IMLs are a renewable source of biological material representing an interesting *in vitro* model system to study the genetics of gene expression, drug response, and other traits in a controlled laboratory setting. Moreover, IMLs offer major advantages: their several passages during cell culture free them from previous neurohormonal, medication and environmental influences that could mask genetically-based differences in RNA expression [113, 114], while genetic characteristics and basal differential expression are conserved even after prolonged cell culture. [115, 116] Convincing relationships between SNPs and RNA levels (eQTLs) have been reported in IMLs [117-123] including after drug treatments [124, 125]. In the course of attempting to map genes for drug responses in *vitro*, the reproducibility of *in vitro* traits across replicates was evaluated. [126] It was found that responses to drugs and levels of many RNAs can be technically well measured after 48 hours of drug stimulation, but can also vary both across experiments and with nongenetic confounders such as growth rates, Epstein-Barr virus (EBV) levels, and ATP levels. These confounders are intrinsic to each cell lines and can be avoided in the case of a drug treatment by contrasting gene RNA expression of the cell line after drug stimulation to itself in a parallel cell culture without the treatment. These normalized gene RNA expression differences could then be contrasted among the different patient cell lines. It has to be strongly emphasized here that the cell lines have to be derived from those patients that use the drug and carry the necessary disease-related genome, since the response is different in controls than in patients.

3.5 Pharmacoepigenomics Studies

Epigenetic modulations are molecular modifications made to DNA, RNA and proteins that fine-tune genotype into phenotype and do not include DNA base changes. For instance, gene-expression modulation is linked to epigenetic codes in chromatin that consist of post-replication DNA methylation, particularly in gene-promoter regions, and histone protein modifications (methylation, acetylation). Translational silencing capacity of DNA methylation may then occur via gene promoter rejection of the binding of some transcription factors to their DNA binding sites. Epigenetic coding is modulated globally, and in a gene-specific manner by environmental exposures that include nutrition, toxins and drugs. Analysis of epigenetic aberrations in diseases will help to identify dysfunctional genes and pathways, establishing more robust cause-effect relationships than genetic studies alone, and identifying new pharmaceutical targets and drugs. [127]

APS target genes usually express their effects in brain and, because most epigenetic modifications are tissue specific, it could be difficult to identify epigenetic abnormalities induced by APS in living subjects since no access to living brain tissue is allowed. Also, detection of epigenetic abnormalities in more accessible tissues that will represent the brain epigenetic marks is one of the critical steps in developing diagnostic and therapeutic biomarkers for APS effects. One promising example is the observation that a hypo-methylated (w50%) state in the DNA promoter of the catechol-O-methyltransferase gene observed in the brain of SZ and bipolar disorder patients, compared to control subjects [128], was also observed in DNA derived from saliva. [129] A second example comes from the serotonin receptor 2A (HTR2A). DNA methylation of HTR2A at the polymorphic site rs6313 (alias T102C) influences HTR2A expression, and aberrant DNA methylation of HTR2A promoter was reported for SZ and bipolar disorder patients in postmortem brain as well as in DNA derived from saliva. [130] These observations open the door to the analysis in saliva of differential gene methylation following antipsychotic medication use in relation to therapeutic and secondary effects such as weight gain. One important group of genes that should be targeted for methylation study are the CYP450 because of their numerous different forms arising from differential splicing of their RNA modulated by methylation. [131] Several other examples of methylation of genes include the DNA (cytosine-5-)-methyltransferase 1 which is up-regulated in the cortex of SZ and is preferentially expressed in interneuron's secreting GABA where it very likely contributes to promoter CpG island hypermethylation of downstream genes. (132) Histone H3-lysine 4 methylation, a chromatin mark associated with the transcriptional process, is progressively increased at GABAergic gene promoters in human prefrontal cortex from prenatal to peripubertal ages and throughout adulthood. Therefore, chromatin remodeling mechanisms at GABAergic gene promoters operate throughout an extended period of normal human brain development playing a role in the neurobiology of SZ [133] and eventually of APS effects.

Conclusion

It is now well accepted that APS can induce metabolic side effects in addition to the well-known neuromotor side effects such as tardive dyskinesia. The factors involved in these metabolic side effects are less obvious. With the number of studies increasing in the past few years, genetic factors are becoming more recognized as being involved in the APS side effects on body weight. Accordingly, APS side-effects on body weight is probably the most studied metabolic effect in regards to genetics probably because it is a spectacular effect observed in up to 80% of treated patients according to the drug used and the period of treatment. Weight and height are also relatively easy to collect in contrast to more invasive and costly variables such as glucose, lipid or leptin levels from the blood. Actually, the genes most frequently associated with APS-induced body weight gain are the serotonin receptor 2C and the leptin genes. Interestingly, the first one encodes a direct APS receptor, which is also directly related to common obesity, and the second one a hormone central to body weight and energy expenditure controls. An increasing number of metabolic genes have been shown to be related to APS-induced weight likely due to an increasing number of such genes being studied. Given the large number of candidate genes for the control of weight and obesity, as well as the number of APS receptors likely to be involved, with all of these factors interacting and with additional unknown genes, it would be highly desirable to use new genomic tools such as whole-genome RNA expression and whole-genome association, and preferably a combination of them, if we want to be able to define a true genetic model of APS-induced weight gain, and more importantly, to define individual susceptibility. We can expect in the relatively near future, if resources are provided, that the use of pharmacogenetics will allow us to predict and diagnose APS adverse effects individually in treated patients.

References

[1] Doris, A., K. Ebmeier, et al. Depressive illness. *Lancet* 1999;354(9187): 1369-75.

[2] Lazarou, J., B. H. Pomeranz, et al. Incidence of adverse drug reactions in hospitalized patients: a meta-analysis of prospective studies. *Jama* 1998;279(15): 1200-5.

[3] Mjorndal, T., M. D. Boman, et al. Adverse drug reactions as a cause for admissions to a department of internal medicine. *Pharmacoepidemiol. Drug Saf.* 2002;11(1): 65-72.

[4] Pirmohamed, M., S. James, et al. Adverse drug reactions as cause of admission to hospital: prospective analysis of 18 820 patients. *Bmj.* 2004;329(7456): 15-9.

[5] Budnitz, D. S., D. A. Pollock, et al. National surveillance of emergency department visits for outpatient adverse drug events. *Jama* 2006;296(15): 1858-66.

[6] Davies, M. A., Y. Conley, et al. (2011). "Functional SNPs in genes encoding the 5-HT2A receptor modify the affinity and potency of several atypical antipsychotic drugs." Biol Res Nurs **13**(1): 55-60.

[7] Stanton, J. M. Weight gain associated with neuroleptic medication: a review. 1995;*Schizophr. Bull.* 21(3): 463-72.

[8] Yusufi, B., S. Mukherjee, et al. Prevalence and nature of side effects during clozapine maintenance treatment and the relationship with clozapine dose and plasma concentration. *Int. Clin. Psychopharmacol,* 2007;22(4): 238-43.

[9] Malhotra, A. K., T. Lencz, et al. Genomics and the future of pharmacotherapy in psychiatry. *Int. Rev. Psychiatry,* 2007;19(5): 523-30.

[10] Arranz, M. J. and Kapur, S. Pharmacogenetics in psychiatry: are we ready for widespread clinical use? *Schizophr. Bull.* 2008;34(6): 1130-44.

[11] Allison, D. B., J. L. Mentore, et al. Antipsychotic-induced weight gain: a comprehensive research synthesis. *Am. J. Psychiatry,* 1999;156(11): 1686-96.

[12] Baptista, T., D. Reyes, et al. Antipsychotic drugs and reproductive hormones: relationship to body weight regulation. *Pharmacol. Biochem. Behav.* 1999;62(3): 409-17.

[13] Basson, B. R., B. J. Kinon, et al. Factors influencing acute weight change in patients with schizophrenia treated with olanzapine, haloperidol, or risperidone. *J. Clin. Psychiatry,* 2001;62(4): 231-8.

[14] Fontaine, K. R., M. Heo, et al. Estimating the consequences of anti-psychotic induced weight gain on health and mortality rate. *Psychiatry Res.* 2001;101(3): 277-88.

[15] Czobor, P., J. Volavka, et al. Antipsychotic-induced weight gain and therapeutic response: a differential association. *J. Clin. Psychopharmacol.* 2002;22(3): 244-51.

[16] Homel, P., D. Casey, et al. Changes in body mass index for individuals with and without schizophrenia, 1987-1996. *Schizophr. Res.* 2002;55(3): 277-84.

[17] Ratzoni, G., D. Gothelf, et al. Weight gain associated with olanzapine and risperidone in adolescent patients: a comparative prospective study. *J. Am. Acad. Child. Adolesc. Psychiatry,* 2002;41(3): 337-43.

[18] Ader, M., W. T. Garvey, et al. Ethnic heterogeneity in glucoregulatory function during treatment with atypical antipsychotics in patients with schizophrenia. *J. Psychiatr. Res.* 2008;42(13): 1076-85.

[19] Fleischhaker, C., P. Heiser, et al. Weight gain in children and adolescents during 45 weeks treatment with clozapine, olanzapine and risperidone. *J. Neural. Transm.* 2008;115(11): 1599-608.

[20] Fraguas, D., J. Merchan-Naranjo, et al. Metabolic and hormonal side effects in children and adolescents treated with second-generation antipsychotics. *J. Clin. Psychiatry,* 2008;69(7): 1166-75.

[21] Cohen, J. A. and J. M. Perel Adolescent weight loss during treatment with olanzapine. *J. Child Adolesc. Psychopharmacol.* 2004;14(4): 617-20.

[22] Leadbetter, R., M. Shutty, et al.Clozapine-induced weight gain: prevalence and clinical relevance. *Am. J. Psychiatry,* 1992;149(1): 68-72.

[23] Falloon, I., D. C. Watt, et al. A comparative controlled trial of pimozide and fluphenazine decanoate in the continuation therapy of schizophrenia. *Psychol. Med.* 1978;8(1): 59-70.

[24] Jones, B., B. R. Basson, et al. Weight change and atypical antipsychotic treatment in patients with schizophrenia. *J. Clin. Psychiatry,* 2001;62(Suppl 2): 41-4.

[25] Bromley, C. M., S. Close, et al. Designing pharmacogenetic projects in industry: practical design perspectives from the Industry Pharmacogenomics Working Group. *Pharmacogenomics J.* 2009;9(1): 14-22.

[26] Rauch, A., D. Nolan, et al. Prospective genetic screening decreases the incidence of abacavir hypersensitivity reactions in the Western Australian HIV cohort study. *Clin. Infect. Dis.* 2006;43(1): 99-102.

[27] Crow, T. J. 'The missing genes: what happened to the heritability of psychiatric disorders?' *Mol. Psychiatry,* 2011;16(4): 362-4.

[28] Brady, K. T. Weight gain associated with psychotropic drugs. *South Med. J.* 1989;82(5): 611-7.

[29] Bymaster, F. P., D. O. Calligaro, et al. Radioreceptor binding profile of the atypical antipsychotic olanzapine. *Neuropsychopharmacology* 1996;14(2): 87-96.

[30] Richelson, E. and T. Souder Binding of antipsychotic drugs to human brain receptors focus on newer generation compounds. *Life Sci.* 2000;68(1): 29-39.

[31] Roth, B. L., D. J. Sheffler, et al. Magic shotguns versus magic bullets: selectively non-selective drugs for mood disorders and schizophrenia. *Nat. Rev. Drug Discov.* 2004;3(4): 353-9.

[32] Ellingrod, V. L., D. Miller, et al. CYP2D6 polymorphisms and atypical antipsychotic weight gain. *Psychiatr. Genet.* 2002;12(1): 55-8.

[33] Reynolds, G. P., Z. J. Zhang, et al. Association of antipsychotic drug-induced weight gain with a 5-HT2C receptor gene polymorphism. *Lancet* 2002;359(9323): 2086-7.

[34] Reynolds, G. P., Z. Zhang, et al. Polymorphism of the promoter region of the serotonin 5-HT(2C) receptor gene and clozapine-induced weight gain. *Am. J. Psychiatry,* 2003;160(4): 677-9.

[35] Basile, V. S., M. Masellis, et al. 759C/T genetic variation of 5HT(2C) receptor and clozapine-induced weight gain. *Lancet,* 2002;360(9347): 1790-1.

[36] Buckland, P. R., B. Hoogendoorn, et al. Low gene expression conferred by association of an allele of the 5-HT2C receptor gene with antipsychotic-induced weight gain. *Am. J. Psychiatry,* 2005;162(3): 613-5.

[37] Reynolds, G. P., M. J. Hill, et al. The 5-HT2C receptor and antipsychoticinduced weight gain - mechanisms and genetics. *J. Psychopharmacol.* 2006;20(4 Suppl): 15-8.

[38] Hill, M. J. and G. P. Reynolds 5-HT2C receptor gene polymorphisms associated with antipsychotic drug action alter promoter activity. *Brain Res.* 2007;1149: 14-7.

[39] Tecott, L. H., L. M. Sun, et al. Eating disorder and epilepsy in mice lacking 5-HT2c serotonin receptors. *Nature* 1995;374(6522): 542-6.

[40] Vickers, S. P., K. R. Benwell, et al. Comparative effects of continuous infusion of mCPP, Ro 60-0175 and d-fenfluramine on food intake, water intake, body weight and locomotor activity in rats. *Br. J. Pharmacol.* 2000;130(6): 1305-14.

[41] Bundo, M., K. Iwamoto, et al. Mutation screening and assessment of the effect of genetic variations on expression and RNA editing of serotonin receptor 2C in the human brain. *Psychiatry Clin. Neurosci.* 2010;64(1): 57-61.

[42] Flomen, R., J. Knight, et al. Evidence that RNA editing modulates splice site selection in the 5-HT2C receptor gene. Nucleic Acids Res 2004;32(7): 2113-22.

[43] Black, D. L. Mechanisms of alternative pre-messenger RNA splicing. *Annu. Rev. Biochem.* 2003;72: 291-336.

[44] Matlin, A. J., F. Clark, et al. Understanding alternative splicing: towards a cellular code. *Nat. Rev. Mol. Cell Biol.* 2005;6(5): 386-98.

[45] Wang, E. T., R. Sandberg, et al. Alternative isoform regulation in human tissue transcriptomes. *Nature* 2008;456(7221): 470-6.

[46] Wang, Y., H. R. Krishnan, et al. Drug-induced epigenetic changes produce drug tolerance. *PLoS Biol.* 2007;5(10): e265.

[47] Okada, M., J. K. Northup, et al. Modification of human 5-HT(2C) receptor function by Cys23Ser, an abundant, naturally occurring amino-acid substitution. *Mol. Psychiatry,* 2004;9(1): 55-64.

[48] Kuhn, K. U., B. B. Quednow, et al. Allelic variants of the serotonin(2C) receptor and neuroendocrinological responses to the serotonin(2C) receptor agonist m-chlorophenylpiperazine in healthy male volunteers. *Pharmacopsychiatry* 2002;35(6): 226-30.

[49] Quested, D. J., R. Whale, et al. Allelic variation in the 5-HT2C receptor (HTR2C) and functional responses to the 5-HT2C receptor agonist, m-chlorophenylpiperazine. *Psychopharmacology* (Berl) 1999;144(3): 306-7.

[50] Polesskaya, O. O. and B. P. SokolovDifferential expression of the "C" and "T" alleles of the 5-HT2A receptor gene in the temporal cortex of normal individuals and schizophrenics. *J. Neurosci. Res.* 2002;67(6): 812-22.

[51] Fukuda, Y., M. Koga, et al. Monoallelic and unequal allelic expression of the HTR2A gene in human brain and peripheral lymphocytes. *Biol. Psychiatry* 2006;60(12): 1331-5.

[52] Polesskaya, O. O., C. Aston, et al. Allele C-specific methylation of the 5-HT2A receptor gene: evidence for correlation with its expression and expression of DNA methylase DNMT1. *J. Neurosci. Res.* 2006;83(3): 362-73.

[53] Salomon, L., C. Lanteri, et al. Paradoxical constitutive behavioral sensitization to amphetamine in mice lacking 5-HT2A receptors. *Psychopharmacology* (Berl) 2007;194(1): 11-20.

[54] Prado-Lima, P. S., I. B. Cruz, et al. Human food preferences are associated with a 5-HT(2A) serotonergic receptor polymorphism. *Mol. Psychiatry* 2006;11(10): 889-91.

[55] Teff, K. L. and S. F. Kim Atypical antipsychotics and the neural regulation of food intake and peripheral metabolism. *Physiol. Behav.* 2011;104(4): 590-8.

[56] Lambe, E. K., S. G. Fillman, et al. Serotonin receptor expression in human prefrontal cortex: balancing excitation and inhibition across postnatal development. *PLoS One* 2011;6(7): e22799.

[57] Masellis, M., V. S. Basile, et al. Lack of association between the T-->C 267 serotonin 5-HT6 receptor gene (HTR6) polymorphism and prediction of response to clozapine in schizophrenia. *Schizophr. Res.* 2001;47(1): 49-58.

[58] Lane, H. Y., C. C. Lee, et al. (2005). "Pharmacogenetic studies of response to risperidone and other newer atypical antipsychotics." Pharmacogenomics 6(2): 139-149.

[59] Ikeda, M., Y. Yamanouchi, et al. Variants of dopamine and serotonin candidate genes as predictors of response to risperidone treatment in first-episode schizophrenia. *Pharmacogenomics* 2008;9(10): 1437-43.
[60] Vazquez-Bourgon, J., M. J. Arranz, et al. Serotonin transporter polymorphisms and early response to antipsychotic treatment in first episode of psychosis. *Psychiatry Res.* 2010;175(3): 189-94.
[61] Philibert, R. A., H. Sandhu, et al. The relationship of 5HTT (SLC6A4) methylation and genotype on mRNA expression and liability to major depression and alcohol dependence in subjects from the Iowa Adoption Studies. *Am. J. Med. Genet. B. Neuropsychiatr. Genet.* 2008;147B(5): 543-9.
[62] Morimoto, T., Y. Yamamoto, et al. Involvement of the histaminergic system in leptin-induced suppression of food intake. *Physiol. Behav.* 1999;67(5): 679-83.
[63] Kroeze, W. K., S. J. Hufeisen, et al. H1-histamine receptor affinity predicts short-term weight gain for typical and atypical antipsychotic drugs. *Neuropsychopharmacology* 2003;28(3): 519-26.
[64] Eiermann, B., G. Engel, et al. The involvement of CYP1A2 and CYP3A4 in the metabolism of clozapine. *Br. J. Clin. Pharmacol.* 1997;44(5): 439-46.
[65] Brockmoller, J., J. Kirchheiner, et al. The impact of the CYP2D6 polymorphism on haloperidol pharmacokinetics and on the outcome of haloperidol treatment. *Clin. Pharmacol. Ther.* 2002;72(4): 438-52.
[66] Berecz, R., P. Dorado, et al. The role of cytochrome P450 enzymes in the metabolism of risperidone and its clinical relevance for drug interactions. *Curr. Drug Targets* 2004;5(6): 573-9.
[67] Roh, H. K., J. Y. Chung, et al. Plasma concentrations of haloperidol are related to CYP2D6 genotype at low, but not high doses of haloperidol in Korean schizophrenic patients. *Br. J. Clin. Pharmacol.* 2001;52(3): 265-71.
[68] Han, Z., S. C. Heath, et al. Candidate genes involved in cardiovascular risk factors by a family-based association study on the island of Kosrae, Federated States of Micronesia. *Am. J. Med. Genet.* 2002;110(3): 234-42.
[69] Gennari, L., L. Masi, et al. A polymorphic CYP19 TTTA repeat influences aromatase activity and estrogen levels in elderly men: effects on bone metabolism. *J. Clin. Endocrinol. Metab.* 2004;89(6): 2803-10.
[70] Baghaei, F., R. Rosmond, et al. The CYP19 gene and associations with androgens and abdominal obesity in premenopausal women. *Obes. Res.* 2003;11(4): 578-85.
[71] Tworoger, S. S., J. Chubak, et al. The effect of CYP19 and COMT polymorphisms on exercise-induced fat loss in postmenopausal women. *Obes. Res*. 2004;12(6): 972-81.
[72] Theisen, F. M., M. Haberhausen, et al. No evidence for binding of clozapine, olanzapine and/or haloperidol to selected receptors involved in body weight regulation. *Pharmacogenomics J.* 2007;7(4): 275-81.
[73] Chagnon, Y. C., A. Bureau, et al. Possible association of the pro-melanin-concentrating hormone gene with a greater body mass index as a side effect of the antipsychotic olanzapine. *Am. J. Med. Genet. B. Neuropsychiatr. Genet.* 2007;144B: 1063-1069.
[74] Kuo, P. H., C. F. Kao, et al. Polymorphisms of INSIG2, MC4R, and LEP Are Associated With Obesity- and Metabolic-Related Traits in Schizophrenic Patients. *J. Clin. Psychopharmacol.* 2011;31(6): 705-711.

[75] Herran, A., M. T. Garcia-Unzueta, et al. Effects of long-term treatment with antipsychotics on serum leptin levels. *Br. J. Psychiatry,* 2001;179: 59-62.

[76] McIntyre, R. S., D. A. Mancini, et al. Antipsychotic-induced weight gain: bipolar disorder and leptin. *J. Clin. Psychopharmacol.* 2003;23(4): 323-7.

[77] tmaca, M., M. Kuloglu, et al. Weight gain, serum leptin and triglyceride levels in patients with schizophrenia on antipsychotic treatment with quetiapine, olanzapine and haloperidol. *Schizophr. Res.* 2003;60(1): 99-100.

[78] Atmaca, M., M. Kuloglu, et al. Serum leptin and triglyceride levels in patients on treatment with atypical antipsychotics. *J. Clin. Psychiatry,* 2003;64(5): 598-604.

[79] Zhang, Z. J., Z. J. Yao, et al. Effects of antipsychotics on fat deposition and changes in leptin and insulin levels. Magnetic resonance imaging study of previously untreated people with schizophrenia. *Br. J. Psychiatry,* 2004;184: 58-62.

[80] Melkersson, K. I. and A. L. Hulting Insulin and leptin levels in patients with schizophrenia or related psychoses--a comparison between different antipsychotic agents. *Psychopharmacology* (Berl) 2001;154(2): 205-12.

[81] Hoffstedt, J., P. Eriksson, et al. A polymorphism in the leptin promoter region (-2548 G/A) influences gene expression and adipose tissue secretion of leptin. *Horm. Metab. Res.* 2002;34(7): 355-9.

[82] Ben Ali, S., A. Kallel, et al. Association of G-2548A LEP polymorphism with plasma leptin levels in Tunisian obese patients. *Clin. Biochem.* 2009;42(7-8): 584-8.

[83] Zhang, Z. J., Z. J. Yao, et al. Association of -2548G/A functional polymorphism in the promoter region of leptin gene with antipsychotic agent-induced weight gain]. Zhonghua Yi Xue Za Zhi 2003;83(24): 2119-23.

[84] Ben Ali, S., A. Kallel, et al. LEPR p.Q223R Polymorphism influences plasma leptin levels and body mass index in Tunisian obese patients. *Arch. Med. Res.* 2009;40(3): 186-90.

[85] Tiwari, A. K., C. C. Zai, et al. Association study of polymorphisms in insulin induced gene 2 (INSIG2) with antipsychotic-induced weight gain in European and African-American schizophrenia patients. *Hum. Psychopharmacol.* 2010;25(3): 253-9.

[86] Herbert, A., N. P. Gerry, et al. A common genetic variant is associated with adult and childhood obesity. *Science* 2006;312(5771): 279-83.

[87] Le Hellard, S., F. M. Theisen, et al. Association between the insulin-induced gene 2 (INSIG2) and weight gain in a German sample of antipsychotic-treated schizophrenic patients: perturbation of SREBP-controlled lipogenesis in drug-related metabolic adverse effects? *Mol. Psychiatry.* 2009;14(3): 308-17.

[88] Siffert, W., D. Rosskopf, et al. Association of a human G-protein beta3 subunit variant with hypertension. *Nat. Genet.* 1998;18(1): 45-8.

[89] Baumgart, D., C. Naber, et al. G protein beta3 subunit 825T allele and enhanced coronary vasoconstriction on alpha(2)-adrenoceptor activation. *Circ. Res.* 1999;85(10): 965-9.

[90] Naber, C., B. L. Hermann, et al. Enhanced epinephrine-induced platelet aggregation in individuals carrying the G protein beta3 subunit 825T allele. *FEBS Lett.* 2000;484(3): 199-201.

[91] Hegele, R. A., C. Anderson, et al.G-protein beta3 subunit gene splice variant and body fat distribution in Nunavut Inuit. *Genome Res.* 1999;9(10): 972-7.

[92] Siffert, W., P. Forster, et al. Worldwide ethnic distribution of the G protein beta3 subunit 825T allele and its association with obesity in Caucasian, Chinese, and Black African individuals. *J. Am. Soc. Nephrol.* 1999;10(9): 1921-30.
[93] Jonsson, E. G., M. M. Nothen, et al. Polymorphisms in the dopamine D2 receptor gene and their relationships to striatal dopamine receptor density of healthy volunteers. *Mol. Psychiatry,* 1999;4(3): 290-6.
[94] Lencz, T., D. G. Robinson, et al. DRD2 promoter region variation as a predictor of sustained response to antipsychotic medication in first-episode schizophrenia patients. *Am. J. Psychiatry,* 2006;163(3): 529-31.
[95] Rankinen, T., A. Zuberi, et al. The human obesity gene map: the 2005 update. *Obesity* (Silver Spring) 2006;14(4): 529-644.
[96] Chagnon, Y. C., C. Merette, et al. A genome wide linkage study of obesity as secondary effect of antipsychotics in multigenerational families of eastern Quebec affected by psychoses. *Mol. Psychiatry,* 2004;9(12): 1067-74.
[97] Qu, D., D. S. Ludwig, et al. A role for melanin-concentrating hormone in the central regulation of feeding behaviour. *Nature* 1996;380(6571): 243-7.
[98] Shimada, M., N. A. Tritos, et al. Mice lacking melanin-concentrating hormone are hypophagic and lean. *Nature* 1998;396(6712): 670-4.
[99] Chagnon, Y. C. A second genome scan for obesity as a side effect of antipsychotics in new multigenerational pedigrees. *Pharmacogenetics in Psychiatry Meeting*,;NewYork;2006.
[100] Aberg, K., D. E. Adkins, et al. Genomewide association study of movement-related adverse antipsychotic effects. *Biol. Psychiatry,* 2010;67(3): 279-82.
[101] Adkins, D. E., K. Aberg, et al. A genomewide association study of citalopram response in major depressive disorder-a psychometric approach. *Biol. Psychiatry,* 2010;68(6): e25-7.
[102] Adkins, D. E., K. Aberg, et al. Genomewide pharmacogenomic study of metabolic side effects to antipsychotic drugs. *Mol. Psychiatry,* 2011;16(3): 321-32.
[103] McClay, J. L., D. E. Adkins, et al. Genome-wide pharmacogenomic analysis of response to treatment with antipsychotics. *Mol. Psychiatry,* 2011;16(1): 76-85.
[104] Chagnon, Y. C. Association study of 17 candidate genes with obesity phenotypes in schizophrenia patients taking antipsychotics and in controls. *Pharmacogenetics in Psychiatry Meeting*; New-York:2009.
[105] Kirkwood, S. C., D.-J. Fu, et al. Genome-wide association study for olanzapine treatment-emergent weight gain. *Pharmacogenetics in Psychiatry Meeting*; New-York:2005.
[106] Yang, Y., C. K. Hwang, et al. Three-amino acid extension loop homeodomain proteins Meis2 and TGIF differentially regulate transcription. *J. Biol. Chem.* 2000;275(27): 20734-41.
[107] Alizadeh, A. A., M. B. Eisen, et al. Distinct types of diffuse large B-cell lymphoma identified by gene expression profiling. *Nature* 2000;403(6769): 503-11.
[108] Gunther, E. C., D. J. Stone, et al. Prediction of clinical drug efficacy by classification of drug-induced genomic expression profiles in vitro. *Proc. Natl. Acad. Sci. U S A* 2003;100(16): 9608-13.

[109] Gunther, E. C., D. J. Stone, et al. A quantitative genomic expression analysis platform for multiplexed in vitro prediction of drug action. *Pharmacogenomics J.* 2005;5(2): 126-34.

[110] Sun, X., L. T. Young, et al. Identification of lithium-regulated genes in cultured lymphoblasts of lithium responsive subjects with bipolar disorder. *Neuropsychopharmacology* 2004; 29(4): 799-804.

[111] Chagnon, Y. C. Biomarkers of the effects of antipsychotics on obesity by differential gene expression in immortalized lymphocytes. Pharmacogenetics in Psychiatry Meeting;New-York:2007.

[112] Chagnon, Y. C. Differential RNA expression in immortalized lymphocytes between schizophrenic patients and controls for 26 neurotransmitter receptors showing various affinities for the antipsychotic olanzapine. Pharmacogenetics in Psychiatry Meeting; New York:2008.

[113] Karege, F., M. Schwald, et al. Drug-induced decrease of protein kinase a activity reveals alteration in BDNF expression of bipolar affective disorder. *Neuropsychopharmacology* 2004;29(4): 805-12.

[114] Leek, J. T. and J. D. Storey Capturing heterogeneity in gene expression studies by surrogate variable analysis. *PLoS Genet.* 2007;3(9): 1724-35.

[115] Siffert, W., D. Rosskopf, et al. Enhanced G protein activation in immortalized lymphoblasts from patients with essential hypertension. *J. Clin. Invest.* 1995;96(2): 759-66.

[116] Spielman, R. S., L. A. Bastone, et al. Common genetic variants account for differences in gene expression among ethnic groups. *Nat. Genet.* 2007; 39(2):226-31.

[117] Deutsch, S., R. Lyle, et al. Gene expression variation and expression quantitative trait mapping of human chromosome 21 genes. *Hum. Mol. Genet.* 2005;14(23): 3741-9.

[118] Stranger, B. E., M. S. Forrest, et al. Genome-wide associations of gene expression variation in humans. *PLoS Genet.* 2005;1(6): e78.

[119] Dixon, A. L., L. Liang, et al. A genome-wide association study of global gene expression. *Nat. Genet.* 2007;39(10): 1202-7.

[120] Stranger, B. E., A. C. Nica, et al. Population genomics of human gene expression. *Nat. Genet.* 2007;39(10): 1217-24.

[121] Duan, S., R. S. Huang, et al. Genetic architecture of transcript-level variation in humans. *Am. J. Hum. Genet.* 2008; 82(5): 1101-13.

[122] Quinn, E. M., M. Hill, et al. Evidence for cis-acting regulation of ANK3 and CACNA1C gene expression. *Bipolar. Disord.* 2010;12(4): 440-5.

[123] Sharma, N. K., K. A. Langberg, et al. Type 2 diabetes (T2D) associated polymorphisms regulate expression of adjacent transcripts in transformed lymphocytes, adipose, and muscle from Caucasian and African-American subjects. *J. Clin. Endocrinol. Metab.* 2011;96(2): E394-403.

[124] Hogarth, P., L. Lovrecic, et al. Sodium phenylbutyrate in Huntington's disease: a dose-finding study. *Mov. Disord.* 2007;22(13): 1962-4.

[125] Jones, T. S., W. Yang, et al. Using HapMap tools in pharmacogenomic discovery: the thiopurine methyltransferase polymorphism. *Clin. Pharmacol. Ther.* 2007;81(5): 729-34.

[126] Choy, E., R. Yelensky, et al. Genetic analysis of human traits in vitro: drug response and gene expression in lymphoblastoid cell lines. *PLoS Genet.* 2008;4(11): e1000287.

[127] Abdolmaleky, H. M., J. R. Zhou, et al.Epigenetic and pharmacoepigenomic studies of major psychoses and potentials for therapeutics. *Pharmacogenomics* 2008;9(12): 1809-23.

[128] Abdolmaleky, H. M., K. H. Cheng, et al. Hypomethylation of MB-COMT promoter is a major risk factor for schizophrenia and bipolar disorder. *Hum. Mol. Genet.* 2006;15(21): 3132-45.

[129] Nohesara, S., M. Ghadirivasfi, et al. DNA hypomethylation of MB-COMT promoter in the DNA derived from saliva in schizophrenia and bipolar disorder. *J. Psychiatr. Res.* 2011;45(11): 1432-8.

[130] Ghadirivasfi, M., S. Nohesara, et al. Hypomethylation of the serotonin receptor type-2A Gene (HTR2A) at T102C polymorphic site in DNA derived from the saliva of patients with schizophrenia and bipolar disorder. *Am. J. Med. Genet. B. Neuropsychiatr. Genet.* 2011;156(5): 536-45.

[131] Ingelman-Sundberg, M., S. C. Sim, et al. Influence of cytochrome P450 polymorphisms on drug therapies: pharmacogenetic, pharmacoepigenetic and clinical aspects. *Pharmacol. Ther.* 2007;116(3): 496-526.

[132] Veldic, M., A. Guidotti, et al. In psychosis, cortical interneurons overexpress DNA-methyltransferase 1. *Proc. Natl. Acad. Sci. U S A* 2005;102(6): 2152-7.

[133] Huang, H. S., A. Matevossian, et al. Prefrontal dysfunction in schizophrenia involves mixed-lineage leukemia 1-regulated histone methylation at GABAergic gene promoters. *J. Neurosci.* 2007;27(42): 11254-62.

In: Antipsychotic Drugs
Editors: T.L. Schwartz, J. Megna and M.E. Topel
ISBN: 978-1-62100-071-6

Chapter 11

MANAGEMENT OF ANTIPSYCHOTIC-INDUCED EXTRAPYRAMIDAL MOTOR DISORDERS: REGULATORY ROLES OF THE SEROTONERGIC NERVOUS SYSTEM

Yukihiro Ohno**, *Saki Shimizu, Junta Imaki, Atsushi Masui andAyaka Tatara
Laboratory of Pharmacology, Osaka University of Pharmaceutical Sciences, Osaka, Japan

ABSTRACT

Introduction: Antipsychotic-induced extrapyramidal motor disorders such as parkinsonian symptoms (e.g., bradykinesia, tremor and muscle rigidity), akathisia, dystonia and tardive dyskinesia are the most common neurological side effects in the treatment of schizophrenia. It is now known that the serotonergic nervous system modulates the induction of antipsychotic-induced extrapyramidal side effects (EPS) viadiverse mechanisms mediated by multiple 5-HT receptors.

Conclusion: Antagonism of 5-$HT_{2A/2C}$ receptorshas been shown to alleviate antipsychotic-induced EPS by relieving the 5-$HT_{2A/2C}$ receptor-mediated inhibition of nigro-striatal dopaminergic neurons. Many of the second-generation antipsychotics (e.g., clozapine, risperidone, olanzapine, quetiapine, perospirone, ziprasidone, blonanserin and lurasidone) possesspotent 5-$HT_{2A/2C}$ blocking activity, which contributes to their atypical antipsychotic properties. In addition, 5-HT_{1A} receptors also play an important role in modulating EPS induction. Microinjection studies revealed that stimulation of postsynaptic 5-HT_{1A} receptors in the striatum or cerebral cortex, as well as presynaptic 5-HT_{1A}autoreceptors in the raphe nuclei,attenuates antipsychotic-induced EPS. Indeed, several atypical antipsychotics (e.g., perospirone, ziprasidone, aripiprazoleand lurasidone) show a high affinity for 5-HT_{1A} receptors. Furthermore, recent studies demonstrated that antagonism of 5-$HT_3$and 5-HT_6 receptors alleviates antipsychotic-

*Tel:+81-72-690-1052. FAX:+81-72-690-1053. E-mail: yohno@gly.oups.ac.jp.

induced EPS. In this chapter, the functional roles and mechanisms of 5-HT receptors in modulating antipsychotic-induced EPS are reviewed.

1. INTRODUCTION

Schizophrenia is a serious and heterogenous psychotic disorder with a prevalence of about 0.5 to 1% of the population. Patients with schizophrenia show various clinical symptoms such as positive symptoms (e.g., hallucinations, delusions and excitation), negative symptoms (e.g., apathy, flattened affect, social and emotional withdrawal), and cognitive impairments (e.g., inattention, deficits in social recognition, learning and memory). [1-4]Although the precise mechanisms for the pathogenesis of schizophrenia are still uncertain, hyperfunction of dopamine D_2 receptors in the limbic and cortical regions (i.e., the meso-corticolimbic dopaminergic systems) is implicated in the etiology of schizophrenia ("dopamine hypothesis") (Figure 1). [5, 6]Based on the "dopamine hypothesis", various D_2 receptor antagonists have been developed as antipsychotic drugs, which include phenothiazine-(e.g., chlorpromazine), butyrophenone-(e.g., haloperidol) and benzamide- (e.g., sulpiride) derivatives. These first-generation antipsychotics (FGAs) effectively improve schizophrenia symptoms, especially the positive symptoms. However, FGAs frequently induce severe extrapyramidal side effects (EPS) (e.g., akathisia, bradykinesia,akinesia, tremors, muscle rigidity, dystonia and dyskinesia) and are not so effective at improvingnegative symptoms. [1-4, 7, 8]In the 1980's, itwas shown that blockade of 5-HT_{2A} receptors ameliorates negative schizophrenia symptoms and attenuates antipsychotic-induced EPS, and a line of second-generation antipsychotics (SGAs) (e.g., risperidone, olanzapine,quetiapine, perospirone, ziprasidone and lurasidone) were developed over the past two decades (Figure 2). [1,2, 7-10]These agents commonly exhibita higher affinity to 5-$HT_{2A/2C}$ receptors than to D_2 receptors. In addition, the dopamine D_2 partial agonist aripiprazole was also developed as an SGA (Figure 2). [11] These SGAs are differentiated from FGAs based on their pharmacological features, high efficacy for negative symptoms and reduced EPS liability, and are now widely used as first line drugs for schizophrenia treatment.

Antipsychotic treatments often cause a variety of neurological complications, including extrapyramidal motor disorders, neuroleptic malignant syndrome, seizures and cerebrovascular events. [12] Among them, antipsychotic-induced EPS are the most common and frequently-observed side effects which significantly disrupt the patient's quality of life. Even though SGAs have lower EPS liability than FGAs, they are not free of EPS and produce all the features of EPS associated with FGAs. [12, 13] On the other hand, it is now evident that the serotonergic nervous system plays an important role in modulatingextrapyramidal motor functions. [1, 2, 4, 7] In this chapter, the functional roles and mechanisms of 5-HT receptors in modulating antipsychotic-induced extrapyramidal motor disorders are reviewed.

2. ANTIPSYCHOTIC-INDUCED EXTRAPYRAMIDAL MOTOR DISORDERS

Antipsychotic-induced extrapyramidal motor disorders are brought about by the blockade of dopaminergic neurotransmission in the basal ganglia (Figure 1).

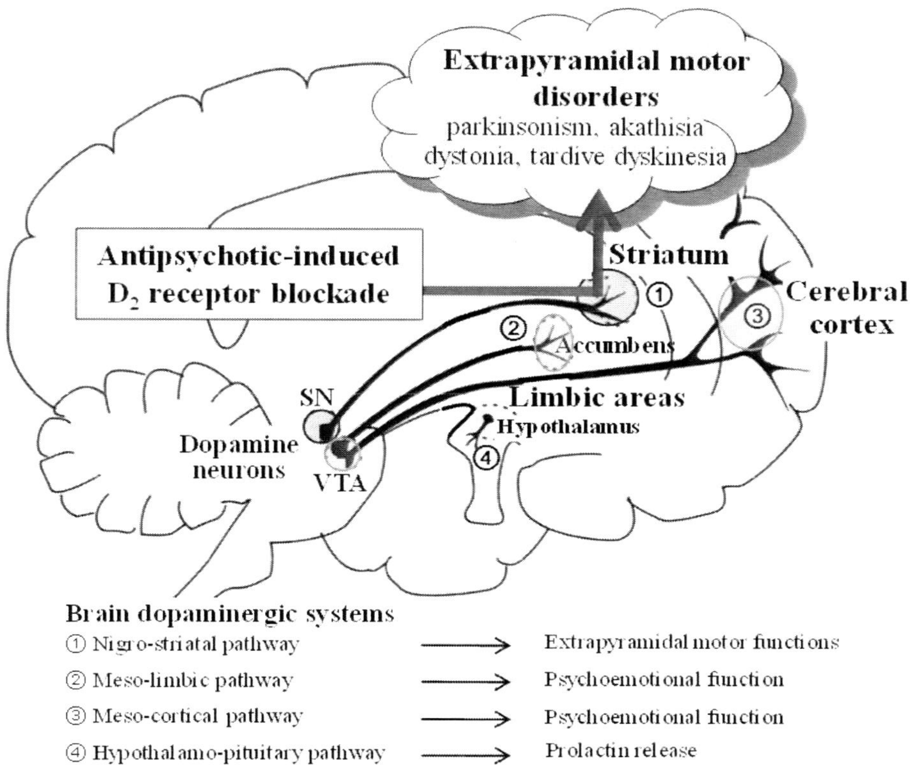

Figure 1. Brain dopaminergic system and extrapyramidal motor disorders.SN:Substantianigra (pars compacta), VTA:Ventral tegmental area.

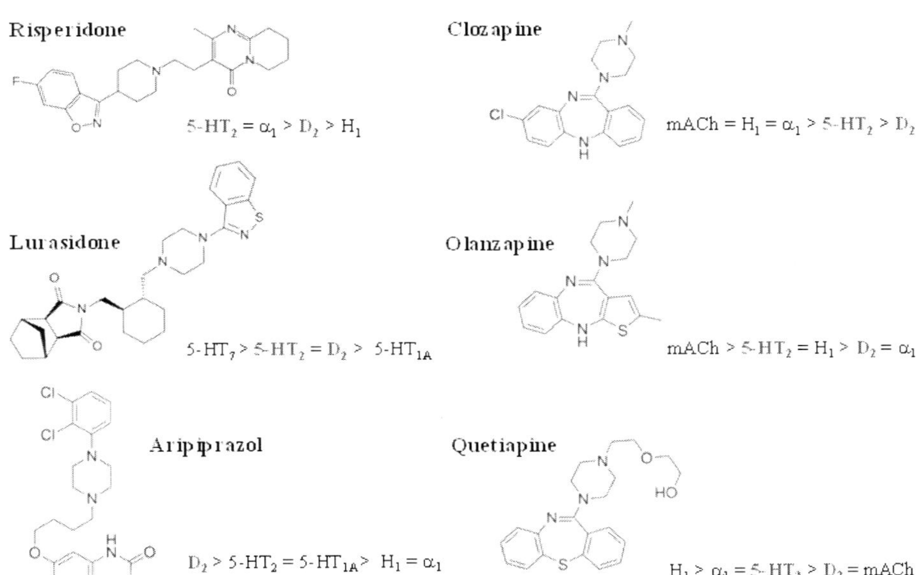

Figure 2.Chemical structures and receptor-binding properties of the second generation antipsychotics.

The basal ganglia consists of structures including the striatum (caudate-putamen), globuspallidus, subthalamic nucleus and substantianigra. These structures form the "cerebral cortex-basal ganglia-thalamus" neural circuit and control the extrapyramidal motor functions (Figure 3).

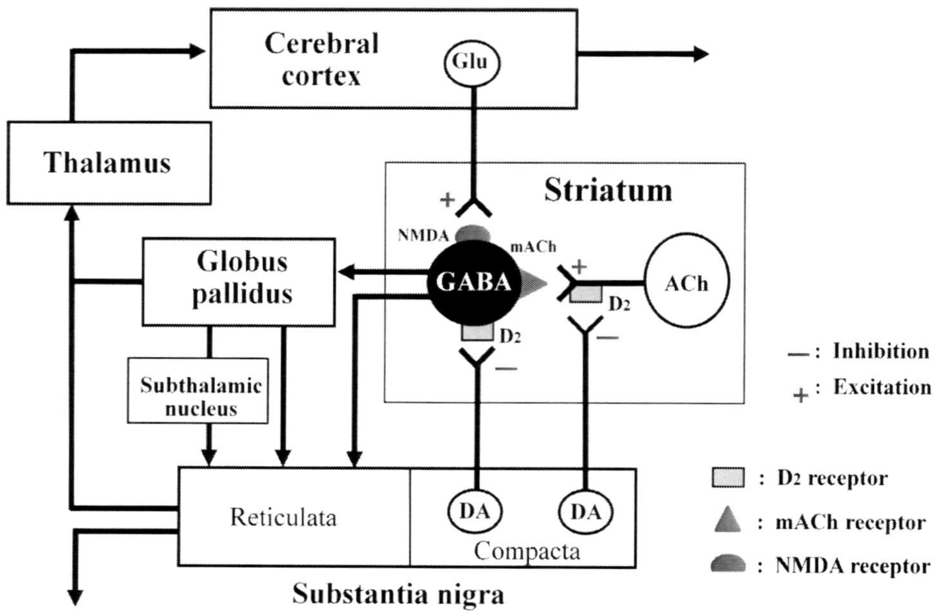

Figure 3.Regulation of extrapyramidal motor functions in the striatum. DA: Dopaminergic neuron, ACh: Acetylcholinergic neuron, Glu: Glutamatergic neuron.

The striatum, in particular, which receives dopaminergic input from the substantianigra (pars compacta) and contains a high density of D_2 receptors, is a core nucleus which regulates the induction of antipsychotic-associated EPS. [7] Striatal neurons are negatively controlled by nigral dopaminergic neurons and positively regulated by glutamatergic neurons from the cerebral cortex, as well asbyacetylcholinergic interneurons within the striatum (Figure 3). Extrapyramidal motor disorders are manifested by the antipsychotic-induced blockade of striatal D_2 receptors (i.e., drug-induced parkinsonism) or the degeneration of nigrostriatal dopaminergic neurons (i.e., Parkinson's disease). [14] Thus, most antipsychotics, even SGAs, often induce EPS during the treatment of schizophrenia. Major EPS symptoms associated with antipsychotic treatments include 1)parkinsonism, 2)akathisia, 3)dystonia and 4)tardive dyskinesia.

(1) Parkinsonism

Parkinsonian symptoms associated with antipsychotic treatments include bradykinesia, akinesia, tremor, muscle rigidity and impaired postural reflex. [12, 14] These disturbances tend to have an insidious onset usually starting a few weeks after starting the antipsychotic treatments. Bradykinesia refers to reduced and impaired motor activity and manifests as slowing and/or interrupted flow of voluntary movements. Antipsychotic-induced tremor is prominent at rest and is low frequency, affecting the hands, head and other parts of the body.

Patients suffering from parkinsonism often exhibit a stooped posture with increased muscle tone (rigidity), a slow gait with lack of arm swing and/or a mask-like face.

Antipsychotic-induced parkinsonism can be controlled by antiparkinsonian agents such as trihexyphenidyl and biperidene, which act as central muscarinic antagonists.

(2) Akathisia

Patients with akathisia complain of inner restlessness, distress and dysphoria, which are a subjective component of this disorder. Akathisia also manifests as objective symptoms such as repetitive movements of the legs and feet, rocking from foot to foot, and walking on the spot. Thus, patients with akathisia sometimes cannot keep sitting and frequently stand or shift their body position. [12, 13, 15]Akathisia usually appears soon after starting or increasing the dose of antipsychotics. Akathisia also occurs during long-term antipsychotic treatments (i.e., tardive akathisia) or upon withdrawal of the antipsychotic treatments (i.e., withdrawal akathisia). Antipsychotic-induced akathisia can be controlled by antiparkinsonian agents (e.g., trihexyphenidyl and biperidene) or adrenergic antagonists (e.g., propranolol).

(3) Dystonia

Dystonia is manifested as intensive and sustained contraction of voluntary muscles, which often leads to a postural distortion. [12, 16] The contractions attack the neck, tongue, trunk or limbs and may last from minutes to hours. Acute dystonia usually appears in the first week after starting or increasing the dose of antipsychotics. Antipsychotic-induced dystonia can be controlled by antiparkinsonian agents (e.g., trihexyphenidyl and biperidene).

(4) Tardive Dyskinesia

Tardive dyskinesia consists of involuntary movements which often appear in oro-facial muscles such as the tongue, lips, mouth or face. However, any parts of the body can be affected and it manifests as various movement disorders including myoclonic jerks, tics, chorea and dystonia. [12, 15] These symptoms are prominent when the patients are alert or excited and disappear during sleep. Tardive dyskinesia typically occurs after months or years of antipsychotic treatment, especially upon reduction of the dose or cessation of the antipsychotic medication. Slow reduction of the antipsychotic dosage can prevent the incidence of tardive dyskinesia, and low doses of antipsychotics ameliorate tardive dyskinesia.

3. Serotonergic Modulation of Antipsychotic-Induced EPS

Serotoninneurons are located in the raphe nuclei and send axons to various brain regions including the cerebral cortex, limbic regions, basal ganglia, diencephalon and the spinal cord.[4, 17]

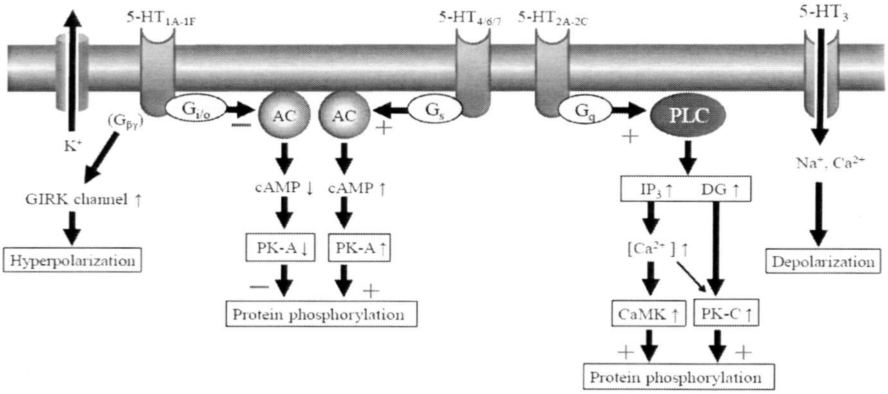

Figure 4.5-HT receptor subtypes and their signal transduction pathways. AC: Adenylatecyclase, PK-A:Protein kinase A, PLC: Phospholipase C,IP_j:Inositol triphosphate, DG: Diacylglycerol, CaMK: Ca^{2+}/calmodulin-dependent protein kinase, PK-C: Protein kinase C, GIRK: G protein-coupled inwardly rectifying potassium channel.

Serotonergic neurotransmissions are mediated by various 5-HT receptor subtypes, which consist of 7 families (5-HT_1 to 5-HT_7) and 14 subtypes (5-$HT_{1A, 1B, 1D, 1E, 1F}$, 5-$HT_{2A, 2B, 2C}$, 5-HT_3, 5-HT_4, 5-$HT_{5A, 5B}$, 5-HT_6 and 5-HT_7) based on their signal transduction pathways (Figure 4). [18]. 5-HT_1-type receptors, 5-HT_{1A}, 5-HT_{1B}, 5-HT_{1D}, 5-HT_{1E} and 5-HT_{1F} receptors, are coupled to $G_{i/o}$ protein and inhibit adenylatecyclase, c-AMP formation and protein kinase A (PK-A) activity. 5-HT_2-type receptors, 5-HT_{2A}, 5-HT_{2B} and 5-HT_{2C} receptors are G_q-coupled and enhance phosphatidilinositol (PI) turnover by activating phospholipase C, which consequently stimulates protein kinase C (PK-C)-and/or Ca^{2+}/calmodulin-cascades.5-HT_4 to 5-HT_7 receptors areG_s-coupled receptors and activate the adenylatecyclase and PK-A cascades.In addition, 5-HT_3 receptors function as channel-type receptors which elicit cation (e.g., Na^+ and Ca^{2+}) influx upon activation (Figure 4).

All 5-HT receptors act as postsynaptic receptors and regulate the neural activity of target neurons. Furthermore, 5-HT_{1A}, 5-HT_{1B} and 5-HT_{1D} receptors also act as presynaptic 5-HT autoreceptors, which inhibit 5-HT neuron activity as a kind of self-feedback regulation. Specifically, 5-HT_{1A} receptors are located on the cell bodies or dendrites of 5-HT neurons in the raphe nuclei and negatively regulate the firing of 5-HT neurons. 5-HT_{1B} or 5-HT_{1D} receptors are located on the nerve terminals of 5-HT neurons in the projected regions, where they inhibit 5-HT release and synthesis of 5-HT.It is now known that the serotonergic nervous system plays an important role in regulating not only psycho-emotional functions, but also motor functions that involve extrapyramidal motor disorders. [3, 4, 17, 18] Specifically, 5-HT_{1A}, 5-$HT_{2A/2C}$, 5-HT_3 and 5-HT_6receptorshave a crucial role in modulating antipsychotic-induced EPS.

(1) 5-HT_{1A}Receptors

5-HT_{1A} receptors are $G_{i/o}$ protein-coupled receptors that,when stimulated,inhibit adenylatecyclase activity, which leads to inhibition of the c-AMP-PK-A cascade (Figure 4). [4, 18, 19] In addition, 5-HT_{1A} receptors activate G protein-gated inwardly rectifying K^+ (GIRK) channels, which consequently hyperpolarize the target neurons and inhibit their firing. [20-25]

Brain regions which contain a high density of 5-HT_{1A} receptors include the raphe nuclei and the limbic regions such as the hippocampus, amygdala and lateral septum. 5-HT_{1A} receptors are also expressed in the cerebral cortex, basal ganglia (e.g., striatum) and diencephalon (e.g., thalamus and hypothalamus) at low to moderate densities. [4, 18, 19] As described previously, 5-HT_{1A} receptors exist not only as postsynaptic receptors, but also as presynaptic autoreceptors which are located on the cell bodies and dendrites of 5-HT neurons in the raphe. To date, numerous 5-HT_{1A} ligands with different intrinsic activities have been synthesized, including 5-HT_{1A} full agonists (e.g., 8-OH-DPAT, flesinoxan and F-11440), 5-HT_{1A} partial agonists (e.g., buspirone, tandospirone, ipsapirone and gepirone) and 5-HT_{1A}antagonists (e.g., WAY-100135, WAY-100635, NAD-299 and lecozotan). [3, 4]

Several lines of studies have shown that stimulation of 5-HT_{1A}receptors improvesantipsychotic-induced EPS and motor disabilities in animal models of Parkinson's disease. [26-32] In our previous studies, 5-HT_{1A} agonists (e.g., 8-OH-DPAT and tandospirone) amelioratedhaloperidol-induced bradykinesia and catalepsy with potencies similar to those of the antiparkisonian agents (e.g., trihexyphenidyl and L-DOPA) (Figure 5). [30, 31] Supporting these anti-EPS actions, 8-OH-DPAT and tandospirone significantly reversed the striatal Fos protein expression due to haloperidol, indicating that 5-HT_{1A}receptors can counteract the antipsychotic-induced D_2 receptor blockade in the striatum. [31, 32] In addition, inhibition of both antipsychotic-induced EPS and striatal Fos expression by 5-HT_{1A} agonistswas antagonized by 5-HT_{1A} antagonists(e.g., WAY-100135). Interestingly, 5-HT_{1A} agonists reversed haloperidol-induced Fos expression region-specifically in the striatum, which is the site closely associated with EPS induction. [31] In contrast, 5-HT_{1A} agonists failed to affect haloperidol-induced Fos expression in the nucleus accumbens (shell region), which is responsible for the therapeutic action of antipsychotics.Thus, it is conceivable that 5-HT_{1A} agonists preferentially alleviate antipsychotic-induced EPS without interrupting the therapeutic actions of antipsychotic drugs.Earlier studies showed that microinjection of 5-HT_{1A}agonists into the raphe nuclei attenuated antipsychotic-induced catalepsy, suggesting that activation of presynaptic 5-HT_{1A}autoreceptors can reduce EPS (Figure 6).[27]

On the other hand, a line of studies demonstrated that the anti-EPS actions of 5-HT_{1A}agonists were resistant against the denervation of 5-HT neurons by 5-HT neurotoxins (e.g., *p*-chlorophenylalanine), indicating that postsynaptic 5-HT_{1A}receptors also play a crucial role in ameliorating EPS. [26, 30, 33, 34] In addition, it is now evident from microinjection studies that local stimulation of 5-HT_{1A}receptors in the striatum or cerebral cortex (i.e., motor cortex) attenuates antipsychotic-induced EPS. [35] It is therefore likely that 5-HT_{1A}agonists ameliorate antipsychotic-induced EPS in three brain regions, the striatum, motor cortex and raphe nuclei, by stimulating postsynaptic 5-HT_{1A}receptors in the former two structures and presynaptic 5-HT_{1A}autoreceptors in the latter (Figure 6). Since the inhibition of cortico-striatal glutamatergic neurotransmission by blocking NMDA receptors has been shown to counteract the striatal D_2 blocking action (i.e., Fos expression) of antipsychotics and reduce their EPS. [36, 37] It is possible that stimulation of cortical 5-HT_{1A}receptors may alleviate EPS by inhibiting activity of cortico-striatal glutamatergic neurons (Figure 6 and Table 1). Furthermore, 5-HT_{1A}agonists are known to improve the extrapyramidaldisorders elicited by dopaminergic neurotoxins (e.g., MPTP and 6-hydroxydopamine), indicating that 5-HT_{1A}receptors alleviate EPS via non-dopaminergic mechanisms. [29, 38]

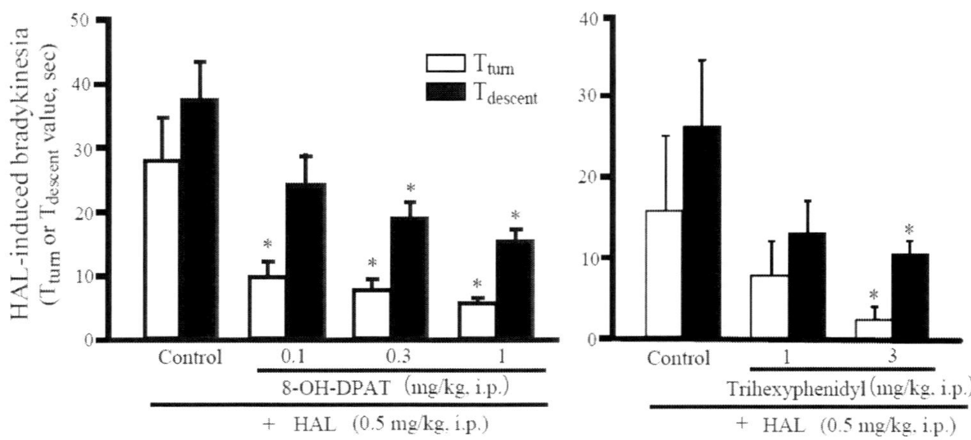

Figure 5.Ameliorative actions of the 5-HT_{1A}agonist 8-OH-DPAT on haloperidol (HAL)-induced bradykinesia in the mouse pole-test.T_{turn} and $T_{descent}$ values are the time required for mice to rotate on the pole and to descent to the floor, respectively. Actions of the antiparkinsonian drug trihexyphenidyl are also shown for comparison.

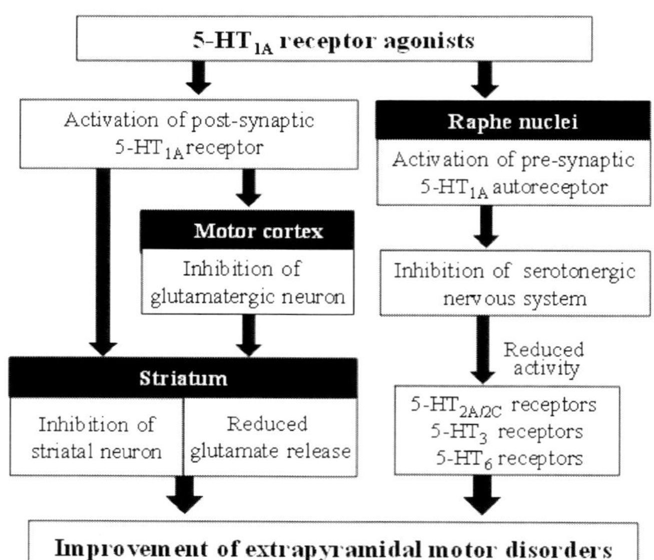

Figure 6.Action mechanisms of 5-HT_{1A} agonists in regulating extrapyramidal motor disorders.

(2) 5-$HT_{2A/2C}$Receptors

Among 5-HT_2receptor subtypes, 5-HT_{2A} and 5-HT_{2C} receptors are highly expressed in the brain, while 5-HT_{2B} receptors mainly exist in the peripheral tissues (e.g., stomach fundus) [18]. Specifically, 5-HT_{2A} receptors are expressed at a high density in the forebrain regions such as the cerebral cortex (e.g., neocortex, entorhinal and piriform cortex), caudate nucleus, olfactory tubercle and limbic regions (e.g., nucleus accumbens, hippocampus). 5-HT_{2C} receptors are distributed in various brain regions including the cortex (e.g., neocortex, cingulate and pyriform cortex), limbic regions (e.g., nucleus accumbens, hippocampus and amygdala), and basal ganglia (e.g., striatum and substantianigra).Both 5-HT_{2A} and 5-HT_{2C} receptors are G_q protein-coupled, and their stimulation activates phospholipase C, yielding IP_3 and diacylglycerol (Figure 4).Thus, 5-HT_{2A} and 5-HT_{2C} receptors activate Ca^{2+}/calmodulin- and/or protein kinase C- cascades, which consequently cause a slow excitation of neurons in various regions of the brain. [18] It is well documented that 5-$HT_{2A/2C}$ antagonists attenuate antipsychotic-induced EPS (Figure 7). [1, 2, 7, 39] The ameliorative effects of 5-$HT_{2A/2C}$ antagonists (e.g., ritanserin and ketanserin) on haloperidol-induced bradykinesia were almost equipotent to those of an anti-muscarinic drug (i.e., trihexyphenidyl) in the mouse pole-test. [39] It is known that 5-$HT_{2A/2C}$ antagonists reverse various responses of striatal neurons to antipsychotics (D_2 antagonists) such as increases in acetylcholine release, metabolic turnover of dopamine and Fosexpression in the striatum (Figure 7), supporting the EPS-ameliorating actions of 5-$HT_{2A/2C}$ antagonists. [40-42]

Table 1. Serotonergic strategies for alleviation of extrapyramidal motor disorders

5-HT Receptor	Proposed functions	Therapeutic Strategy	Related Compounds
5-HT_{1A} receptor	Inhibition of cortico-striatal glutamatergic neuron Reduced glutamine release in the striatrum	Agonist (Partial agonist)	8-OH-DPAT Buspirone Tandospirone Osemozotan PRX-00023 U93385
5-$HT_{2A/2C}$ receptor	Inhibition of dopamine release in the striatum Inhibition of dopamine neron firing in the substantia nigra Activation of Ach interneurons in the striatum (5-HT_{2C})	Antagonist (Inverse agonist)	Ritanserin MDL100907 SR46349B
5-HT3 receptor	Activation of cortico-striatal glutamatergic neuron Glutamine release in the striatum	Antagonist	Ondansetron Granisetron Azasetron Tropisetron
5-HT_6 receptor	Activation of Ach interneurons in the striatum	Antagonist	SB-742457 BGC20-761 LY-483518 PRX-07034

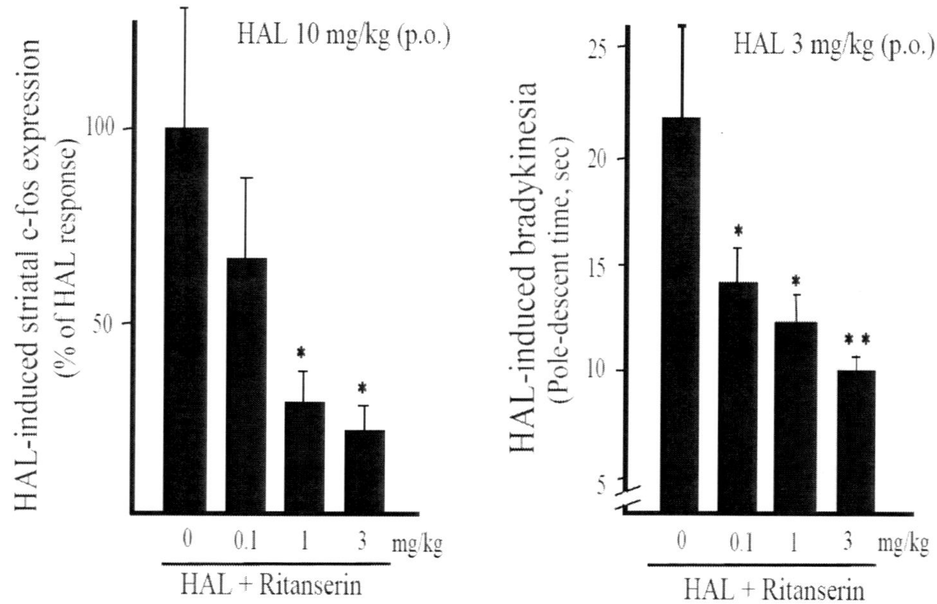

Figure 7.Effects of the 5-$HT_{2A/2C}$antagonist ritanserin on haloperidol (HAL)-induced c-fos mRNA expression in the striatum (left) and bradykinesia in the mouse pole-test (right).

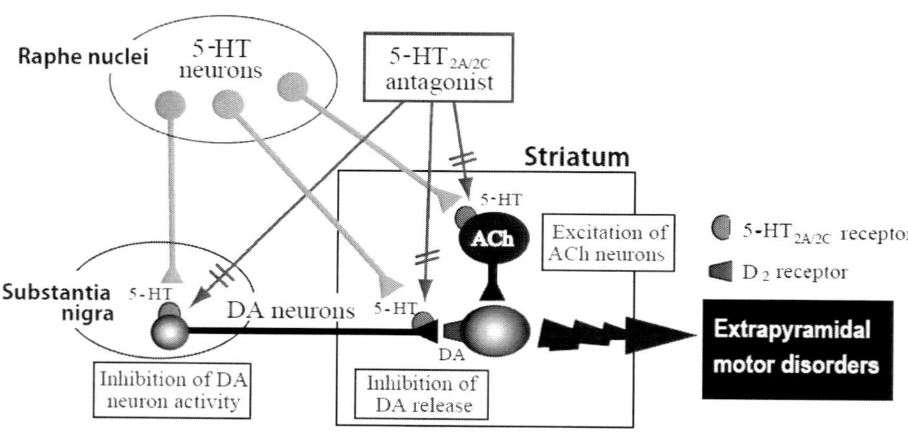

Figure 8. Potential mechanisms of 5-$HT_{2A/2C}$ receptors and 5-$HT_{2A/2C}$ antagonists underlying the regulation of extrapyramidal motor disorders. ACh: Acetylcholine, DA: Dopamine.

It is now postulated that blockade of 5-$HT_{2A/2C}$ receptors alleviates EPS by relieving the 5-$HT_{2A/2C}$ receptor-mediated inhibition of dopamine release in the striatum,and of neural firing of the nigral dopamine neurons (Figure 8 and Table 1). [2, 7, 43, 44] In addition, although the precise subtype(s) of 5-HT_2 receptors in modulating extrapyramidal motor functions are still uncertain, several studies suggest that 5-HT_{2C} receptors have a crucial role in modulating EPS. [45, 46] Supporting this possibility, a recent electrophysiological study using a combined single cell PCR technique [47] showed that 5-HT_{2C} receptors are expressed in the striatal cholinergic interneurons and mediate 5-HT-elicited excitation, leading to EPS induction (Figure 8 and Table 1).

(3) 5-HT$_3$ Receptors

5-HT$_3$receptors are composed of a hetero-pentamer consisting of 5-HT$_{3A}$ to 5-HT$_{3E}$ subunits and function as Na^+ and Ca^{2+}-permeable cation channels (Figure 4). [17, 18, 48]

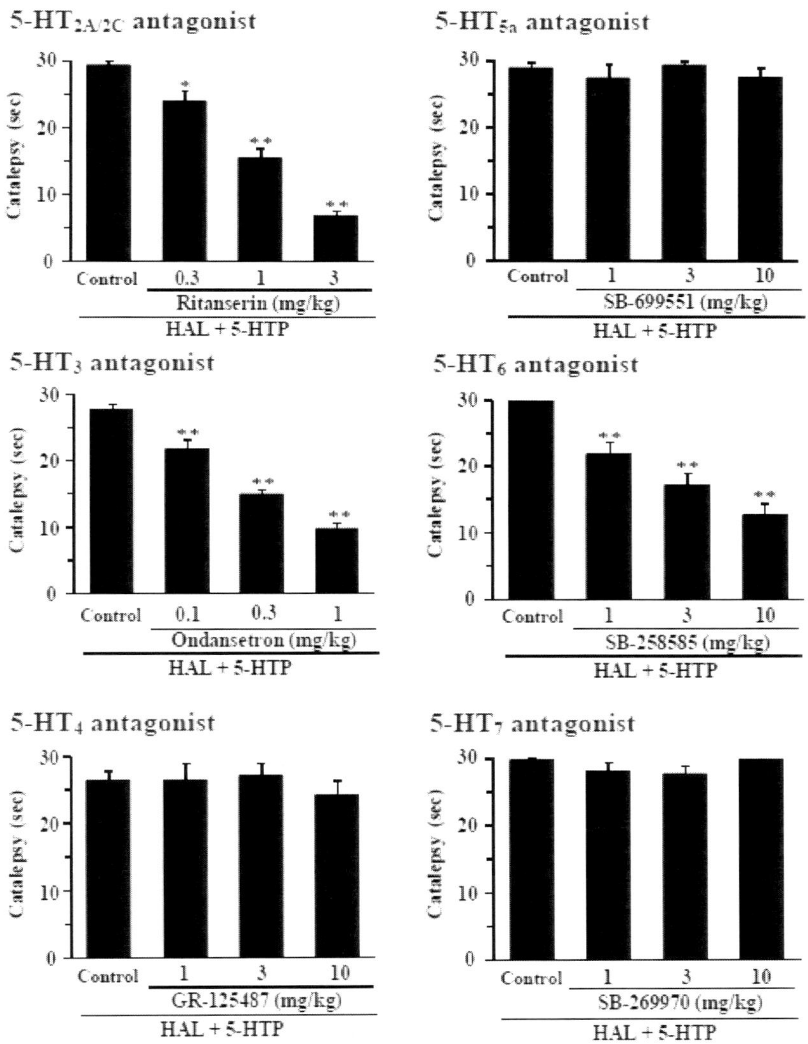

Figure 9. Effects of various 5-HT antagonists on haloperidol (HAL:0.3mg/kg, i.p.)-induced extrapyramidal symptom (catalepsy) in mice. 5-Hydroxytryptophan (5-HTP: 100 mg/kg, i.p.) was pretreated with 5-HT antagonists 60 min before HAL injection to facilitate the serotonergic activity.

Therefore, activation of 5-HT_3receptors depolarizes the postsynaptic membranes and excites the target neurons. 5-HT_3receptors are also located on the nerve terminals of acetylcholinergic and glutamatergic neurons and regulate neurotransmitter release.

Previous studies showed that 5-HT_3 receptor antagonists (e.g., ondansetron and granisetron) reduced haloperidol-induced EPS (e.g., catalepsy and bradykinesia). [49, 50] In our studies, activation of the serotonergic system by 5-hydroxytryptophan (5-HTP) significantly potentiatedhaloperidol-induced catalepsy and this 5-HTP-potentiated EPS was also suppressed by systemic treatments or intrastriatal microinjections of ondansetron (Figure 9). [50]These findings indicate that postsynaptic 5-HT_3 receptors in the striatum are involved in potentiating antipsychotic-induced EPS.

Although the precise mechanisms for the anti-EPS actions of 5-HT_3 antagonists arestill uncertain, previous studies showed that 5-HT_3 antagonists stimulate glutamate release in various regions of the brain. [51-53]Since the cortico-striatal glutamatergic neurons are implicated ininduction of antipsychotic-associated EPS [36, 37], 5-HT_3 antagonists may reduce EPS by inhibiting glutamate release (Table 1).

(4) 5-HT_6 Receptors

5-HT_6receptors are coupled to Gs protein, and their activation stimulates c-AMP formation and the PK-A cascade (Figure 4). 5-HT_6receptors are predominantly expressed in the brain, specifically in the basal ganglia (e.g., striatum and nucleus accumbens), limbic regions (e.g., olfactory tubercles and hippocampus) and cerebral cortex. [17, 18]

5-HT_6receptors are implicated in psychoemotional disorders (e.g., schizophrenia and depression), eating disorders, cognitive deficits in schizophrenia and Alzheimer's disease. Besides these functions, 5-HT_6receptors may modify the extrapyramidal motor functions since they are highly expressed in the striatum. Although an early study reported that the 5-HT_6antagonist Ro 04-6790 failed to affect haloperidol-induced catalepsy [54], we recently demonstrated that the 5-HT_6antagonist SB-258585 alleviated haloperidol-induced bradykinesia and catalepsy. [50] In addition, the EPS potentiating actions of 5-HTPwas also blocked by systemic injection of SB-258585 or its microinjection into the striatum (Figure 9), implying that blockade of the striatal 5-HT_6 receptors is at least partly involved in alleviating antipsychotic-induced EPS. [50] The anti-EPS actions of 5-HT_6antagonistswere further supported by electrophysiological studies [47]showing that 5-HT_6 receptors, as well as 5-$HT_{2A/2C}$receptors, are expressed in the striatal acetylcholine interneurons, where 5-HT_6 receptors excite acetylcholine neurons. Since activation of striatal acetylcholine neurons evokes extrapyramidal disorders, it is conceivable that 5-HT_6 antagonists alleviate antipsychotic-induced EPS by inhibiting the acetylcholinergic activity in the striatum (Table 1).

(5) Other 5-HTReceptors

Although the information is limited, other 5-HT receptor subtypes seem to have only limited roles in modulating extrapyramidal motor disorders. [50] As shown in Figure 9, neither the 5-HT_4 (i.e., GR-125487), 5-HT_{5a}(SB-699551) nor 5-HT_7(SB-269970) antagonistaffectedhaloperidol-induced extrapyramidal symptoms (i.e., catalepsy).

4. Roles of 5-HT Receptors in Atypical Antipsychotic Actions

As described previously, the serotonergic systemmodulates extrapyramidal motor functions via multiple 5-HT receptor subtypes, 5-HT_{1A} receptors reducing EPS, and 5-$HT_{2A/2C}$, 5-HT_3 or 5-HT_6 receptors enhancing it. Among these mechanisms, antagonism of 5-$HT_{2A/2C}$ receptors is implicated in the common mechanism of SGAs (e.g., risperidone, olanzapine,quetiapine, perospirone, ziprasidone and lurasidone) which exhibit reduced EPS liability (Figure 2). [1, 2, 7, 8, 44] Some of the SGAs (e.g., ziprasidone, perospirone, lurasidone and aripiprazole) possess a partial agonistic activity at 5-HT_{1A} receptors, which may also contribute to their atypical antipsychotic properties (Figure 2). [4, 55, 56] It should be noted that the mechanisms underlying the anti-EPS actions of 5-HT_{1A} agonists are distinct from those of 5-$HT_{2A/2C}$ antagonists. Namely, 5-$HT_{2A/2C}$ antagonists reverse antipsychotic-induced EPS by activating dopaminergic neurons via antagonizing the 5-$HT_{2A/2C}$receptor-mediated inhibition of dopamine neurons in the substantianigra and of dopamine release in the striatum (Figure 8).However, the anti-EPS actions of 5-HT_{1A} agonists are independent of the dopaminergic activity, since the antiparkinsonian actions of 5-HT_{1A} agonists are resistant against D_2 antagonists and are effective for extrapyramidal disorders elicited by dopaminergic denervation. [29, 35, 38] Therefore, it seems likely that 5-HT_{1A}agonism and 5-HT_{2A} antagonism can work in an additive fashion in alleviating EPS.Furthermore, a partial agonistic action of 5-HT_{1A} receptors reportedly improved cognitive impairments in patients with schizophrenia, providing benefits in the schizophrenia treatment.

5-HT_3antagonists (e.g., ondansetron, granisetron, azasetron and tropisetron) seem to be useful as an adjunctive treatment for antipsychotic-induced EPS (Table 1). Interestingly, 5-HT_3antagonists are known to enhance cognitive functions or alleviate cognitive deficits associated with aging or drug treatment in various animal models (e.g., Morris water maze test and novel object recognition test). [51, 52, 57, 58] Thus, 5-HT_3receptors may serve as a novel therapeutic target for schizophrenia. Indeed, recent double-blind and randomized studies using patients with chronic schizophrenia have shown that add-on treatments of ondansetron with haloperidol or risperidone for 8-12 weeks significantly reduced the incidence and severity of antipsychotic-induced EPS (e.g., akathisia and parkinsonism). [59, 60] In addition, ondansetron significantly improved cognitive impairments and negative symptoms in schizophrenia.

5-HT_6receptors are one of the action sites of clozapine, the prototype of SGAs, which exhibits very weak EPS liability. [8, 10, 61] The clozapine-derivatives (e.g., olanzapine) also show high affinity to 5-HT_6receptors, which are implicated in their atypical antipsychotic properties .[8, 61, 62] In addition, 5-HT_6antagonists are known to ameliorate cognitive impairments. [63-66] Thus, similar to 5-HT_3receptors, blockade of 5-HT_6receptors provides benefits in terms of both reduction of antipsychotics-induced EPS and improvement in cognitive deficits, in schizophrenia treatment. Several new 5-HT_6antagonists (e.g., BGC20-761, LY-483518, PRX-07034 and SB-742457) are now being developed (Table 1).

CONCLUSION

Extrapyramidal motor disorders are the most common and frequently-observed side effects of antipsychotics. Although SGAs have been developed as an advanced medication for schizophrenia, they are not free of EPSs and still significantly disrupt the patient's quality of life. This chapter reviewed the functional roles and mechanisms of the serotonergic system in modulating extrapyramidal motor functions and introduced potential strategies for the management of antipsychotic-induced EPS. Among 5-HT receptor subtypes, stimulation of 5-HT_{1A} and blockade of 5-$HT_{2A/2C}$, 5-HT_3 or 5-HT_6 receptors are promising strategies to reducing EPS liability. These serotonergic strategies, such as add-on therapy with 5-HT_{1A} agonists or 5-HT_3 antagonists and drug discovery research to design new 5-HT_{1A}, 5-HT_3 or 5-HT_6 receptorligands possessing combined actions on the current therapeutic targets (e.g., $D_2$and 5-HT_{2A}receptors), will contribute to future therapy for schizophrenia.

REFERENCES

[1] H. Y. Meltzer,*Schizophr. Bull.*17,263 (1991).
[2] S. Kapur and G. Remington,*Ann. Rev. Med.*52, 503 (2001).
[3] Y. Ohno, *Cent. Nerv. Syst. Agents Med. Chem.*10, 148 (2010).
[4] Y. Ohno, *CNS Neurosci. Ther.*17,58 (2011).
[5] H. Y. Meltzer and S. M. Stahl, *Schizophr Bull.* 2, 19 (1976).
[6] P. Seeman, *Synapse.*1,133 (1987).
[7] Y. Ohno, K. Ishida-Tokuda, T. Ishibashi, H. Sakamoto, R. Tagashira, T. Horisawa, et al. *Pol. J. Pharmacol.*49,213 (1997).
[8] H. Y. Meltzer, Z. Li, Y. Kaneda and J. Ichikawa, *Prog. Neuro-Psychopharmacol. Biol. Psychiatry* 27,1159 (2003).
[9] A. Bleich, S. L. Brown, R. Kahn and H. M. van Praag, *Schizophr. Bull.* 14,297 (1988).
[10] A. Breier, *Schizophr. Res.* 14, 187 (1995).
[11] M. Wood and C. Reavill, *Expert. Opin. Investig. Drugs*16,771 (2007).
[12] P. M. Haddad and S. M. Dursun, *Hum. Psychopharmacol.* 23, 15 (2008).
[13] R. Kumar and P. S. Sachdev, *Curr. Opin. Psychiatry*22, 293 (2009).
[14] A. Samii, J. G. Nutt and B. Ransom,*Lancet* 363,1783 (2004).
[15] T. R. E. Barnes and W. M. Braude, *Arch. Gen. Psychiatry* 42, 874 (1985).
[16] C. Swett Jr. *Am. J. Psychiatry* 132, 532 (1975).
[17] B. L. Roth, *Ann.Clin. Psychiatry.*6,67 (1994).
[18] N. M. Barnes and T. Sharp, *Neuropharmacology.*38,1083 (1999).
[19] T. J. Pucadyil,S. Kalipatnapu and A.Chattopadhyay,*Cell. Mol.Neurobiol.* 25,553 (2005).
[20] A. Hirose, M. Sasa,A. Akaike and S. Takaori,*Neuropharmacology* 29,93 (1990).
[21] P. Van den Hooff, and M. Galvan, *Br. J. Pharmacol.* 106,893 (1992).
[22] V. Hadrava, P. Blier, T. Dennis, C. Ortemann and de Montigny C, *Neuropharmacology.* 34, 1311 (1995).

[23] Y. Ohno, K. Ishida,T. Ishibashi, H. Tanaka,H. Shimizu and M. Nakamura, In "*Serotonin in the Central Nervous System and Periphery*." edited by A. Takada and G, Curzon, pp. 159, *Elsevier Science BV*, Amsterdam (1995).
[24] J. R. Raymond,Y. V. Muklin,T. W. Gettys, and M. N.Garnovskaya,*Br. J. Pharmacol.*127,1751 (1999).
[25] K. Tada,K. Kasamo,N. Ueda,T. Suzuki,T. Kojima, andK. Ishikawa,*J.Pharmacol. Exp.Ther.*288,843 (1999).
[26] B. S. Neal-Beliveau, J. N. Joyce andI. Lucki,*J.Pharmacol. Exp.Ther.*265,207 (1993).
[27] M. L. WadenbergK. A. Young,J. T. Richter andP. B. Hicks,*Neuropharmacology*38,151 (1999).
[28] E. P. Prinssen,F. C. Colpaert and W. Koek,*Eur. J.Pharmacol.*453,217 (2002).
[29] T. Ishibashi and Y. Ohno, *Biog. Amines.*8,329,(2004).
[30] Y. Ohno,S. Shimizu,J. Imaki,S. Ishihara,N. Sofue M. Sasa et al. *Prog.Neuro-Psychopharmacol. Biol. Psychiatry* 32, 1302 (2008).
[31] Y. Ohno,S. Shimizu,J. Imaki,S. Ishihara,N. Sofue,M. Sasa et al.*Neuropharmacology*55,717 (2008).
[32] Y. Ohno,S. Shimizu and J. Imaki,*J.Pharmacol. Sci.*109,593 (2009).
[33] L. Mignon andW. A. Wolf,*Psychopharmacology*163,85 (2002).
[34] A. Zazpe, I. Artaiz, A. Innerarity, E. del Olmo, E. Castro, L. Labeaga, et al. *Neuropharmacology*51,129 (2006).
[35] S. Shimizu, A. Tatara, J. Imakiand Y. Ohno,*Prog. Neuro-Psychopharmacol. Biol. Psychiatry* 34,877 (2010).
[36] E. H. Chartoff, R. P. Ward andD. M. Dorsa,*J.Pharmacol. Exp.Ther.*291,531 (1999).
[37] N. Hussain, B. A. Flumerfelt and N. Rajakumar, *Neuroscience*102, 391 (2001).
[38] K. Matsubara, K. Shimizu, M. Suno, K. Ogawa, T. Awaya, T. Yamada, et al. *Brain Res.*1112,126 (2006).
[39] Y. Ohno,K. Ishida, K. Ikeda, T. Ishibashi, K. Okada andM. Nakamura,*Pharmacol.Biochem. Behav.*49,19 (1994).
[40] T. Ishibashi,K. Ikeda, K. Ishida, J.Yasui, R. Tojima, M. Nakamura, et al. *Eur. J. Pharmacol.*303, 247 (1996).
[41] K. Ishida,Y.Ohno, T. Ishibashi andM. Nakamura, *Gen. Pharmacol.*27, 1203 (1996).
[42] K.D.Alex and E.A.Pehek, *Pharmacol. Ther.*113, 296, (2007).
[43] G. Remington and S. Kapur, *J. Clin. Psychiatry 60*(Suppl 10),15 (1999).
[44] J.Horacek, V.Bubenikova-Valesova, M.Kopecek, T. Palenicek, C. Dockery, P. Mohr,et al.*CNS Drugs*20,389(2006).
[45] C. Reavill, A. Kettle, V. Holland. G. Riley and T. P. Blackburn, *Br. J. Pharmacol.* 126, 572 (1999).
[46] M. Creed-Carson, A. Oraha and J. N. Nobrega, *Behav. Brain Res.*219, 273 (2011).
[47] P.Bonsi, D.Cuomo, J. Ding, G.Sciamanna, S. Ulrich, A. Tscherter, et al. *Neuropsychopharmacology*32, 1840 (2007).
[48] M. R. Livesey,M. A. Cooper, T. Z. Deeb, J.E. Carland, J. Kozuska, T.G. Hales, et al.*J. Biol. Chem.*283,19301 (2008).
[49] S.R.Silva, H.A.Futuro-Neto and J.G.Pires, *Neuropharmacology*34, 97(1995).
[50] Y.Ohno, J.Imaki, Y. Mae, T. Takahashi and A.Tatara, *Neuropharmacology*60, 201 (2010).

[51] H. Hodges,P. Sowinski,J. J. Turner and A. Fletcher,*Psychopharmacology (Berl).*125,146 (1996).
[52] F. J. Gil-Bea,J. Domínguez,M. García-Alloza,B. Marcos, B. Lasheras and M.J. Ramirez, *Neuropharmacology* 47,225 (2004).
[53] M. G. Giovannini,I. Ceccarelli, B. Molinari,M. Cecchi, J. Goldfarb and P. Blandina, *J. Pharmacol. Exp. Ther.*285,1219 (1998).
[54] A. Bourson,F. G. Boess, M.Bös and A. J. Sleight, *Br. J. Pharmacol.*125, 1562 (1998).
[55] M. J. Millan,*J.Pharmacol. Exp.Ther.*295,853 (2000).
[56] T. Ishibashi and Y. Ohno, *Biog. Amines.*18, 307 (2004).
[57] J. M. Barnes,B. Costall, J. Coughlan,A. M. Domeney, P.A. Gerrard, M.E. Kelly, et al.*Pharmacol. Biochem. Behav.*35,955 (1990).
[58] A. F. Arnsten,C. H. Lin,C. H. Van Dyck,and K.J. Stanhope,*Neurobiol. Aging.*18,21 (1997).
[59] Z. J. Zhang,W. H. Kang,Q. Li,X. Y. Wang, S. M. Yao and A.Q. Ma, *Schizophr. Res.*88,102 (2006).
[60] S. Akhondzadeh,N. Mohammadi,M. Noroozian, N. Karamghadiri, A. Ghoreishi, A.H. Jamshidi, et al. *Schizophr. Res.*107,206 (2009).
[61] R. Kohen,M. A. Metcalf,N. Khan, T. Druck, K. Huebner, J. E. Lachowicz, et al.*J. Neurochem.*66,47 (1996).
[62] F. Bymaster, K. W. Perry, D. L. Nelson, D. T. Wong, K. Rasmussen, N. A. Moore and D. O. Calligaro, *Br. J. Psychiatry Suppl.* 37, 36 (1999).
[63] M. L. Woolley,C. A. Marsden,A. J. Sleight,C. A. Marsden and K. C. Fone, *Psychopharmacology (Berl).*170,358 (2003).
[64] M. V. King,A. J. Sleight, M. L. Woolley,I. A. Topham, C. A. Marsden and K. C. Fone, *Neuropharmacology*47,195 (2004).
[65] C. K. Lieben,A. Blokland, A. Sik, E. Sung, P. van Nieuwenhuizen and R. Schreiber,*Neuropsychopharmacology*30,2169 (2005).
[66] W. D. Hirst,T. O. Stean, D. C. Rogers, D. Sunter, P. Pugh, S.F. Moss, et al. *Eur. J. Pharmacol.*553,109 (2006).

In: Antipsychotic Drugs
Editors: T.L. Schwartz, J. Megna and M.E. Topel

ISBN: 978-1-62100-071-6

Chapter 12

TARDIVE DYSKINESIA

***Nisha Warikoo*[1], *Thomas L. Schwartz*[1,*] *and Leslie Citrome*[2]**
[1]SUNY Upstate Medical University, Department of Psychiatry, Syracuse, NY, US
[2]New York Medical College, Valhalla, NY, US

ABSTRACT

Introduction: The treatment of schizophrenia was revolutionized by the introduction of first-generation antipsychotics (FGAs) in the 1950s. FGAs have now been largely replaced by second-generation antipsychotics (SGAs), which have a lower propensity for acute extrapyramidal symptoms (EPS)[1,2] and perhaps tardive dyskinesia (TD).[3] There remains a need however to be able to accurately detect and manage motoric side effects of antipsychotics as these problems persist in clinical practice.

Conclusion: Tardive dyskinesia rates appear to be lower with newer antipsychotic agents but still a problematic side effect that requires astute clinical skills for detection and mitigation. This chapter will review all aspects of this side effect to aid clinicians' ability to provide safe patient care while prescribing second generation antipsychotics.

MOTORIC SIDE EFFECTS OF ANTIPSYCHOTIC MEDICATIONS

Motoric side effects can be broadly divided into acute and chronic categories. Acute side effects are usually dose dependent and are known to occur within first the few hours, days or weeks of antipsychotic medication administration. These include acute akathisia, acute dystonia, and Parkinsonism.[4-8] Akathisia is characterized by somatic restlessness that manifests as pacing and inability to sit still and is often mistaken for psychotic agitation.[9] Effective treatments for akathisia include lowering the dose or switching antipsychotic [9] and use of centrally acting beta blockers or benzodiazepines.[9] Dystonias are disturbances in muscle tone characterized by spastic contraction of discrete skeletal muscle groups e.g. neck, face, tongue or back that respond dramatically to the administration of anticholinergic medication. Parkinsonism includes tremor, muscle rigidity and a generalized loss of energy

* Tel:315 464-3100. FAX:315 464-3163. E-mail:schwartt@upstate.edu.

and spontaneity. Symptoms of Parkinsonism usually resolve with reduction of the dose of antipsychotic medication and administration of an anticholinergic agent, though cases of persisting symptoms have been reported.[8]All antipsychotics may can cause potentially fatal neuroleptic malignant syndrome (NMS), characterized by diffuse muscular rigidity, tremors, fever, labile blood pressure, and cognitive disturbances.[5,10] Removal of the antipsychotic, symptomatic measures and use of dantrolene or bromocriptine are warranted.

Chronic motoric side effects can occur after months and years of antipsychotic medication administration, are not clearly dose dependent, and may persist after medication discontinuation. These adverse effects include tardive dystonia and tardive dyskinesia (TD). Dystonias that have been observed to persist 20 months after discontinuation of antipsychotic medications were first described as tardive dystonia in 1962.[11] Tardive dystonia is characterized by spastic muscle contractions, resulting in dystonic postures, abnormal gait or head position and is often associated with great distress and physical discomfort. [12] In contrast to tardive dyskinesia (TD), tardive dystonia often begins after a relatively short period of exposure to antipsychotics i.e. months. In a review by Harten et al, mean prevalence of tardive dystonia was estimated to be 3%.[13] About one-fifth of these cases are known to occur in the first year, and half of the cases in the first 5 years of exposure.[14] Dopamine depleters like tetrabenazine, reserpine, anticholinergic medications such as trihexyphenidyl, clozapine, clonazepam, or the combination of clozapine plus clonazepam, have been found to be helpful in some cases.[15,16] There is also limited evidence of the effectiveness of electroconvulsive therapy (ECT) in this condition, and this may be considered if pharmacological treatments and treatments like deep brain stimulation (DBS) or botulinum toxin have failed.[17] Some dyskinesias have been noted to appear after abrupt discontinuation of antipsychotic medications and remit in a few weeks to a few months. This is known as a withdrawal dyskinesia and these symptoms reflect the ability of neuroleptic agents to mask dyskinesia. [18,19] A persistent form of late-onset akathisia has been referred to as tardive akathisia. It was suggested that tardive akathisia may be a preliminary stage of TD in some patients receiving long-term antipsychotic treatment. Unlike acute akathisia, tardive akathisia can worsen when the antipsychotic dose is lowered and can present with emergent TD. [20] In a retrospective study of 52 patients, most patients developed tardive akathisia after years of antipsychotic treatment (mean = 4.5 years) but 34% developed it within 1 year. Akathisia persisted for several years in 50% of the patients who discontinued antipsychotic medications. Only 33% of patients had complete abatement of their symptoms on follow-up.[21] The remainder of this paper will focus on TD in regards to epidemiology, diagnosis and treatment.

HISTORY OF TARDIVE DYSKINESIA

Tardive dyskinesia (TD) has been intricately linked to antipsychotics since their introduction in the 1950s. The syndrome was described as early as in 1959 by Sigwald et al.[22] Faurbye et al, first coined the term in 1964 and recognized that the incidence of TD increased with chronic exposure.[23] TD is also known as rhythmical chorea, oral-buccal-lingual dyskinesias, facial myochymia, classical tardive dyskinesia and tardive stereotypy because of its late onset and repetitive, rather than random nature. It was described in early reports that TD may persist long after the discontinuation of the antipsychotic medication.[11] Since the 1990s, SGAs have largely replaced the use of FGAs. The interest in TD from a clinical standpoint may have decreased of recent as it may occur at a lower rate with the SGAs or may be less severe in nature, as compared to what has been experienced with FGAs. However, it is important to recognize that TD tends to be persistent and can be irreversible in up to 50% of affected patients. Moreover, TD has been shown to increase mortality and is associated with a more severe and treatment refractory illness course.[24]

INCIDENCE AND PREVALENCE

The incidence and prevalence rates of TD vary widely depending upon the population, study design and diagnostic criteria used. It is important to note that some of these studies have not controlled for certain factors, which may confound the results, for example, age, gender, diagnosis, length of illness, exposure to different antipsychotics, or presence of acute EPS. In addition, spontaneous abnormal involuntary movements identical to neuroleptic-induced tardive dyskinesia have been described in schizophrenia for over a century, even before the availability of antipsychotics.[25,26] A report using data from 14 studies of neuroleptic-naive patients with schizophrenia, reported a spontaneous dyskinesia rate of approximately 4% in first-episode schizophrenic patients, 12% for patients ill several years but below age 30, 25% for those aged between 30 and 50, and 40% for those aged 60 or older.[25] A recent systematic review identified 13 studies which suggests a spontaneous dyskinesia median rate of 9% and a spontaneous parkinsonism median rate of 17%.[27] Investigators have proposed that spontaneous movement disorders may be intrinsic to the pathophysiology of schizophrenia and that antipsychotic medication might be acting by modifying the expression of disease-based motor dysfunctions.[28,29] Furthermore, non-adherence rate to antipsychotic medications in patients with schizophrenia has been reported to be about 50%. In the context of non-adherence, patients may thus be developing TD with less exposure to antipsychotics than assumed.[30,31]. Additionally, not only are antipsychotics known to worsen TD, but also can mask TD, possibly owing to bradykinesia and rigidity effects. Severity of TD is known to fluctuate depending on the level of emotional or behavioral arousal and spontaneously as well. These factors can contribute to erroneous underestimation of prevalence rates of TD.[32,33]

In a literature analysis of 56 studies involving approximately 35,000 antipsychotic treated patients the prevalence of TD averaged 20%. The rate of TD in approximately 11,000 antipsychotic naïve patients was found to be 5% and the corrected rate for neuroleptic induced TD was calculated to be about 15%.[34,35] In a recent systematic review that included four adult studies of 2088 patients, TD prevalence rates were 13.1% for patients on SGAs, 15.6% for antipsychotic-free patients, and 32.4% for those on FGAs [36] This review also estimated annual TD incidence rates across twelve trials in 58,021 patients: 2.98% with SGAs versus 7.7% with FGAs in adults, and 0.35% with SGAs in children.[36] A relationship between longer exposure and a steadily rising cumulative risk of developing TD is supported by a prospective study; rates suggest an annual incidence of about 5% overall, including transient (less than three months) and persistent TD (greater than 3 months).The rate of persistent TD was about 3%, suggesting early spontaneous remission in about 2% of cases annually. [37] Other prospective studies of TD incidence are consistent, yielding estimates of annual new cases of TD ranging from 4% to 8%. [38-40] Age has been the most consistent risk factor for TD. Higher incidence and lower remission rates are noted in older patients, especially among females.[41,42] In one study, 23% of a subgroup of patients older than 55 years developed TD within 2.2 years.[37] Incidence rate of TD was found to be 56.5% in another prospective study of elderly patients exposed to typical antipsychotics for 3 years.[43]

RISK FACTORS

Demographic Risk Factors

Age: As noted, age is one of the most robust risk factors found to be associated with TD. Both higher incidence rate and lower remission rates are reported with patients older than 50 years of age. [31,34,35,40,43,44,45-49] Prospective trials in elderly patients on FGAs found incidence rates of TD to be 26-31% within 1 year of exposure.[40,43] The Hillside Study group prospectively examined 261 drug-naive patients older than 55 years, who were examined quarterly for 2.2 years, during which time 23% developed TD that persisted for at least 6 months in 67% of cases. In those over age 65, the prevalence of TD was five to six times greater than among younger patients exposed to antipsychotic medications.[40,43] However, in a recent meta analysis of 8 prospective studies in patients with schizophrenia, the association of age with TD was found to be suggestive but not conclusive.[50] A history of electroconvulsive therapy has also been found to be a strong predictor of TD in the elderly.[40] Study results may also be confounded by mistaking spontaneous dyskinesia for TD, especially in the elderly.[37]

Gender: Female gender has also been reported to be a risk factor for TD. [35,38,39,40,45,51-53]

An analysis of 19 studies before 1981 showed a weighted mean prevalence 41% higher in women than in men. However, in some of the studies, women received longer and/or higher dose treatment than the men.[31] Some incidence [46] and prevalence studies [54,55] have not supported an increased risk of TD in women. In a recent meta-analysis, gender did not qualify as a risk factor for TD in patients diagnosed with schizophrenia.[50] Thus, the evidence is inconclusive. Some of the discrepancies may be related to differences in age/sex demographics and methodology in older studies.[54] This data is largely regarding patients with schizophrenia and not with patients diagnosed with affective illnesses (bipolar affective disorder or major depression) receiving antipsychotics.

Race/ethnicity: In a recent pooled analysis of eleven studies of patients treated with antipsychotics, race did not have a significant association with incidence of TD.[56] However, limited data does suggest higher risk in patients of African descent.[55] In a recent meta-analysis, non-white ethnic group qualified as a risk factor for the emergence of TD in schizophrenia.[44,50] In another study, non-white patients (mostly African Americans) were almost twice as likely to develop TD.[38] African descent has also predicted poorer TD outcomes.[49] However, most of these associations are tentative and based on time-limited studies of prevalence, rather than prospective longitudinal studies of TD.[57]

Clinical Factors

Antipsychotic drug exposure: Possible contributions of drug exposure by dose to TD are challenging to evaluate. [37,58] Overall difference in TD prevalence has been reported to be little between moderate and high doses of chlorpromazine in a retrospective study.[32] It has been suggested that the risk of TD is already maximal at chlorpromazine equivalent doses of 300 mg or more, which is considered within a lower range for FGA doses. [59] However, the incidence of new cases of TD was approximately halved by reducing the dose of injected long-acting fluphenazine decanoate by 10-fold, from an approximate daily equivalent of about 500 mg to 50 mg of orally administered chlorpromazine, pointing in the favor of a possible risk plateau above moderate doses.[32,60,61] Although, association between antipsychotic dose and TD has been suggested by some studies,[51] systematic reviews,[3] and a recent meta-analysis found no association. [50] Furthermore, there is little evidence comparing the incidence of TD with low versus high-potency FGAs.[46]

Because TD appears to be related to duration of treatment,[19,31,47,48] clinicians should become more vigilant about TD over time with antipsychotic use. TD can take from months to years to appear. The wide variation in onset may relate in part to variations in cumulative antipsychotic exposure because of dosing variations and intermittent versus continuous treatment. One study found duration of prior neuroleptic use at baseline and cumulative amount of high-potency neuroleptics increased risk of TD by factors of 2.4 and 1.7, respectively.[43] However, evidence for cumulative drug exposure as a risk factor for TD is equivocal.[19,62] The problem is made more difficult due to the complex natural history of TD and the difficulty of accurate drug recording in patients with chronic schizophrenia.[62]

It is generally accepted that long term FGA use bears a risk for TD. Trials of SGA efficacy and safety have suggested an incidence of approximately 1% per year with SGAs versus approximately 5% per year with FGAs.[63] The Mount Sinai Conference on the Pharmacotherapy of Schizophrenia issued the consensus opinion, "There is sufficient evidence to conclude that SGAs are less likely to cause TD than FGAs are."[64] This opinion is widely supported, but nonetheless TD does occur with the SGAs and can become permanent and disfiguring. [3,46-48,65-67] Recent evidence suggests that the difference may be modest at best. Correll and colleagues at Hillside Medical Center have reviewed the risk of TD during clinical trials of SGA use. A total of 23 reports that included 17,896 patients with exposures to SGAs for up to 12 months were assessed.[3,36] Estimated TD incidence averaged 4%/year for SGAs versus 5.5%/year for FGAs. TD rates for SGAs by age group ranked as follows: 0.35%/year in juveniles, 3%/year in adults and 5.2%/year in the elderly, thus indicating a modest sparing of TD risk with SGAs and an important age-risk relationship as demonstrated earlier with FGAs [36] The same group of investigators also suggested that perphenazine (FGAs) had an identified TD risk of 17.3%/year, compared to haloperidol having an identified risk of only 5.3%/year in other studies.[36] These unexpected findings may indicate use of relatively low doses of SGAs in some trials,[68] inclusion of relatively few elderly,[3,36] some being evaluated by retrospective chart analysis.

It is important to be aware of various factors that may confound the results. One factor is the medication history of patients who have been exposed to various types and combinations of antipsychotics agents.[69] Studies involving patients who have been on a single SGAs are rare. TD can arise from years of FGAs treatment even after discontinuation of the drugs. Since this factor can confound results of SGAs studies, in patients previously treated with

FGAs, longitudinal studies of patients who never received FGAs would be necessary to determine the true risk of TD with SGAs.[37] Interpretation of prevalence estimates is also confounded by studies involving large, unrepresentative samples of chronic and severely ill patients, with medical and neurological comorbidities, and at risk of treatment resistance.[36] Most recent findings are based on short-term studies, which were not specifically designed to address the question of TD risk.[3,36] Additionally, SGAs have not been available for as long as the FGAs and most SGAs studies have lasted less two years, not long enough to conclude definitively that the risk of TD is truly low with long-term SGAs treatment. There are few randomized, double blind trials and naturalistic studies may not adequately control for nonadherent patients or switch of antipsychotic medications.[70] Few studies included specific assessments designed to rate dyskinesia; this is important as the clinical implications between mild and severe dyskinesia must be weighed.

It is also important to consider that the risk of TD may be related to the cumulative-dose exposure. A meta-analysis of 31 randomized controlled trials comparing SGAs with low-potency FGAs found that “optimum” doses of these FGAs were no more likely to induce EPS than the SGAs were; the risk was significantly lower only with clozapine.[37,71] This could also hold true theoretically for TD. Most studies used haloperidol as a standard comparator, a high-potency antipsychotic with high risk of TD, sometimes in higher doses. Results are thus not generalizable to those of low potency antipsychotics on relatively lower cumulative doses.[37,71] Suppression of dyskinetic movements with atypical antipsychotic agents likely by reducing emotional and behavior arousal, and/or direct bradykinetic actions and possibility of spontaneous remission of TD may also influence prevalence estimates.[72-74]

Anticholinergic medication use and EPS: A few studies have shown that anticholinergic medications used to treat EPS, may worsen TD.[19,47] As TD may not be detected, it may advance and become challenging to treat. However, a recent study suggested no association between concomitant anticholinergic medication use and TD.[51] Other medications like tricyclic antidepressants, psychostimulants and antihistaminics have also been associated with dyskinesias. [45,75]

Several studies have found an association of EPS with TD.[3,37,40,44,47,49,51] A prospective, naturalistic study of 10000 patients with schizophrenia indicated that early EPS doubled the risk of developing TD in a year. [76] In the Hillside Studies of both young and elderly patients, those with a history of early EPS developed TD more frequently than those without a history of early EPS.[40,41] Early EPS emerged as a significant risk factor for TD in a recent meta-analysis.[50] However, it is unclear whether EPS is an independent risk factor for TD or merely represents greater use of potent neuroleptics at relatively higher doses, which in itself is a risk factor for TD. It has not been determined whether EPS or its treatment with anticholinergics constitutes the greater risk.[46]

Because SGAs have a lower risk of EPS,[37] it may follow that SGAs carry a lower risk of TD.[44] Meta-analyses have shown that all SGAs at recommended doses have significantly lower rates of EPS and levels of antiparkinsonian medication use.[74] Three SGAs demonstrate ES rates no different from placebo: clozapine, quetiapine and iloperidone. More often than not, studies have supported the idea of lower TD risk with SGAs. [68,70,73]

Mood disorders: The presence of a mood disorder (major depressive disorder, bipolar disorder) may increase the risk of developing TD, compared to schizophrenia [40,45,49,62,77,78] and may also predict poorer outcomes, with less chances of reversal of TD.[49] Prevalence of TD in studies of patients with mood disorders was found to range from

26% to 64%. Prevalence was 26% and 42% in patients with affective disorders compared to 18% and 25% in those with schizophrenia in 2 of the studies, respectively.[77,78] Patients with schizophrenia and with depression or with a family history of mood disorders have a higher risk of developing TD as well.[78]

Substance use: Several studies have suggested that a comorbid diagnosis of substance abuse may increase the risk of TD. [40,44,47,49,58] In a study of older patients, TD risk was increased by a factor of 1.7 in those with history of alcohol abuse.[43] However, a newer study suggested no association.[51] Diabetes mellitus: Diabetes Mellitus has been considered to be as a risk factor. In patients treated with antipsychotics, an association has been suggested between pre-existing diabetes or insulin resistance and emergence of TD.[79-82] However, the evidence is equivocal as more recently, a few newer studies, did not find this as a risk factor for development of TD.[47,48,51]

Genetic factors: Potential susceptibility genes associated with risk of TD have been identified. It has been suggested that deficiency of isoenzymes, CYP 2D6 and 1A2, might lead to a "poor drug metabolizing" phenotype, leading to elevated levels of some cumulatively dosed antipsychotic drugs. This may contribute to increased risk for TD. However, studies of association between the CYP2D6 genotype and risk of EPS or TD have led to inconsistent results.[83,84] Additionally weak associations between TD and expression of genes controlling synthesis of DRD2 and DRD3 (Dopamine Receptor proteins) have been identified.[85,86] Additional details are provided in in the pathophysiology section found below. Other factors: In a longitudinal study of 8,620 patients of schizophrenia, incidence of TD was longitudinally associated with a worsening of the Clinical Global Impressions Scale (CGI) overall symptom severity in the months preceding TD onset.[87] Other reported risk factors include baseline movement disorder or tremor,[44] brain damage,[88] mental retardation,[52] and history of electroconvulsive therapy.[37,89] In another recent study, a strong positive correlation was found between the increase in cigarette consumption and severity of TD. 90]

PATHOPHYSIOLOGY

The etiology and pathophysiology of TD have not been conclusively established. Several theories have been proposed to explain the underlying mechanisms, but the evidence is equivocal.

The weight of evidence favors the notion that chronic blockade of D2 receptors by antipsychotics can lead to an up regulation of dopamine receptors in the brain striatum, leading to spontaneous, random muscle contractions or movements, the hallmarks of TD [52,66] and ultimately increased sensitivity to dopamine over time. [8,91-93] In animal models of TD, after two weeks of antipsychotic treatment, the affinity and number of dopamine receptors were noted to increase.[93] Recently a case report suggested increased dopamine transporter uptake to be associated with improvement of TD, as demonstrated by a DAT scan using SPECT imaging.[94] However, till date there is lack of unequivocal evidence supporting the hypersensitivity hypothesis in human studies[93]

A predictive relationship between variation in the DRD2 gene, which codes for D2 receptor synthesis (located on chromosome 11q22) and antipsychotic-induced side effects has been examined in a few studies. The minor (T) allele (also called the A1 allele) at rs1800497 has been associated with a 40% reduction in striatal D2 receptor density based on in vitro assays [95] and in vivo imaging studies[96] and appears to be protective against TD. Two recent meta-analyses have demonstrated increased rates of TD in A2 (C) allele carriers (odds ratio (OR) of 1.30).[86,97] However, it is important to note that the A2 allele is the common allele, and A1/A1 homozygotes represent <10% of the Caucasian. Several pharmacogenetic studies in schizophrenia have examined the DRD3 gene, located on chromosome 3q13.3. To date, only one functional SNP (rs6280), a missense variant that results in a Ser to Gly substitution at amino acid position 9, has been validated for DRD3, the D3 receptor protein.[98] The Gly variant has been associated with 4-fold greater dopamine binding affinity in vitro,[99] and concordant with this finding, three recent meta-analytic studies [85,100,101] indicate that this effect is detectable across a large pooled sample including patients of multiple ethnicities. However, the effect size for TD risk is quite small (OR=1.16 in the largest meta-analysis. This includes the recent CATIE cohort study showing no effects of either DRD3 Ser9Gly or DRD2 Taq1A.[102] In a recent meta-analysis that included thirteen eligible studies, no or little association between DRD3 rs6280 polymorphisms and prevalence of TD existed.[101]

Catechol-o-methyltransferase (COMT) is the third dopamine-related protein that has been investigated in multiple pharmacogenetic studies of TD. Across five studies meta-analyzed by Bakker and colleagues,[86] the valallele of the COMT gene (that leads to reduced synaptic dopamine due to more rapid clearance) was associated with a small increased risk for TD (OR=1.19).

Reduced activity in a subgroup of striatal GABA neurons has also been suggested as a basis of TD.[103] Altered GABA function or decreased GABA-synthesizing enzymes with antipsychotic treatment has been supported by some animal [104,105] and human studies [103] but not by others in regards to TD onset.[93] A recent study in Japanese patients with schizophrenia suggested that the GABA receptor signaling pathway may be involved in the pathophysiology of TD Associations with antipsychotic-induced TD were replicated in the confirmation samples for SNPs in SLC6A11 (GABA transporter 3), GABRB2 ([beta]-2 subunit of GABA-A receptor), and GABRG3 ([gamma]-3 subunit of GABA-A receptor) among 8 SNPs.[106]

Reduced availability of the serotonin 5-HT2A receptor has also been proposed to be a risk factor for TD. 5-HT2A receptors are strongly expressed in the caudate and putamen,[107] and recent evidence obtained from dopamine-depleted rodents suggests a complex interplay of subcortical dopamine and 5-HT in the regulation of motor behavior.[108] The 5-HT2A receptor gene (HTR2A) has been examined in several pharmacogenetic studies of TD; in particular, a promoter region SNP (rs6313). The C allele has been associated with significantly increased risk for TD. A recent meta-analysis reported an odds ratio of about 1.6 for C allele carriers across six studies; effects were strongest in older patients (age >47 years), and were specifically associated with limb-truncal (but not orofacial) TD.[109]

Metabolic problems may also contribute to TD. This is supported by increased risk of TD in diabetics and some treatment success with branched chain amino acids.[93]

Neurotoxicity and neuronal cell loss could also be related to the pathophysiology of TD. Some brain imaging studies have shown differences between patients with and without TD,[110] but others have not.[93] Oxidative stress (OS) mediated neurotoxic damage is also an important hypothesis proposed to explain the development of TD. Considerable support to

OS hypothesis comes from the observations of increased lipid peroxidation in cerebrospinal fluid in patients with TD and that antioxidants such as vitamin E may alleviate some TD symptoms.[111] In a recent meta-analysis of NADPH quinine oxidoreductase 1 (NQO1) and superoxide dismutase 2 (SOD2, MnSOD), no significant association of NQO1 Pro187Ser or SOD2 Ala9Val alleles or genotypes with TD occurrence emerged.[112]

Reduced CYP2D6 activity can be expected to result in higher plasma drug concentration with potential for increased dose-dependent side effects. A recent meta-analysis of eight studies demonstrated a moderate effect of (any) loss of function alleles on risk for TD (OR=1.43), while homozygotes (poor metabolizers) had 1.64-fold greater odds of suffering TD.[113] Results were confirmed by another recent small study.[114]

The point prevalence of spontaneous, non-drug induced dyskinesias has ranged widely from 3.7% to 77%, averaging at 5%33 and is known to increase with age.[33,35] Spontaneous dyskinesias have been documented in about 40% of antipsychotic-naïve patients [25] and may represent underlying cerebral pathology in such patients.[25,115] Spontaneous dyskinesias possibly unrelated to antipsychotic medications or possibly worsened or suppressed by them, may occur coincidentally in patients with TD and thus confound incidence or prevalence estimates of TD.[116] It has been suggested that in psychotic patients who do not experience spontaneous dyskinesias, chronic antipsychotic treatment may be the "final straw" that induces TD. [93]

Clinical Manifestations of TD

Involuntary, repetitive, and purposeless movements that primarily involve the tongue, lips, and jaw characterize TD.[66] Three possible types of movements have been described: chorea (variable, rapid, jerky or fidgety), athetoses (slow, writhing, irregular), or ballismus (sudden, fast, flinging [eg, of arms]).[117,118] In addition to orofacial movements, TD is also known to involve the limbs and the trunk.

Orofacial dyskinesias can lead to impairment of chewing swallowing and dental problems in addition to tooth infections. The involuntary mouth movements may be readily suppressed by the patient when asked to do or by voluntary actions such as putting food in the mouth or talking. It is usually more distressing to the family or physician but can cause social embarrassment to the patient or could lead to dysphagia or dysarthria.

Nutritional intake, especially in the elderly, may become insufficient. [44,89] Orofacial and truncal TD may be associated with unintelligible speech.[44] Severe limb or truncal dyskinesia may lead to gait disturbances and can result in falls.[44,89] Respiratory dyskinesias resulting from involvement of the diaphragm are known to occur and may result in hypo or hyperventilation.[119]

Severe TD can add considerably to the stigma, social and employment obstacles faced by persons with psychiatric disorder. According to a 2002 consensus conference assembled to develop recommendations for physical health monitoring of patients with schizophrenia, "Movement disorders… add to the stigmata associated with schizophrenia and can provide unnecessary obstacles to optimum social and vocational adjustment."[74]

Table 1.

Orofacial	Limbs	Trunk
Mouthing movements, chewing, sucking, licking Lip smacking Grimacing, tongue protrusion, lip Puckering and pursing Rapid eye blinking, brow wrinkling Likelihood of oral-lingual movements increasing with age	Rapid movements of arms, legs, or trunk Flexion-extension movements in fingers, toes, ankles, or wrists Finger movements evoking guitar or piano playing Symptoms in extremities more common in younger patients	Shoulder shrugging Pelvic rocking (if abdominal involvement) Grunting or other sounds with each breath (if diaphragmatic involvement)

TD is not only associated with increased morbidity and poor quality of life,[3] but also increased mortality, according to a recent study.[24] TD imposes costs of medical care, disability, lost productivity, in addition to costs of human suffering for patients and their families. With the increased use of antipsychotics, including off-label use for non-psychotic conditions, TD and its burdens may continue to rise. With the increased use of antipsychotics, including off-label use, the costs and frequency of lawsuits that allege inappropriate prescribing have increased.[120] Failure to understand TD, to detect its early signs, or failure to intervene to prevent progression when those signs appear, may risk legal action [120].

TD can become chronic and irreversible in about 50% patients who develop it. Hence, early detection of TD is important as it may enable possible reversal by discontinuing or reducing the dose of the antipsychotic.[121] The diagnosis of TD is simple in some cases but can be quite challenging in others and is based on a complete neuropsychiatric history and examination. There is no single clinical or laboratory test that can diagnose or rule TD out. Although persistent TD usually takes several years of antipsychotic treatment to appear, some cases have been documented after only two months.[88]

Nature and severity of TD is known to fluctuate depending on the level of emotional or behavioral arousal and sometimes spontaneously. Studies have shown the natural course of TD to persist,[74] to usually improve,[31,62] or to have an unpredictable course.18 Clinicians should be vigilant because patients may not complain of TD symptoms; many are unaware of their own dyskinesias.[12]

Some authors refer to an "induction period" of exposure to antipsychotics, followed by a "latent period" when the pathology has begun, and finally a "clinical period" when TD becomes detectable.[46] During the course of treatment, clinicians may increase the dose of antipsychotics to maintain efficacy, which might raise the risk for TD development,[46,63] It is important to keep in mind that TD could remain latent, its symptoms masked by the antipsychotics for months to years.[122]

Table 2.

Conditions that may resemble Tardive Dyskinesia
Primary movement disorders
Spontaneous dyskinesias occurring in the elderly
Oral movements from ill-fitting dentures and other dental problems
Senile chorea
Tourette syndrome
Meige's syndrome
Restless legs syndrome
Secondary movement disorders
Neurodegenerative conditions like Huntington's disease, Wilson's disease
Infectious conditions like Sydenham's chorea
Psychiatric conditions like schizophrenia, autism, Rett's syndrome
Drug-induced dyskinesias from antiparkinsonian drugs or stimulants

TD needs to be carefully distinguished from other disorders that resemble it and some that are also known to coexist with TD.[8] TD is a diagnosis of exclusion (Table II); that requires ruling out of many other syndromes that also cause abnormal movements.[46] When in doubt, it is prudent to consult a neurologist.

Clinical Diagnosis of TD

A panel of experts (see Mount Sinai consensus statement) reviewed the quality and quantity of data regarding the development of TD and recommended the following regarding the management of TD risk [74,]

- Before initiating FGAs or SGAs treatment, examine all patients for baseline neurologic status, including parkinsonian signs and involuntary movements.
- When initiating treatment or increasing dose, monitor for EPS weekly until the dose has been stabilized for two weeks.
- With FGAs, examine for TD at least every six months.
- With SGAs and no concomitant FGAs, examine for TD annually.
- With patients at high risk for EPS (eg, older age, history of dystonic reactions, akathisia, clinically significant parkinsonism), examine every three months with FGAs or six months with SGAs.

In 1982 Schooler and Kane developed three diagnostic criteria for TD [12,121,123]

- At least three months cumulative exposure to neuroleptics.
- Presence of at least moderate abnormal involuntary movements in one or more body area(s) or mild movements in two or more body areas.
- Absence of other conditions that might produce involuntary movements.

Brief interruptions of neuroleptic treatment can unmask latent TD, thereby aiding early detection.[124] However, in vulnerable patients, a diagnostic drug-free interval long enough to unmask TD may risk relapse into psychosis.[124] Moreover, evidence suggests that drug holidays or other drug-free intervals may possibly increase the risk for TD due to fluctuating antipsychotic blood levels allowing for fluctuating D2 receptor occupancy in the nigrostriatal pathways .[31,45,89]

Rating Scales

The National Institute of Mental Health developed the Abnormal Involuntary Movements Disorder Scale (AIMS) as a research tool.[121] By itself, AIMS does not diagnose TD,[121] but identifies the presence and severity of choreoathetoid and other movements typical of TD. AIMS is a reliable instrument for measurement of TD severity and is widely recommended for clinical screening for TD and follow-up of patients diagnosed with TD.[121] Recently, in patients with intellectual disability, the Matson Evaluation of Drug Side-effects (MEDS) and the Dyskinesia Identification System: Condensed User Scale (DISCUS) have been reported to have validity and significant clinical utility useful in measuring TD.[125] Tongue dyskinesia is often under diagnosed or misdiagnosed. Recently, an instrument measurement of lingual force variability has been developed as a valid and reliable method for assessing tardive tongue dyskinesia. [126]

COURSE

It is challenging to determine the natural history of TD as the antipsychotic agents that tend to cause it may also suppress it. Studies have shown the natural course of TD to persist,[74] to usually improve,[31,63] or to have an unpredictable course.[18] Variability in TD's course among patients may be explained by variable length of follow-up and the differences in study populations. [127] In a thirteen year follow-up study of 53 long-term psychiatric inpatients, 33 of 53 patients had complete resolution of TD. However, a significant worsening of parkinsonism occurred, suggesting that TD was being masked. Furthermore, the worsening of parkinsonism was significantly greater in patients whose TD resolved versus those whose did not.[128] In a long-term follow up study of ten patients with TD, AIMS score severity improved in five, worsened in four and remained unchanged in one patient, supporting the view that under continuous treatment with antipsychotics there is an equal chance for improvement as for deterioration.[129] Results from a large prospective naturalistic study indicated that persons with TD have a significantly more severe and more refractory course of illness than those without TD.[130]

Prevention and Treatment

In up to 50% of affected patients, TD becomes chronic and irreversible.[18] Prevention is the best strategy, as no treatment has been shown to be uniformly effective. Antipsychotics should be used only for compelling and evidence-based indications. Prolonged off label use should thus be avoided whenever possible. For patients who do not have a psychotic illness, treatment alternatives other than antipsychotics should be considered.[31] Since recent data suggests that risk of TD with SGAs is lower, although modest, they should be considered the first-line treatment. Patients should be forewarned of the risk of TD before being placed on a drug for maintenance treatment exceeding three months. Prevention strategies should include: using a single antipsychotic at the lowest effective dose,[15,19,37,38] for the shortest term possible19 with regular documented re-evaluations of antipsychotic need, efficacy, and possible dose reduction,[19,31,38,89] and regular examination for specific signs of dyskinesia.[19,37] Extra caution should be exercised when treating special groups like the elderly, who have a higher risk of developing TD and lower dosages should be used. In all patients receiving antipsychotics, some authors have recommended avoidance of anticholinergic medications.[131] The American Psychiatric Association (APA) Task Force on Late Neurological Effects of Antipsychotic Drugs called discontinuing antipsychotics the "theoretical treatment of choice" for TD.[8] Some studies have shown that when TD was identified early, up to 90% of younger patients achieved TD remission after discontinuing the antipsychotic.[11] In most cases, TD remission can be predicted to occur within three months of withdrawal or not at all. TD may be mild and reversible by withdrawing antipsychotics in one third of patients, with higher rates in younger patients.[11,31,52] For those patients with chronic schizophrenia, where antipsychotics cannot be reduced or discontinued, several options have been recommended. Switching to an SGAs is suggested [48,88,89] for those on an FGAs. If TD emerges when the patient is already on SGAs, lowering the dose to that least effective can be helpful, as shown by several studies when TD is identified early enough.[8,88,89]

Switching to another SGA is another option. Clozapine and quetiapine have the lowest reported incidence of TD and, in general, have not been convincingly reported to cause TD among patients who were never exposed to other neuroleptics.[57,132] Iloperidone, another SGA with placebo-level motoric effects can also be considered, although it is relatively new to the marketplace and is thus less well studied. If signs of TD appear during treatment with antiparkinsonian agents, they should be tapered gradually to the minimum necessary to control parkinsonism, or ideally discontinued.[45,48,53,88] TD may improve in up to 60% of patients after ceasing anticholinergics.[131] A systematic review of the TD treatment literature shows no definitive treatment in stringently performed studies;[132] however, the review did not include all possible interventions, such as branched-chain amino acids (BCAAs). As suggested by some studies, owing to neuroprotective properties, lithium may protect against TD,[133] however controlled studies have not supported this.[19,45,134] Several studies have demonstrated some efficacy of tetrabenazine in the treatment of TD.[45,135,136]

However, much work remains to be done to determine its full therapeutic potential[137] as it is associated with numerous adverse effects, several important drug-drug interactions and effects are known to reverse with discontinuation.[88] Cholinergic agents - deanol, lecithin, and meclofenoxate were compared with placebo in eleven randomized trials.[132] No statistically significant differences were observed for greater than 50% improvement in any validated scale for TD in those trials and in meta-analysis.[138] Evidence of the effects gama-hydroxybutyric acid agonists - baclofen, progabide, sodium valproate, or THIP for people with antipsychotic-induced TD is inconclusive and unconvincing. Any possible benefits are likely to be outweighed by the adverse effects associated with their use.[139] Small trials of limited quality suggest that vitamin E may protect against deterioration of TD, but there is no evidence that vitamin E improves TD symptoms.[140] Evidence is also limited, mixed, or anecdotal regarding benzodiazepines,[141] vitamin B6,[142] botulinum toxin,[143,144] donepezil,[145] levatiracetam,[146] piracetam,[147] amantadine,[148] galantamine,[116] kampo medicine,[149] yi-gan,[150] deep brain stimulation[151,152] melatonin, levodopa, reserpine, ondansetron, insulin, phenylalanine, and estrogen.[45,53] Evidence has suggested an association between TD and impaired clearance of the large neutral amino acid phenylalanine, particularly in men. BCAAs, a "medical food" (designed for oral or enteral administration under physician supervision for a specific condition with nutritional requirements), was approved for TD in males. BCAAs might improve TD by decreasing availability of phenylalanine to the brain. In one study, men with long histories of antipsychotic treatment and TD were randomized to receive BCAAs or placebo. TD movements decreased 36.5% in the BCAA group but increased 3.4% in the placebo group. One third of the BCAA group had TD movement reductions of 60%.[153] Results were replicated in a small uncontrolled trial of children and adolescents, with resulting decreases of 40% to 65% in TD symptoms.[154] BCAAs were shown to be safe and tolerable in both studies. [153,154] BCAA formulations have not been tested in women of childbearing age and are not recommended in patients with diabetes and other metabolic disorders, renal disease, and certain other disorders.[153] There continues to be a strong need for future studies of therapeutic options for TD. Ideally, new randomized trials should include larger sample sizes; be of double blind, parallel-group design, and have longer follow-up at least 1 year. [132] Study methodology should include examining for TD at three-month intervals using AIMS as well as a final reassessment to confirm diagnosis in patients and should include adherence assessments to minimize the effects of intermittent treatment and potential withdrawal dyskinesia.

Medico-Legal Considerations

Most long-term incidence studies have focused on FGAs and have clearly linked TD with FGAs use. With the higher TD risk posed by FGAs, using SGAs as first-line treatment for antipsychotic- naïve patients is recommended.[48,66] Furthermore, it is now clear that sparing of risk of TD with SGAs is surprisingly modest and less than was generally assumed. It is important to continue to maintain awareness of TD as a potential risk with SGAs, maintain vigilance of new cases and continue to train young physicians to recognize adverse neurological effects of this class of medications. Managed care programs usually require patients to seek care through primary care providers.[89] As more individuals are covered by managed care plans, more antipsychotic prescriptions are now issued by primary care physicians.[89] There is lack of adequate training in the use of antipsychotics and the need for periodic examination for TD amongst primary care providers.[89] With the increased use of antipsychotics, including off-label use, the costs and frequency of lawsuits that allege inappropriate prescribing have increased.[120] In two classic malpractice cases involving TD after antipsychotic treatment, the defense lacked two elements of good care: informed consent and documentation of valid medical reasons for the antipsychotic treatment decision, including adequate consideration of TD.[155] Therefore, documentation of the rationale not to change the treatment or the decision to change it should be carefully documented. Negligence can also occur after good informed consent is issued, but there is poor or absent ongoing monitoring i.e. AIMS is not performed or documented. Physicians, patients, and families need education on TD risks, symptoms, management, and outcomes. Clinicians should employ appropriate preventive measures to minimize the chances of occurrence of TD. Clinicians should consider TD before prescribing antipsychotics, review the need for neuroleptic medications periodically whether or not signs of TD exist, prescribe the lowest amount needed to achieve the desired effect and be prepared to withdraw the medication at the earliest opportunity.[156]

REFERENCES

[1] Fleischhacker WW, Hummer M. Drug treatment of schizophrenia in the 1990s. Achievements and future possibilities in optimising outcomes. *Drugs*. 1997; 53:915–929.

[2] Emsley R, Oosthuizen P. Evidence-based pharmacotherapy of schizophrenia. *Int. J. Neuropsychopharmacol*. 2004; 7:219–238.

[3] Correll CU, Leucht S, Kane JM. Lower risk for tardive dyskinesia associated with second-generation antipsychotics: a systematic review of 1-year studies. *Am. J. Psychiatry*. 2004; 161:414–425.

[4] Braude WM, Barnes TR, Gore SM: Clinical characteristics of akathisia: a systematic investigation of acute psychiatric inpatient admissions. *Br. J. Psychiatry*. 1983; 143:139–150.

[5] Caroff SN: The neuroleptic malignant syndrome. *J. Clin. Psychiatry*. 1980; 41:79–83.

[6] Rupniak NM, Jenner P, Marsden CD: Acute dystonia induced by neuroleptic drugs. *Psychopharmacology (Berl)*. 1986; 88:403–419.

[7] Goetz CG, Klawans HL: Drug-induced extrapyramidal disorders: a neuropsychiatric interface. *J. Clin. Psychopharmacol*. 1981; 1:297–303.

[8] Task Force on Late Neurological Effects of Antipsychotic Drugs. Tardive dyskinesia: summary of a task force report of the American Psychiatric Association. *Am. J. Psychiatry*. 1980; 137:1163-1172.

[9] Miller CH, Fleischhacker WW: Managing antipsychotic-induced acute and chronic akathisia. *Drug Saf*. 2000; 22:73–81.

[10] Strawn JR, Keck PE, Caroff SN. Neuroleptic malignant syndrome. *Am. J. Psychiatry*. 2007;164:870-876.

[11] Tarsy D. History and definition of tardive dyskinesia. *Clin. Neuropharmacol.* 1983;6:91-99.

[12] Germer CK, Seraydarian L, McBrearty JF. Training hospital clinicians to diagnose tardive dyskinesia. *Hosp. Community Psychiatry.* 1984; 35:769-783.

[13] Harten PN, Kahn RS. Tardive Dystonia. *Schizophr. Bull.* 1999; 25(4): 741-748.

[14] Kang, UJ, Burke, RE, Fahn, S. Tardive dystonia. In: Fahn, S, Marsden, CD, and Calne, DB, eds. *Advances in Neurology*. Dystonia 2. Vol. 50. New York, NY: Raven Press, 1988; 415-429.

[15] Simpson GM. The treatment of tardive dyskinesia and tardive dystonia. *J. Clin. Psychiatry.* 2000;61(suppl 4):39-44.

[16] Shapleske J, Mickay A, Mckenna PJ. Successful treatment of tardive dystonia with clozapine and clonazepam. *Br. J. Psychiatry.* 1996;168:516-518.

[17] Adityanjee, Aderibigbe YA, Jampala VC, Mathews T. The current status of tardive dystonia. *Biol. Psychiatry.* 1999;45(6):715-30.

[18] Cummings JL, Wirshing WC. Recognition and differentiation of tardive dyskinesia. *Int. J. Psychiatry Med.* 1989;19:133-144.

[19] Klawans HL, Goetz CG, Perlik S. Tardive dyskinesia: review and update. *Am. J. Psychiatry.* 1980; 137: 900-908.

[20] Dufresne RL, Wagner RL. Antipsychotic-withdrawal akathisia versus antipsychotic-induced akathisia: further evidence for the existence of tardive akathisia. *J. Clin. Psychiatry.* 1988;49:435-438.

[21] Burke RE, Kang UJ, Jankovick J, Miller LG, Fahn S. Tardive akathisia: An analysis of clinical features and response to open therapeutic trials. *Movement Disorders.* 1989; 4(2):157-175.

[22] Sigwald J, Bouttier D, Raymondeaud C, Piot C. Quatre cas de dyskinesie facio-bucco-linguo-masticatrice a l'evolution prolongee secondaire a un traitement par less neuroleptiques. *Rev. Neurol.* (Paris) 1959;100:751–755.

[23] Faurbye A, Rasch P, Peterson P, Brandborg G, Pakkenberg H. Neurological symptoms in pharmacotherapy of psychoses. *Acta Psychiatr. Scand.* 1964;40:10–27.

[24] Chong SA, Tay JA, Subramaniam M, et al. Mortality rates among patients with schizophrenia and tardive dyskinesia. *J. Clin. Psychopharmacol.* 2009;29:5-8.

[25] Fenton WS. Prevalance of spontaneous dyskinesia in schizophrenia. *J. Clin. Psychiatry.* 2000;61 (4):4-10.

[26] Fenn DS, Moussaoui D, Hoffman WF, Kadri N, Bentounssi B, Tilane A, Khomeis M, Casey DE. Movements in never-medicated schizophrenics: a preliminary study. *Psychopharmacology.* (Berl). 1996;123(2):206-10.

[27] Pappa S, Dazzan P. Spontaneous movement disorders in antipsychotic-naive patients with first-episode psychoses: a systematic review. *Psychol. Medicine.* 2009; 39: 1065-1076.

[28] Yarden PE, DiScipio WJ. Abnormal movements and prognosis in schizophrenia. *Am. J. Psychiatry.* 1971;128:317–323.

[29] Crow TJ, Cross AJ, Johnstone EC, Owen F, Owens DG, Waddington JL. Abnormal involuntary movements in schizophrenia : are they related to the disease process or its treatment ? Are they associated with changes in dopamine receptors ? *J. Clin. Psychopharm.* 1982; 2: 336–340.

[30] Thieda P, Beard S, Richter A. An economic review of compliance with medication in the treatment of schizophrenia. *Psychiatr. Services.* 2003;54:508-515.

[31] Jeste DV, Wyatt RJ. Changing epidemiology of tardive dyskinesia; An overview. *Am. J. Psychiatry.* 1981;138:297-309.

[32] Baldessarini RJ, Cole JO, James JM, Gardos G, Prescorn HS, Simpson GM, Tarsy D. Tardive dyskinesia: American psychiatric association taskforce on late effects of antipsychotic drugs. *Am. J. Psychiatry.* 1980;137: 1163-1172.

[33] Lohr JB. Commentary: Is tardive dyskinesia disappearing? In Factor SA Lang AE, Weiner WJ, editors. Drug-induced movement disorders. *Malden MA Futura-blackwell*; 2004: 302-312.

[34] Smith JM, Baldessarini RJ. Changes in prevalence, severity, and recovery in tardive dyskinesia with age. *Arch. Gen. Psychiatry.* 1980; 37: 1368–1373.

[35] Kane JM, Smith JM. Tardive dyskinesia: prevalence and risk factors, 1959 to 1979. *Arch. Gen. Psychiatry.* 1982; 39: 473–481.

[36] Corell CU, Schenk EM. Tardive dyskinesia and new antipsychotics. *Curr. Opin. Psychiatry.* 2008;21(2):151-6.

[37] Tarsy D, Baldessarini RJ. Epidemiology of tardive dyskinesia: is risk declining with modern antipsychotics? Mov Disord. 2006;21:589-598.

[38] Morgenstern H, Glazer WM. Identifying risk factors for tardive dyskinesia among long-term outpatients maintained with neuroleptic medications: results of the Yale tardive dyskinesia study. *Arch. Gen. Psychiatry.* 1993; 50: 723–733.

[39] Glazer WM, Morgenstern H, Doucette JT. Predicting the long-term risk of tardive dyskinesia in outpatients maintained on neuroleptic medications. *J. Clin. Psychiatry.* 1993; 54: 133–139.

[40] Woerner MG, Alvir JMJ, Saltz BL, Lieberman JA, Kane JM. Prospective study of tardive dyskinesia in the elderly: rates and risk factors. *Am. J. Psychiatry.* 1998;: 1521–1528.

[41] Kane JM, Woerner M, Borenstein M, et al. Integrating incidence and prevalence of tardive dyskinesia. *Psychopharmacol. Bull.* 1986;22:254–258.

[42] Muscettola G, Pampallona S, Barbato G, Casiello M, Bolini P. Persistent tardive dyskinesia: demographic and pharmacological risk factors. *Acta Psychiatr. Scand.* 1993;87:29–36.

[43] Jeste DV, Carigiuri NP, Paulsen JS, et al. Risk of tardive dyskinesia in older patients: a prospective longitudinal study of 266 outpatients. *Arch Gen. Psychiatry.* 1995;52:756 – 765.

[44] Jeste DV. Tardive dyskinesia in older patients. *J. Clin. Psychiatry.* 2000; 65:21-24.

[45] Simpson GM, Pi EH, Sramekk JJ. An update on tardive dyskinesia. *Hosp. Community Psychiatry.* 1986;37:362-369.

[46] Glazer WM. Review of incidence studies of tardive dyskinesia associated with typical antipsychotics. *J. Clin. Psychiatry.* 2000;61(suppl 4):15-20.

[47] Miller DD, McEvoy JP, Davis SM, et al. Clinical correlates of tardive dyskinesia in schizophrenia: baseline data from the CATIE schizophrenia trial. *Schizophr. Res.* 2005;80:33-43.

[48] Margolese HC. Psychopharmacology for the clinician. Management of conventional antipsychotic-induced tardive dyskinesia. *Rev. Psychiatr. Neurosci.* 2007;32:72.

[49] Wonodi I, Adami HM, Cassady SL, Sherr JD, Avila MT, Thaker GK. Ethnicity and the course of tardive dyskinesia in outpatients presenting to the Motor Disorders Clinic at the Maryland Psychiatric Research Center. *J. Clin. Psychopharmacol.* 2004;24:592-598.

[50] Tenback DE, Van Harten PN, Van Os J. Non-therapeutic risk factors for onset of tardive dyskinesia in schizophrenia: a meta analysis. *Mov. Disord.* 2009;24(16):2309-2315.

[51] Go CL, Rosales RL, CaraoS RJ, Fernandez HH. The current prevalence and factors associated with tardive dyskinesia among Filipino schizophrenic patients. *Parkinsonism Relat. Disord.* 2009;15(9):655-9.

[52] Nasrallah HA. Tardive dyskinesia. NAMI National Alliance on Mental Illness. 2003. Available at: http://www.nami.org/Content/ContentGroups/Helpline1/Tardive_Dyskinesia.htm. Accessed March 19, 2007.

[53] Brasic JR. Tardive dyskinesia. Emedicine from WebMD. March 12, 2007. Available at: http://www.emedicine.com/neuro/topic362.htm.Accessed March 19, 2007.

[54] Kasper S, Lowry AJ, Hodge A, Bitter I, Dossenbach M. Tardive dyskinesia: analysis of outpatients with schizophrenia from Africa and the Middle East, Asia, Central and Eastern Europe, and Latin America. *Schizophr. Res.*2006;81:139-143.

[55] Van Harten PN, Hoek HW, Matroos GE,van Os J. Incidence of tardive dyskinesia and tardive dystonia in African Caribbean patients on long-term antipsychotic treatment: the Curacao Extrapyramidal Syndromes Study V. *J. Clin. Psychiatry.* 2006;67:1920-1927.

[56] Ormerod S, Mcdowell SE, Coleman JJ, Ethnic differences in risks of adverse reactions to drugs used in the treatment of psychosis and depression: a systematic review and meta-analysis. *Drug safety.* 2008;31:597-607.

[57] Tarsy D, Lungu C, Baldessarini R. Epidemiology of tardive dyskinesia before and during the era of modern antipsychotic drugs. *Handbook of clinical neurology.* 2011. 100;601-615.

[58] Oosthuizen PP, Emstley R, Stephanuz MJ. Incidence of tardive dyskinesia in first dose psychosis treated with low dose haloperidol. *J. Clin. Psychiatry.*2003;64:1075-1080.

[59] Gardner DM, Baldessarini RJ, Waraich P. Modern antipsychotic drugs: a critical overview. *Can. Med. Assoc. J.* 2005; 172: 1703–1711.

[60] Schooler NR, Keith SJ, Severe JB, et al. Relapse and rehospitalization during maintenance treatment of schizophrenia: effects of dose reduction and family treatment. *Arch. Gen. Psychiatry.* 1997; 54: 453–463.

[61] Kane J. Antipsychotic drug effects: their relationship to dose. *J. Clin. Psychiatry.* 1985; 46(Suppl. 5): 16–21.

[62] Kane JM, Woerner M, Weinhold P, Kinon B, Lieberman J, Wegner J. Epidemiology of tardive dyskinesia. *Clin. Neuropharmacol.* 1983;6:109-115.

[63] Remington G. Tardive dyskinesia: eliminated, forgotten, or overshadowed? *Curr. Opin. Psychiatry.* 2007;20:131-137.

[64] Marder SR, Essock SM, Miller AL, et al.The Mount Sinai Conference on the Pharmacotherapy of Schizophrenia. *Schizophr. Bull.* 2002;28:5-16.

[65] Kasper S, Lowry AJ, Hodge A, Bitter I, Dossenbach M. Tardive dyskinesia: analysis of outpatients with schizophrenia from Africa and the Middle East, Asia, Central and Eastern Europe, and Latin America. *Schizophr. Res.* 2006;81:139-143.

[66] Glazer WM. Managing the risk of tardive dyskinesia [interview]. *Behav. Health Management.*2005;25:SS1-SS6.
[67] Dolder CR, Jeste DV. Incidence of tardive dyskinesia with typical versus atypical antipsychotics in very high risk patients. *Biol. Psychiatry.*2003;53:1142-1145.
[68] Lee PE, Sykora K, Gill SS. Antipsychotic medications and drug-induced movement disorders other than parkinsonism, a population based cohort study in older adults. *J. Am. Geriatr. Society.*2005;53:1374-1379.
[69] Centorrini F, Cincotta SL, Talamo A. Hospital use of antipsychotic drugs:polytherapy. *Comp. Psychiatry.*2008;49:65-69.
[70] De Leon J. The effect of atypical versus typical antipsychotics on tardive dyskinesia. A naturalistic study. *Eur. Arch. Psychiatry. Clin. Neurosci.* 2006;257:169-172.
[71] Leucht S, Walbeck K, Harmann J.New generation antipsychotics versus low potency conventional:a systematic review and meta-analysis. *Lancet.*2003;361:1581-1589.
[72] Caroff SN, Mann SC, Cabrina CE. Movement disorders associated with atypical antipsychotics. *J. Clin. Psychiatry.* 2002;63:12-19.
[73] Tarsy D, Baldessarini RJ, Tarazi FI. Effects of newer antipsychotics on extrapyramidal function. *CNS Drugs.*2002;16: 23-45.
[74] Marder SR, Essock SM, Miller AL, et al. Physical health monitoring of patients with schizophrenia. *Am. J. Psychiatry.* 2004;161:1334-1349.
[75] Damier P. Drug-induced dyskinesias. *Curr. Opin. Neurol.* 2009;22(4):394-9.
[76] Tenback DE, Van Harten PN, Sloof CJ. Evidence that early extrapyramidal symptoms predict later tardive dyskinesia: a prospective analysis of 10000 patients in European schizophrenia outpatient health outcomes study. *Am. J. Psychiatry.* 2006;163: 1438-1440.
[77] Kane JM, Woerner M, Weinhold P, Wegner J, Kinon B. Incidence of tardive dyskinesia: five-year data from a prospective study. *Psychopharmacol. Bull.* 1984;20:39-40.
[78] Keck PE, McElroy SL, Strakowski SM, Soutullo CA. Antipsychotics in the treatment of mood disorders and risk of tardive dyskinesia. *J. Clin. Psychiatry.* 2000;61(suppl 4):33-38.
[79] Ganzini L, Heintz RT, Hoffman WF, Casey DE. The prevalence of tardive dyskinesia in neuroleptic-treated diabetics. A controlled study. *Arch. Gen. Psychiatry.* 1991;48:259-263.
[80] Woerner MG, Saltz BL, Kane JM, Lieberman JA, Alvir JMJ. Diabetes and development of tardive dyskinesia. *Am. J. Psychiatry.* 1993;150:966-968.
[81] Schultz SK, Arndt S, Ho BC, Oliver SE,Andreasen NC. Impaired glucose tolerance and abnormal movements in patients with schizophrenia. *Am. J. Psychiatry.* 1999;156:640-642.
[82] Caligiuri MP, Jeste DV. Association of diabetes with dyskinesia in older psychosis patients. *Psychopharmacology.* (Berl). 2004;176:281-286.
[83] Schimada , Yamazaki H, Mimura M. Inter individual variations in human liver cytochrome P 450 enzymes involved in oxidation of drugs, carcinogens and toxic chemicals: studies with liver microsomes of 30 japanese and 30 caucasians. *J. Pharmaco. Exp. Ther.*1994. 270;414-423.
[84] Bertilsson L, Dahl ML, Dalen P. Molecular genetics of CYP2D6: clinical relevance with focus on psychotropic drugs. `2002;53:111-122.

[85] Bakker PR, Van Harten PN, Van Os J. Antipsychotic induced tardive dyskinesia and the Ser9Gli polymorphism in the DRD3 gene: a meta-analysis. *Schizophre. Res.* 2006;83:195-192.
[86] Bakker PR, Van Harten PN, Van Os J. Antipsychotic induced tardive dyskinesia and polymorphic variations in COMT, DRD2, CYP1A2 and mnsod gene: a meta-analysis of pharmacogenetic interactions. *Mol. Psychiatry*. 2008;13:544-556.
[87] Tenback DE, van Harten PN, Slooff CJ, van Os J, SOHO Study Group. Worsening of psychosis in schizophrenia is longitudinally associated with tardive dyskinesia in the european schizophrenia outpatient health outcomes study. *Compr. Psychiatry*. 2007;48(5):436-440.
[88] Margolese HC, Chouinard G, Kolivakis TT, Beauclair L, Miller R. Tardive dyskinesia in the era of typical and atypical antipsychotics. Part 1: pathophysiology and mechanisms of induction. *Can. J. Psychiatry*. 2005;50:541-547.
[89] Saltz BL, Robinson DG, Woerner MG. Recognizing and managing antipsychotic drug treatment side effects in the elderly. *Prim. Care Companion J. Clin. Psychiatry*. 2004;6(suppl 2):14-19.
[90] Diehl A, Reinhard I, Schmitt A, Mann K, Gattaz WF. Does the degree of smoking effect the severity of tardive dyskinesia? A longitudinal clinical trial. *Eur. Psychiatry*. 2009;24(1):33-40.
[91] Hitri A, Weiner W, Borison R, et al. Dopamine binding following prolonged haloperidol pretreatment. *Ann. Neurol*. 1978;3:134–140.
[92] Klawans HL, Tanner CM, Goetz CG. Epidemiology and pathophysiology of tardive dyskinesia. Adv Neurol. 1988;49:185–197.
[93] Casey DE. Tardive dyskinesia: pathophysiology and animal models. *J. Clin. Psychiatry*. 2000;61(suppl 4):5-9.
[94] Rizos EN, Chatziioannou S, Douzenis A, et al. Signs of striatal dopamine transporter density increase in association with improvement of tardive dyskinesia in a patient with schizophrenia, as demonstrated by a DAT scan. *Eur. Neuropsychopharmacol*. 2010;20(2):132-136.
[95] Thompson J, Thomas N, Singleton A, et al. D2 dopamine receptor gene (DRD2) Taq1A polymorphism: reduced dopamine D2 receptor binding in the human striatum associated with the A1 allele. *Pharmacogenetics.*1997;7:479-484.
[96] Pohjalainen T, Rinne JO, Någren K, et al. The A1 allele of the human D2 dopamine receptor gene predicts low D2 receptor availability in healthy volunteers. *Mol. Psychiatry*. 1998;3:256-260.
[97] Zai CC, De Luca V, Hwang RW, et al. Meta-analysis of two dopamine D2 receptor gene polymorphisms with tardive dyskinesia in schizophrenia patients. *Mol. Psychiatry*. 2007;12:794-795.
[98] Schwartz JC, Levesque D, Martres MP, Sokoloff P. Dopamine D3 receptor: basic and clinical aspects. *Clin. Neuropharmacol*. 1993;16:295-314.
[99] Lundstrom K, Turpin MP. Proposed schizophrenia-related gene polymorphism: expression of the Ser9Gly mutant human dopamine D3 receptor with the Semliki forest virus system. *Biochem. Biophys. Res. Commun.*1996;23:225:1068-1072.
[100] Lerer B, Segman RH, Fangerau H, et al. Pharmacogenetics of tardive dyskinesia: combined analysis of 780 patients supports association with dopamine D3 receptor gene Ser9Gly polymorphism. *Neuropsychopharmacology*. 2002;27:105-119.

[101] Tsai HT, North KE, West SL, Poole C. The DRD3 rs6280 polymorphism and prevalence of tardive dyskinesia: A meta-analysis. Am J Med Genet B.Neuropsychiatr Genet. 2010;153B(1):57-66.
[102] Tsai HT, Caroff SN, Miller DD, et al. A candidate gene study of tardive dyskinesia in the CATIE schizophrenia trial. *Am. J. Med. Genet. B Neuropsychiatr. Genet.* 2010;153B(1):336-40.
[103] Kulkarni SK, Naidu PS. Pathophysiology and drug therapy of tardive dyskinesia: current concepts and future perspectives. *Drugs Today.* 2003; 39:19–49.
[104] Gunne LM, Haggstrom JE, Sjoquist B. Association with persistent neuroleptic-induced dyskinesia of regional changes in brain GABA synthesis. *Nature.* 1984; 309:347–349.
[105] Delfs JM, Ellison GD, Mercugliano M, Chesselet MF. Expression of glutamic acid decarboxylase mRNA in striatum and pallidum in an animal model of tardive dyskinesia. *Exp. Neurol.* 1995; 133:175–188.
[106] Inada T, Koga M, Ishiguro H, et al. Pathway-based association analysis of genome-wide screening data suggest that genes associated with the gamma-aminobutyric acid receptor signaling pathway are involved in neuroleptic-induced, treatment-resistant tardive dyskinesia. *Pharmacogenet. Genomics.* 2008;18(4):317-323.
[107] Waeber C, Palacios JM. Binding sites for 5-hydroxytryptamine-2 receptor agonists are predominantly located in striosomes in the human basal ganglia. *Brain Res. Mol. Brain Res.* 1994;24:199-209.
[108] Bishop C, Tessmer JL, Ullrich T, Rice KC, Walker PD. Serotonin 5-HT2A receptors underlie increased motor behaviors induced in dopaminedepleted rats by intrastriatal 5-HT2A/2C agonism. *J. Pharmacol. Exp. Ther.* 2004;310:687-694.
[109] Lerer B, Segman RH, Tan EC, et al. Combined analysis of 635 patients confirms an age-related association of the serotonin 2A receptor gene with tardive dyskinesia and specificity for the non-orofacial subtype. *Int. J. Neuropsychopharmacol.* 2005;8:411-425.
[110] Bai YM, Chou KH, Lin CP, et al. White matter abnormalities in schizophrenia patients with tardive dyskinesia: A diffusion tensor image study. *Schizophr. Res.* 2009;109(1-3):167-181.
[111] Adler LA, Rotrosen J, Edson R, Lavori P, Lohr J, Hitzemann R, Raisch D, Caligiuri M, Tracy K. Vitamin E treatment for tardive dyskinesia. Veterans Affairs Cooperative Study #394 Study Group. *Arch. Gen. Psychiatry.* 1999;56(9):836-41.
[112] Zai CC, Tiwari AK, Basile V, et al. Oxidative stress in tardive dyskinesia: Genetic association study and meta-analysis of NADPH quinine oxidoreductase 1 (NQO1) and superoxide dismutase 2 (SOD2, MnSOD) genes. *Prog. Neuropsychopharmacol. Biol. Psychiatry.* 2010;34(1):50-56.
[113] Patsopoulos NA, Ntzani EE, Zintzaras E, Ioannidis JP. CYP2D6 polymorphisms and the risk of tardive dyskinesia in schizophrenia: a meta-analysis. *Pharmacogenet. Genomics.* 2005;15:151-158.
[114] Kobylecki CJ, Jakobsen KD, Hansen T, Jakobsen IV, Rasmussen HB, Werge T. CYP2D6 genotype predicts antipsychotic side effects in schizophrenia inpatients: a retrospective matched case-control study. *Neuropsychobiology.*2009;59:222-226.
[115] Caroff SN, Walker P, Campbell C, Lorry A, et al. Treatment of tardive dyskinesia with galantamine: a randomized controlled crossover trial. *J. Clin. Psychiatry.* 2007;68:410-415.

[116] Friedman JH. Historical perspective on movement disorders. *J. Clin. Psychiatry.* 2004;65:3-8.
[117] Wolf ME, Mosnaim AD. Identifying subtypes of tardive dyskinesia. *Hosp. Community Psychiatry.* 1984;35:822-830.
[118] Goetz CG. Diagnosis of tardive dyskinesia. *Clin. Neuropharmacol.* 1983;6:101-107.
[119] Jankovic J. Tardive syndromes and other drug-induced movement disorders. *Clin. Neuropharmacol.* 1995;18:197–214.
[120] Slovenko R. Update on legal issues associated with tardive dyskinesia. *J. Clin. Psychiatry.* 2000;61(suppl 4):45-57.
[121] Munetz MR, Benjamin S. How to examine patients using the Abnormal Involuntary Movement Scale. *Hosp. Community Psychiatry.* 1988;39:1172-1177.
[122] Glazer WM. Expected incidence of tardive dyskinesia associated with atypical antipsychotics. *J. Clin. Psychiatry.* 2000;61(suppl 4):21-26.
[123] Schooler NR, Kane JM. Research diagnoses for tardive dyskinesia [letter]. *Arch. Gen. Psychiatry.* 1982;39:486-487.
[124] Davis JM, Schyve PM, Pavkovic I.Clinical and legal issues in neuroleptic use. *Clin. Neuropsychopharmacol.* 1983;6:117-128.
[125] Matson JL, Fodstad JC, Rivet TT. The convergent and divergent validity of the matson evaluation of drug side-effects (MEDS) and the dyskinesia identification system: Condensed user scale (DISCUS). *J. Intellect. Dev. Disabil.* 2008;33(4):337-344.
[126] Koning JP, Tenback DE, Kahn RS, Van Schelven LJ, Van Harten PN. Instrument measurement of lingual force variability reflects tardive tongue dyskinesia. *J. Med. Eng. Technol.* 2010;34(1):71-77.
[127] Gardos G, Cole JO, Haskell D, et al. The natural history of tardive dyskinesia. *J. Clin. Psychopharmacol.* 1988;8(suppl):31S–37S.
[128] Fernandez HH, Krupp B, Friedman JH. The course of tardive dyskinesia and parkinsonism in psychiatric inpatients:14-year follow-up. *Neurology* 2001;56:805–807.
[129] Rittmannsberger H. Ten year outcome of tardive dyskinesia during continuous treatment with first generation antipsychotics. *Psychiatr. Danub.* 2008;20(4):461-465.
[130] Ascher-Svanum H, Zhu B, Faries D, Peng X, Kinon BJ, Tohen M. Tardive dyskinesia and the 3-year course of schizophrenia: Results from a large, prospective, naturalistic study. *J. Clin. Psychiatry.* 2008;69(10):1580-1588.
[131] Egan MF, Apud J, Wyatt RJ. Treatment of tardive dyskinesia. *Schizophr. Bull.* 1997;23:583-609.
[132] Soares-Weiser K, Fernandez HH. Tardive dyskinesia. *Semin. Neurol.* 2007;27:159-169.
[133] Van Harten PN, Hoek HW, Matroos GE, van Os J. Evidence that lithium protects against tardive dyskinesia: The curacao extrapyramidal syndromes study VI. *Eur. Neuropsychopharmacol.* 2008;18(2):152-155.
[134] Mackay AV, Sheppard GP, Saha BK, Motley B, Johnson AL, Marsden CD. Failure of lithium treatment in established tardive dyskinesia. *Psychol. Med.* 1980;10:583–587.
[135] Leung JG, Breden EL. Tetrabenazine for the treatment of tardive dyskinesia. *Ann. Pharmacother.* 2011 Apr;45(4):525-31.
[136] Ondo WG, Hanna PA, Jankovic J. Tetrabenazine treatment for tardive dyskinesia: assessment by randomized videotape protocol. *Am. J. Psychiatry.* 1999;156:1279-1281.
[137] Guay DR. Tetrabenazine, a monoamine-depleting drug used in the treatment of hyperkinetic movement disorders. *Am. J. Geriatr. Pharmacother.* 2010;8(4):331-373.

[138] Tammenmaa IA, Sailas E, McGrath JJ,Soares-Weiser K, Wahlbeck K. Systematic reviewof cholinergic drugs for neuroleptic-induced tardive dyskinesia: a meta-analysis of randomized controlled trials. *Prog. Neuropsychopharmacol. Biol. Psychiatry*. 2004;28:1099-1107.

[139] Alabed S, Latifeh Y, Mohammad HA, Rifai A. Gamma-aminobutyric acid agonists for neuroleptic-induced tardive dyskinesia. *Cochrane Database Syst. Rev*. 2011;(4)(4):CD000203.

[140] Soares-Weiser K, Maayan N, McGrath J. Vitamin E for neuroleptic-induced tardive dyskinesia. *Cochrane Database Syst. Rev*. 2011;(2)(2):CD000209.

[141] Bhoopathi PS, Soares-Weiser K. Benzodiazepines for neuroleptic-induced tardive dyskinesia. *Cochrane Database Syst. Rev*. 2006;3:CD000205.

[142] Lerner V, Miodownik C, Kaptsan A, et al. Vitamin B6 treatment for tardive dyskinesia: A randomized, double-blind, placebo-controlled, crossover study. *J. Clin. Psychiatry*. 2007;68(11):1648-1654.

[143] Krause E, Gurkov R. Local botulinum neurotoxin A therapy in tardive lingual dyskinesia. *Laryngorhinootologie*. 2009;88(8):508-510.

[144] Tschopp L, Salazar Z, Micheli F. Botulinum toxin in painful tardive dyskinesia. *Clin. Neuropharmacol*. 2009;32(3):165-166.

[145] Ogunmefun A, Hasnain M, Alam A, Osuala T, Regenold WT. Effect of donepezil on tardive dyskinesia. *J. Clin. Psychopharmacol*. 2009;29(1):102-104.

[146] Woods SW, Saksa JR, Baker CB, Cohen SJ, Tek C. Effects of levetiracetam on tardive dyskinesia: A randomized, double-blind, placebo-controlled study. *J. Clin. Psychiatry*. 2008;69(4):546-554.

[147] Libov I, Miodownik C, Bersudsky Y, Dwolatzky T, Lerner V. Efficacy of piracetam in the treatment of tardive dyskinesia in schizophrenic patients: A randomized, double-blind, placebo-controlled crossover study. *J. Clin. Psychiatry*. 2007;68(7):1031-1037.

[148] Pappa S, Tsouli S, Apostolou G, Mavreas V, Konitsiotis S. Effects of amantadine on tardive dyskinesia: A randomized, double-blind, placebo-controlled study. *Clin. Neuropharmacol*. 2010;33(6):271-275.

[149] Lee JG, Shin BS, Lee YC, Park SW, Kim YH. Clinical effectiveness of the kampo medicine kamishoyosan for adjunctive treatment of tardive dyskinesia in patients with schizophrenia: A 16-week open trial. *Psychiatry Clin. Neurosci*. 2007;61(5):509-514.

[150] Miyaoka T, Furuya M, Yasuda H, et al. Yi-gan san for the treatment of neuroleptic-induced tardive dyskinesia: An open-label study. *Prog. Neuropsychopharmacol. Biol. Psychiatry*. 2008;32(3):761-764.

[151] Kefalopoulou Z, Paschali A, Markaki E, Vassilakos P, Ellul J, Constantoyannis C. A double-blind study on a patient with tardive dyskinesia treated with pallidal deep brain stimulation. *Acta Neurol. Scand*. 2009;119(4):269-273.

[152] Welter ML, Grabli D, Vidailhet M. Deep brain stimulation for hyperkinetics disorders: Dystonia, tardive dyskinesia, and tics. *Curr. Opin*. Neurol. 2010;23(4):420-425.

[153] Richardson MA, Bevans ML, Read LL, et al. Efficacy of the branched-chain amino acids in the treatment of tardive dyskinesia in men. *Am. J. Psychiatry*. 2003;160:1117-1124.

[154] Richardson MA, Small AM, Read LL, Chao HM, Clelland JD. Branched chain amino acid treatment of tardive dyskinesia in children and adolescents. *J. Clin. Psychiatry*. 2004;65:92- 96.

[155] Wettstein RM, Appelbaum PS. Legal liability for tardive dyskinesia. *Hosp. Community Psychiatry*. 1984;35:992-994.

[156] Citrome L, Dufresne R, Dyrud JM. Tardive Dyskinesia: Minimizing Risk and Improving Outcomes in Schizophrenia and Other Disorders. *Am. J. Manag. Care*. 2007; 13:1-12.

In: Antipsychotic Drugs
Editors: T.L. Schwartz, J. Megna and M.E. Topel
ISBN: 978-1-62100-071-6

Chapter 13

SEDATING EFFECTS OF SECOND GENERATION ANTIPSYCHOTICS

Kamal Poovalingam and Thomas Schwartz*
Psychiatry Department, SUNY Upstate Medical University, Syracuse, NY, US

ABSTRACT

Introduction: The first generation antipsychotics often were classified as being high or low potency descriptively. The lower potency agents were known to have more anticholinergic and antihistaminergic side effects, as well as, antidopaminergic antipsychotic effectiveness. The newer, second generation antipsychotics are not officially categorized into low versus high potency but amongst the several available second generation agents, there appears to be a wide discrepancy in sedating side effects. Furthermore, there is controversy in that sedating side effects may actually be therapeutic if they treat insomnia or anxiety in specific clinical situations.

Conclusion: This chapter reviews pharmacodynamic and translational information related to the second generation antipsychotics' relative ability to create sedation both therapeutically and in terms of tolerability and adverse effects.

INTRODUCTION

The first generation antipsychotics (FGA) are also known as typical antipsychotics and have been used since the 1950s. Based upon relative affinity for antagonizing the histamine-1 (H1) receptor they were known to produce either a great amount of sedation, fatigue, and somnolence at higher receptor affinities or a lesser amount of these side effects with lower affinities.

Typically, the low *potency* class of FGA was associated with lower affinity for the dopamine-2 (D2) receptor thus requiring high doses to alleviate psychosis, but they also typically had a higher affinity for H1 receptor antagonism causing remarkable sedating side

* E-mail: schwartt@upstate.edu.Tel: 315 464-3100. Fax: 315 464-3163.

effects. [1] In the mid-1990s, the second generation antipsychotics (SGA), also known as, the atypical antipsychotics paired serotonin-2a receptor (5HT-2a) with D2 receptor antagonism allowing much less extrapyramidal syndrome (EPS) side effects, but continued to allow quite a varied amount of sedation depending upon each SGA's individual pharmacodynamic receptor profile. This chapter seeks to review this basic science information about each SGA's pharmacodynamic profile, followed by a review of regulatory trial data concerning sedating and somnolence side effect profiles that are often seen in clinical practice. Finally, commentary regarding these adverse effects as actually being therapeutic effects in certain patients will be provided. [2]

SEDATING PHARMACODYNAMICS OF THE SECOND GENERATION ANTIPSYCHOTICS

The sedative effects of second generation antipsychotics (SGA) are most likely related to the following properties that will be discussed in detail throughout this chapter:

1. Antihistamine 1 receptor (H1) antagonism
2. Anticholinergic muscarinic (AchM) receptor antagonism
3. Dopamine (D2) receptor antagonism

H1 Receptor Antagonism

The relative affinities for H1 receptor antagonism amongst the SGA may explain their potential sedating side effects. [3] *Table 1* below shows the affinity of SGAs for H1 receptor blockade in relation to pKi value. The lower the pki value, the greater the affinity the SGA has in binding and blocking H1 receptors. The net effect results theoretically in greater sedation or fatigue experienced by the patient being treated.

Antagonism of H1 receptors causes a decrease in histaminergic activity in the CNS. The tuberomammilary nucleus (TMN) in the hypothalamus is likely the origin of histamine, and the neuronal fibers from this wakefulness center project to the dorsolateral prefrontal cortex (DLPFC) activating glutamatergic neurons involved in attention, concentration, and alertness. Antagonizing H1 receptors in the DLPFC essentially removes the TMN's histaminergic ability to promote wakefulness. The net result of removing this alertness, arousal-based drive is the onset of fatigue, sedation or even somnolence. [4]

Manipulation of H1 receptors via antagonism may be useful in clinical practice. When prescribing an SGA, it may be wise to choose one based upon how much fatigue, sedation, or somnolence might be beneficial to the patient. Outside of the sedation and somnolence that might be useful for insomnia patients, H1 receptor antagonism might provide anxiolysis similar to that afforded to the approved antihistaminergic hydroxyzine formulations. [3,4]

For example, in those patients with insomnia, agitation, or anxiety, some sedation might be clinically beneficial. Therefore, using an SGA with more H1 receptor antagonism should be a good clinical choice. Conversely, for those patients who are sluggish, tired or hypersomnic, then any sedating effect will be considered a side effect and likely not tolerated, this may eventually hurt medication adherence. Therefore, using an SGA with less H1 receptor antagonism may be beneficial in these situations.

Utilizing pharmacodynamic information, or an affinity table like *Table 1*, may not always provide a guaranteed translation into clinical practice. Some patients will have a greater, or lesser amount of H1 receptors available in their central nervous systems (CNS) and their individual receptors may have a greater, or lesser, inherent sensitivity to H1 receptor binding drugs. [5] Some patients taking asenapine, which theoretically should cause sedation, may be excessively groggy in practice, while others may experience mild sedation which treats their insomnia effectively. Finally, some patients will have no sedation at all.

Some SGAs possess other pharmacodynamic properties which may cause either sedation or arousal, further causing a level of sedation that does not translate directly from the H1 affinity table above. For example, ziprasidone may be sedating due to its H1 receptor blockade, but it also has a serotonin reuptake inhibition (SRI) property that is similar to the selective serotonin-reuptake inhibitor (SSRI) antidepressants. Some patients find SSRIs sedating, while other patients find them stimulating. Ziprasidone may be stimulating as it provides norepinephrine reuptake inhibition (NRI) similar to the ADHD medication atomoxetine and the antidepressant bupropion. Some patients find atomoxetine sedating, while some patients find bupropion stimulating and arousing. [6]

Therefore, sometimes using the SGAs may provide for varying side effects versus good clinical effects depending on each patient and the drug's specific pharmacodynamic variables. Sometimes patients will have sedating side effects and at other times the medication may be more stimulating in nature. However, in hedging clinical intuition and practicing the art of psychopharmacology, quetiapine, olanzapine, and asenapine, more often will have sedating side effects. They will also more often tend to avoid akathisia and stimulating side effects.

The dilemma with these agents occurs in that it is sometimes difficult to predict which patients will be sedated versus those who will not.

Dopamine (D2) Receptor Antagonism

All second-generation agents act as D2 receptor antagonists. This ultimate dampening of presumed limbic dopaminergic hyperactivity in schizophrenia or mania leads to clinical effectiveness and a reduction of psychosis or mania. [7] Some agents have a higher affinity for this action and can loosely be assigned a potency (affinity) level in rank order (low to high D2 affinity) shown in *Table 2*.

Regarding the antagonism of D2 receptors in the nigrostriatal dopamine pathway by the SGA class of medications, this action will reduce dopaminergic activity in the CNS. This may cause psychomotor slowing and the appearance of sedation. Dopamine hyperactivity in the mesolimbic dopamine pathway is thought to induce psychosis, so reducing dopamine activity in this pathway will theoretically alleviate psychotic symptoms. In this manner D2 receptor antagonism may provide clinically needed therapeutic effects, but at same time may cause psychomotor impairment as a side effect.

Table 1. Relative SGA H1 Receptor Antagonism

Asenapine	Quetiapne/ norquetiapine	Paliperidone	Risperidone	Olanzapine	Ziprasidone	Aripiprazole	Iloperidone	Lurasidone	
1	4.41/1.15	3.4	5.2	7	47	61	473	>1000	

←-Lowest pKi value-----------Highest pKi value-→

Values are molar pKi values as reported by approved manufacturers package inserts.

Table reprinted with permission of K. Bedynerman MD, SUNY Upstate Medical University.

The currently available SGA are listed in the table above. As quetiapine has an active metabolite (norquetiapine), it is also listed. The left side of the table shows asenapine as having the lowest pKi value and hence the greatest affinity for H1 receptor antagonism. It should, in theory, have a great deal of sedating side effects (fatigue, sedation, somnolence) in clinical practice. The right side of the table shows lurasidone as having the highest pKi value and hence the poorest affinity for the H1 receptor antagonism. It should have the least amount of sedating side effects.

Table 2. Relative SGA D2 Receptor Antagonism

Aripiprazole	Lurasidone	Asenapine	Paliperidone	Risperidone	Zprasidone	Iloperidone	Olanzapine	Quetiapine	Norquetiapi ne
0.34	0.994	1.3	2.8	3.77	4.8	6.3	11-31	626	489

←-Lowest pKi value---------------Highest pKi value-→

Data are presented as molar pKi values reported by the respective manufacturers. Ki values are inversely proportional to affinity (low Ki value=high affinity, high Ki value=low affinity).

Table reprinted with the permission of Dr. Kristina Bedynerman MD, SUNY Upstate Medical University.

It is evident that aripirazole has the greatest affinity and quetiapine the lowest for D2 receptor antagonism. Therefore in theory, aripiprazole should have the highest in psychomotor slowing with possible sedation. Since it is a partial agonist, its sedating side effects may not be as robust as a fully antagonistic agent. Quetiapine theoretically should have the least D2 blocking sedating effects.

For patients with positive symptoms of schizophrenia, blocking D2 receptors alleviates psychosis and may cause a calming effect in treating anxiety and agitation. In patients who are already agitated and activated, it may be helpful to avoid certain SGAs which do not provide any initial therapeutic calming or sedation.

Agents with greater combined antagonism at H1 and D2 receptors should be helpful. It may also make sense to avoid those that tend to be higher in developing the extrapyramidal syndrome (EPS) of akathisia. More akathisia prone SGA include aripiprazole, iloperidone, asenapine, and lurasidone. Conversely, for those patients with negative symptoms such as affective blunting, loss of drive initiation, or executive dysfunction, giving an SGA may make these symptoms worse. This situation may occur if the chosen SGA increases sedation or psychomotor impairment. In such patients, using an SGA with less H1 and D2 antagonism may be worthwhile to avoid increasing now iatrogenic negative symptoms. [8]

Anticholinergic (AchM) Receptor Antagonism

Antagonism of acethycholinergic muscarinic (AChM) receptors are often associated with the side effects of dry mouth, blurred vision, tachycardia, constipation and urinary retention. In the CNS, these anticholinergic effects may promote difficulty with storing and retrieving memory, cognitive dysfunction, and perhaps the interpretation of being in a fatigued state.

Knowledge of the antagonistic effects of the SGAs on the cholinergic system may be useful in clinical practice. For example, patients who are schizophrenic or even depressed may present as fatigued, feeling as though they are dragging throughout the day and feeling slowed down.

They may also present as forgetful, with poor short term memory and an inability to retain information. As noted above, remarkable H1 and D2 receptor blockade from the SGA may cause sedation and psychomotor impairment as side effects, and additional cognition, memory, and executive dysfunction may occur causing even further fatigue, sedation or somnolence to be experienced by the patient. [2, 9]

Sedation and Somnolence in Clinical Practice: Regulatory Trial Findings

The information in *Table 4* suggests sedation levels based upon pooled analyses in clinical trials for each agent. Instead of bench top lab affinity values and theoretical clinical implications, these are actual numbers from patient trials. However, these may not translate wholly into clinical practice outcomes either. Some SGA are studied only in schizophrenia, others in bipolar disorder, major depressive disorder, or even autism. These different populations likely have different rates of subjective side effect reporting which leaves *Table 4* vulnerable to interpretation. Also, many patients in practice have comorbid psychiatric conditions and experience the practice of polypharmacy by their caregivers. In this case, a patient being on many drugs with sedating profiles could additively increase overall sedation values and experience. Conversely, patients on a sedating psychotropic could be placed simultaneously on a combination or augmentation agent that is more stimulating which might counteract the initial fatigue, sedation, or somnolence. Below, each SGA will be better delineated in regards to its clinical trial adverse effects outcomes.

Olanzapine's tolerability is enumerated in *Table 4.* The FDA reports incidence, rounded to the nearest percent, in treatment-emergent adverse reactions that occurred in 2% or more of patients treated with oral olanzapine (doses ≥2.5 mg/day) and with incidence greater than placebo who participated in an acute phase of placebo-controlled trials is delineated here. Overall, 29% of trial subjects taking olanzapine reported sedating side effects. [10] Therefore olanzapine is considered to have a high sedation profile.

Regarding risperidone, there was 3% sedation experienced with a dose of 2-8 mg/day and 3% sedation in 8-16 mg of risperidone per day. Somnolence occurred in 7% of subjects for 2-8 mg/day and 2% for a dose of 8-16 mg/day. [11] Interestingly, in one study it was evident that risperidone may have actually had less sedating effects even at higher doses. Overall, risperidone is felt to be moderately sedating in nature.

Regarding lurasidone, based on the pooled data from short-term placebo-controlled, fixed-dose studies, the apparent dose-related adverse reactions causing somnolence in patients treated for schizophrenia was 15% with a dose of 20mg perday, 19% with a dose of 80mg per day, and 23% with 120mg per day.

Overall sedation for this drug was 22% compared to placebo which was 10%. [12] The overall sedative nature of lurasidone in trials was actually high second to olanzapine.

Somnolence is a commonly reported adverse event in patients treated with quetiapine especially during the 3-5 day period of initial dose-titration. In schizophrenia trials, somnolence was reported in 18% (89/510) of patients on quetiapine compared to 11% of placebo patients. [13]

In a short-term placebo controlled trial of quetiapine extended release for schizophrenia the most commonly observed adverse reactions associated with its use was somnolence (25%), while the rate in those who were on placebo was only 10%. Comparatively it appeared in this instance that quetiapine extended release had greater sedative effects compared to quetiapine immediate release. [13]

Table 4 enumerates similar data for ziprasidone with side effect incidence, where overall sedation caused from ziprasidone was 14% compared to the placebo group which was 7%. [14]

Sedating adverse reactions associated with use of asenapine that occurred during acute therapy up to 6 weeks in patients with schizophrenia showed 15% sedation in patients treated with a dose of 10mg per day and 13% with a dose of 20mg per day. Overall sedation being 13% with 10mg or 20mg per day, compared to placebo group which caused 7% of sedation. [15]

Iloperidone side effect information was derived from pooled data in schizophrenia at daily doses within a range of 10 to 24 mg. Those patients who received 10-16mg per day, had a rate of sedation and somnolence of 9% and those who received a dose of 20-24 mg/day a rate of sedation was 15% compared to the placebo group whose overall rate of sedation was 5%. [16]

Table 3. Relative SGA AChM Receptor Antagonism

Norquetiapine 38.3	*Olanzapine 32-73*	*Quetiapine >1000*	*Iloperidone >1000*	*Ziprasidone >1000*	*Risperidone >1000*	*Paliperidone >1000*	*Asenapine >1000*	*Lurasidone >1000*	Aripiprazole *>1000*

←-Lowest pKi value------------------Highest pKi value-→

Data are presented as molar pKi values reported by the respective manufacturers. Ki values are inversely proportional to affinity (low Ki value=high affinity, high Ki value=low affinity).

Table reprinted with the permission of Dr. Kristina Bedynerman MD, SUNY Upstate Medical University.

Regarding affinity for muscarinic receptors, olanzapine and norquetiapine have higher affinity for AchM receptor antagonism compared to the other SGAs. Therefore olanzapine and norquetiapine may theoretically allow for more cognitive deficits. Patients who feel cognitively slowed often appear to be tired and report cognitive and motor slowing which can appear as sedation in clinical practice. In theory these should also cause more sedation, but with less EPS side effects. All other SGA have minimal AchM receptor antagonism and should be relatively devoid of these potentially sedating adverse effects.

Table 4. Clinical Rates of Sedating Side Effects

Olanzapine	Lurasidone	Quetiapine	Ziprasidone	Asenapine	Iloperidone	Paliperidone	Aripiprazole	Risperidone
Sedation: 10% Somnolence 29%	Sedation and Somnolence 2% Fatigue 4%	Sedation and Somnolence 18%	Somnolence and sedation 14%	Sedation and Somnolence 13% Fatigue: 4%	Somnolence 9% fatigue4%	Sedation and somnolence: 9%	Sedation 7% Somnolence 5% Fatigue 6%	Sedation 3% Somnolence7% Fatigue 3%

←-Most sedative----------------Least sedative----→

Company published and FDA approved drug package inserts that reflect regulatory trial data are summarized showing the amount of sedating side effects suffered by trial subjects. In practice, clinicians should expect to see this amount of adverse effects in their patients when treated at approved doses.

Table 4 includes adverse reactions for the paliperidone dosed groups. A greater incidence of sedation was seen in paliperidone treated group than in the placebo group. Data were pooled from three studies with doses of 3 mg and 9 mg, the second study included 6 mg, 9 mg, and 12 mg, and the third study included 6 mg and 12mg. Those of whom were treated with 3mg had sedation of 6% sedation from 6 mg, 10% sedation from 9 mg and 11% from a dose of 12 mg paliperidone. [17]

Aripiprazole's pooled adverse effect incidence is noted in *Table 4* as well. The rate of sedation was 7% and somnolence was 5% compared to placebo group which was 4% and 3% respectively. [18]

CONCLUSIONS

This chapter began by reviewing relative affinities for each of the SGA in regards to H1, D2, and AChM receptors and theorizing that antagonism at these sites might create sedating side effects that include a spectrum of fatigue to overt somnolence. Fatigue is sometimes also classified as mental versus physical and somnolence may last minutes to hours, but this was not further delineated. Clinically, this might be important when dealing with a patient and their ability to tolerate sedation as a side effect or to be placated in their symptoms by using sedation as a clinically useful effect. Next, clinical trial data was reviewed to determine which SGA might be the most sedating in patients who suffer from a single diagnosis instead of multiple psychiatric comorbidities and also in those patients taking a single monotherapy drug for treatment of schizophrenia versus bipolar mania or depression versus unipolar depression, versus autism. Therefore, a clinician may predict the risk of sedation as a side effect based upon actual trial data or theoretical pharmacodynamic information.

Interestingly, if one were to overlay the multitude of tables displayed in this chapter, there is not one SGA that is the worst, or strongest, in all areas that might be associated with the promoting of sedating side effects. Perhaps olanzapine and quetiapine occupy the *left handed* side of the tables more often with a greater mixture of sedating pharmacodynamics and clinical side effect data to correlate the theoretical into actual clinical practice. However, even quetiapine on some tables moves to the *right* suggesting less fatigue risk. As noted, this agent also possesses NRI properties that might in some patients promote wakefulness thus changing what side effects are seen in clinical practice.

Dosing is also important as for many SGAs, higher doses are used to treat psychosis and mania where lower doses may treat depression. Off label uses for anxiety, agitation and insomnia likely utilize even lower dosing strategies. At these low doses, those SGA with higher affinities for H1 for example may provide a great deal of sedation early, but less so as dosing increases and H1 receptors have been occupied and possibly desensitized.

Finally, polypharmacy and comorbid psychiatric diagnostic presentations are likely the norm in clinical practice making clinical trial data less valid in predicting who will become sedated and who will not. This suggests that a psychopharmacologist should understand the pharmacodynamic underpinnings of all prescribed agents (not just SGA) and be aware of additive effects of combining multiple agents with H1, D2, or AChM antagonism that will likely cause more sedation. Clinicians also should read up and review clinical trials and meta-analyses to better determine side effect risks and also compare all of these to findings found in clinical practice when treating patients.

REFERENCES

[1] Handbook of Psychiatric Drug Therapy, 6th ed. Labbate LA, Fava M, Rosenbaum JF, Arana GW(Eds.) Philadelphia:Lippincott Williams and Wilkins; 2012.

[2] Stahl SM. Describing an Atypical Antipsychotic:Receptor Binding and Its Role in Pathophysiology. *Primary Care Companion J. Clin. Psychiatry*. 2003 ;5[suppl 3]:9–13.

[3] *Stahl SM. Stahl's Essential Psychopharmacology*. 3rd ed. New York: Cambridge University Press; 2008.

[4] Stahl SM. Psychopharmacology of wakefulness:pathways and neurotransmitters. *J. Clin. Psych*. 2002:55(7); 551-552.

[5] Lin JS. Brain structures and mechanisms involved in the control of cortical activation and wakefulness, with emphasis on the posterior hypothalamus and histaminergic neurons. *Sleep Medicine Reviews* 2000:4;471-503.

[6] *Stahl SM. Essential Psychopharmacology:The Prescriber's Guide*. 4th ed. New York: Cambridge University Press; 2011.

[7] Utilizing pharmacodynamics properties of second generation antipsychotics to guide treatment, Kristina Bedynerman., In Press Drugs of Today.

[8] Schwartz TL and Stahl SM. Treatment Strategies for Dosing the Second Generation Antipsychotics. CNS Neuroscience and Therapeutics. *CNS Neuroscience and Therapeutics*. 2011:17 (2);110–117.

[9] Kinon BJ and Lieberman JA. Mechanisms of action of atypical antipsychotic drugs: a critical analysis. *Psychopharmacology*. 1996; 124; 2-34.

[10] Olanzapine FDA Package Insert, Eli Lilly, 1996. Accessed 3.19.12 http://dailymed.nlm.nih.gov/dailymed/drugInfo.cfm?id=46801

[11] Risperidone FDA Package Insert, Janssen Pharmaceuticals, 1993. Accessed 3.19.12 http://dailymed.nlm.nih.gov/dailymed/drugInfo.cfm?id=53550

[12] Lurasidone FDA Package Insert, Sunovion Pharmaceuticals, 2010. Accessed 3.19.12, http://dailymed.nlm.nih.gov/dailymed/drugInfo.cfm?id=58535

[13] Quetiapine (XR) FDA Package Inserts, Astra-Zeneca Pharmaceuticals, 1997-2011. Accessed 3.19.12. http://www1.astrazeneca-us.com/pi/Seroquel.pdf, http://www1.astrazeneca-us.com/pi/seroquelxr.pdf, http://dailymed.nlm.nih.gov/dailymed/drugInfo.cfm?id=60222, http://dailymed.nlm.nih.gov/dailymed/drugInfo.cfm?id=60373

[14] Ziprasidone FDA Package Inserts, Pfizer Pharmaceuticals, 2001-2009. Accessed 3.19.12. http://labeling, http://dailymed.nlm. nih.gov/dailymed/drugInfo.cfm?id=33501

[15] Asenapine FDA Package Inserts, Merck and Co. Pharmaceuticals, 2009-2011. Accessed 3.19.12. http://www.spfiles.com/pisaphrisv1.pdf, http://dailymed.nlm.nih.gov/dailymed/drugInfo.cfm?id=54239

[16] Iloperidone FDA Package Inserts, Novartis Pharmaceuticals,2009. Accessed 3.19.12. http://www.pharma.us.novartis.com/product/pi/pdf/fanapt.pdf, http://dailymed.nlm.nih.gov/dailymed/drugInfo.cfm?id=61550

[17] Paliperidone FDA Package Inserts, Janssen Pharmaceuticals,2006-11. Accessed 3.19.12. http://www.janssencns.com/invega-prescribing-information, http://dailymed.nlm.nih.gov/dailymed/drugInfo.cfm?id=51770
[18] Aripiprazole FDA Package Inserts, Otsuka America Pharmaceuticals,2002-12. Accessed 3.19.12. http://www.abilify.com/pdf/pi.aspx, http://dailymed.nlm.nih.gov/dailymed/drugInfo.cfm?id=40981

In: Antipsychotic Drugs
Editors: T.L. Schwartz, J. Megna and M.E. Topel

ISBN: 978-1-62100-071-6

Chapter 14

ANTIPSYCHOTIC SIDE EFFECTS: IDENTIFICATION AND MANAGEMENT

***Danielle S. Cha*[3] *and Roger S. McIntyre*[1, 2, 3, 4*]**

[1] Department of Psychiatry, University of Toronto, Toronto, ON, Canada
[2] Department of Pharmacology, University of Toronto, Toronto, ON, Canada
[3] Mood Disorders Psychopharmacology Unit, University Health Network, Toronto, ON, Canada
[4] Institute of Medical Science, University of Toronto, Toronto, ON, Canada

ABSTRACT

Introduction: Second generation antipsychotics (SGAs) provide broad-spectrum effectiveness for the acute and/or preventative treatment of disparate psychiatric disorders. Second generation antipsychotic agents offer improved efficacy in some psychopathological domains when compared to first-generation antipsychotics. Notwithstanding these assets, SGAs are not a catholicon and are associated with clinically significant and treatment-limiting side effects.

Conclusion: This chapter reviews treatment-emergent adverse events attributable to the use of SGAs with a particular emphasis on adverse events that frequently lead to treatment discontinuation (e.g. neuroleptic malignant syndrome, QTc prolongation, blood dyscrasias). In addition, updates on the pharmacokinetic and pharmacodynamic profiles of recently approved SGAs (e.g. lurasidone, asenapine, iloperidone) as well as commonly encountered drug interactions are addressed. The overarching aim of this chapter is to provide a sketch of how the efficacy and tolerability of SGAs may be obfuscated by accompanying side effect profiles and/or adverse drug interactions. Moreover, with an increasing trend towards polypharmacotherapy in the treatment of comorbid psychiatric and medical disorders, appropriate treatment selection now requires not only a careful understanding of the various SGAs' proven efficacy across psychopathological

* Corresponding Author: Dr. Roger S. McIntyre, MD, FRCPC, Associate Professor of Psychiatry and Pharmacology, University of Toronto; Head, Mood Disorders Psychopharmacology Unit, University Health Network; 399 Bathurst Street – Toronto, ON, Canada M5T 2S8; Telephone: 416 603 5279; Fax: 416 603 5368; Email: roger.mcintyre@uhn.on.ca

syndromes, but also, importantly, their associated drug interactions and adverse event profiles.

INTRODUCTION

Second generation antipsychotics (SGAs) initially emerged as a treatment alternative with a side effect profile preferable to that associated with their therapeutic predecessors – the first-generation antipsychotics. Some SGAs have a lower propensity to engender and/or exacerbate certain treatment-emergent adverse events (e.g. extrapyramidal symptoms, weight gain, changes in metabolic profile). This reduction in side-effect burden has undeniably advanced the pharmacotherapy of mood disorders and their frequently associated comorbidities (e.g. overweight/obesity, diabetes mellitus, metabolic syndrome). The improved tolerability of SGAs has reduced rates of non-adherence and discontinuation of therapy when compared to first-generation antipsychotics. [1-4]

Second generation antipsychotics are capable of mitigating both positive (e.g. hallucinations, delusions, disorganized speech) and negative (e.g. apathy, affective flattening, avolition) symptomatology as well as affective/anxiety symptoms and behavioural disorders. This overall therapeutic profile has led to indications for mood, psychotic, and pervasive developmental disorders for some of these agents. [3;5-9]

This chapter evaluates adverse events attributable to SGAs (with the exception of adverse events relating to weight gain, metabolics, sedation, and extrapyramidal symptoms –which are topics discussed in separate chapters of this book) that are often treatment-limiting and lead to medication discontinuation (Table 1). In addition, the present chapter provides an update on the pharmacokinetic (Table 2 [55]) and pharmacodynamic (Table 3 [55]) profiles of recently approved SGAs (e.g. lurasidone, asenapine, iloperidone) as well as commonly encountered drug interactions. The chapter finishes with recommendations for selecting and sequencing SGAs in clinical practice.

ATYPICAL ANTIPSYCHOTICS: AN OVERVIEW OF ADVERSE EVENTS

Neurologic

Seizures

Few studies have examined the onset of antipsychotic-induced seizures; some studies have, however, implicated clozapine and olanzapine in elevated (dose-dependent) risk for seizures when compared with other SGAs [1;10;11]. *Centorrino* [10] *et al.* analysed electroencephalography (EEG) abnormalities associated with first-generation and second generation antipsychotic use. The greatest risks were associated with 1) clozapine and olanzapine use; 2) hypertension (diastolic pressure >90 mmHg); 3) SGA as compared to first-generation antipsychotic therapy; 4) age (>40 years); 5) bipolarity (as compared to other mood disorders); 6) sustained SGA use (i.e. >1.29 weeks); and 7) absence of substance use disorders, respectively. Quetiapine exhibits the lowest risk for EEG abnormalities when

Table 1. Commonly Encountered Adverse Events Attributed to Second-Generation Antipsychotics*

	Clozapine	Olanzapine	Risperidone	Quetiapine	Ziprasidone	Aripiprazole	Iloperidone	Asenapine	Lurasidone
Neurologic									
Seizure Risk	DD	±	±	±	±	±	±	±	±
Neuroleptic Malignant Syndrome	+	+	+	+	+	+	+	+	+
Cardiovascular									
Myocarditis/Cardiomyopathy	+/0	ISF	ISF	ISF	ISF	ISF	ISF	ISF	ISF
QTc Prolongation	ISF	±	±	±	++	+/0	++	+	ISF
Neuroendocrine									
Hyperprolactinemia	+/0	±	DD	±	±	±	±	±	ISF
Blood Dyscrasias									
Leukopenia/Neutropenia	+	+	+/0	+	ISF	+/0	ISF	ISF	ISF
Agranulocytosis	+	+	±	±	ISF	+/0	ISF	ISF	ISF
Reproductive Health & Safety									
Pregnancy	B	C	C	C	C	C	C	C	B
Lactation	+	+	+/0	+/0	ISF	ISF	ISF	ISF	ISF

*Number of plus symbols represent extent of associated risk for adverse event

+/0 : Minimal Risk

± :Equivocal

DD: Dose Dependent

ISF: Insufficient Data

FDA Pregnancy Categories:

Category A: Controlled studies in humans demonstrate no risk in fetal development

Category B: [a]No evidence for increased risk in fetal development in animal studies; No available human data

[b]Adverse events observed in animal studies; No risk for fetal development in controlled human studies

Category C: [a]Insufficient evidence for risk in fetal development from both animal and human studies

[b]Adverse events observed in animal studies; No available human data

Category D: Evidence for risk in fetal development (benefits > risks)

Category X: Evidence for risk in fetal development (risks > benefits)

Table 2. Pharmacokinetic Properties of Second-Generation Antipsychotics

				P450 Systems		
Generic Names	**Bioavailability (%)**	**Protein Binding (%)**	**Half-Life (h)**	**Substrate of**	**Inhibits**	**Excretion (%)[a]**
Aripiprazole	87	99	75-94	3A4, 2D6		
Clozapine	50-60	95	5-16	1A2, 3A4, 2D6		50 R/30 F
Olanzapine	60	93	21-54	1A2, 2D6		57 R/30 F
Paliperidone	28	74	23	2D6, 3A4		80 R/11 F
Quetiapine	90 ± 9	83	6-7	3A4		73 R/20 F
Risperidone	70	90	20-24	2D6	2D6	70 R/15 F
Ziprasidone	60	99	7	3A4		20 R/66 F
Asenapine	35	95	24	1A2, 1A4, 3A4	2D6	50 R/40 F
Iloperidone	96	95	18	2D6, 3A4		58 R/22 F
Lurasidone	10-20	99	18	3A4		9 R/80 F

[a] F = fecal; R = renal.

Table adapted from: [55]

Table 3. Pharmacodynamics: Relative Neuroreceptor Affinities for Second-Generation Antipsychotics at Therapeutic Doses

Generic Names	D2	H1	α1	α2	5-HT1A	5-HT2A	5-HT2C
Aripiprazole	++++	+	+	0	+++	+++	+++
Clozapine	+	+++	++++	+++	0	+++	+++
Olanzapine	++	+++	0	0	0	+++	+++
Quetiapine	+	++	+	0	0	0	0
Risperidone	+++	+	++	0	0	++++	++++
Ziprasidone	+++	+	+	+	+	++++	++++
Asenapine	++++	+++	0	++	++	++++	++++
Iloperidone	+++	0	+	0	+	++++	+++
Lurasidone	++++	0	+	+++	++	++++	0

Note: + to ++++ = low to marked affinity; 0 = minimal to none.

Table adapted from: [55]

compared to clozapine, olanzapine, and haloperidol. [12] Agents involved in polypharmacotherapy elevate seizure risk by concomitantly producing a lower seizure threshold via heterogeneous factors (e.g. slow drug metabolism, rapid dose titration, drug-drug interactions). [1;11]

Neuroleptic Malignant Syndrome

Neuroleptic Malignant Syndrome (NMS) is a serious adverse event which is less often reported with SGAs when compared to first-generation antipsychotics. Notwithstanding, evidence for an increased susceptibility for developing this potentially lethal condition in persons prescribed polypharmacotherapy (i.e. mood stabilizers and psychotropic agents) have been established. [1,11,13] The classic features of NMS are muscle rigidity, hyperthermia (may be accompanied by extrapyramidal symptoms), changes in mental status, and autonomic disruption. [1,13] In addition, NMS may present with associated laboratory features such as elevated serum creatine kinase levels, leucocytosis, electrolyte disturbance, impaired liver function tests, ECG abnormalities, and renal impairment. [14]

Second generation antipsychotics which have been associated with NMS as a treatment-emergent adverse event includes: clozapine, olanzapine, risperidone, quetiapine, ziprasidone, paliperidone, aripiprazole, and amisulpride. [14] These SGAs typically exhibit clinical presentations aligned with the classic features of NMS (e.g. muscle rigidity, hyperthermia, changes in mental status, autonomic disruption). [1, 13-14] However, a notable exception is made for clozapine-induced NMS which is significantly less likely to manifest with muscle rigidity when compared to other SGAs. [14]

Various factors have been proposed to confer increased risk for NMS; examples include: male sex; comorbid medical/neurological disorders; mental retardation; extrapyramidal syndromes; iron deficiency; depot administration of medication; and rapid escalation of antipsychotic dose. [11, 13-14] Rapid treatment, using first-line NMS management, including adequate hydration, temperature reduction, nutritional support, and pharmacological interventions (i.e. reduction of muscle rigidity using benzodiazepines/dantrolene) is necessary to eliminate NMS. [1, 13-14] As NMS is a medical emergency, prevention is the primary objective and careful surveillance for clinical presentations suggestive of NMS is warranted.

Cardiovascular

Myocarditis/Cardiomyopathy

Myocarditis is normally an asymptomatic autoimmune response provoked by viral infection followed by lymphocytic infiltration. [1,15] The pathoetiology of myocarditis remains largely unknown; case reports have, however, evinced clozapine-treatment in the development of myocarditis with symptoms including chest pain, dyspnea, tachypnea, palpitations, unexplained fatigue, and other anomalies related to heart failure. [1,15-16]

Elevated risk for myocarditis is seen within the first 6 weeks of clozapine therapy in 80% of patients [16] with an incidence estimated to be 10- to 20-fold greater than the general population. [1] The relative risks for myocarditis/cardiomyopathy among other atypical antipsychotic agents have yet to be elucidated. If patients undergoing clozapine therapy are suspected of myocarditis, prompt discontinuation is recommended. [1]

QTc Prolongation

The prolongation of the QTc interval is associated with an increased risk for ventricular tachyarrhythmia, specifically Torsades de Pointes (TdP), which can result in sudden cardiac death. [17-18] Torsades de Pointes is a rare but fatal arrhythmia that may be induced by SGAs. [18] Controlled epidemiological studies evaluating cardiac risk profiles for antipsychotic agents provide a set of risk factors linked to increased incidence of QTc prolongation and TdP including female gender, congenital long QT syndrome, concomitant cardiovascular disease, polypharmacotherapy, substance abuse, electrolyte disorders, bradychardia, and anorexia nervosa. [19] The use of SGAs has been variably reported to elevate the risk for cardiac events, SGAs which have demonstrated a greater propensity for QTc prolongation, ventricular arrhythmia, and cardiac arrest include: clozapine, olanzapine, risperidone, ziprasidone and iloperidone. [1,19-21] Clozapine therapy demonstrates a substantially higher risk for QTc prolongation when compared to other SGAs. [17] Olanzapine- and ziprasidone-induced TdP have also been reported. [19]

Neuroendocrine

Hyperprolactinemia

The physiological function of prolactin in both men and women involves the secretion of gonadotropin-releasing hormone (GnRH) from the hypothalamus to prevent the release of gonadotropins (e.g. luteinising hormone, follicle-stimulating hormone) from the pituitary, which suppresses ovarian or testicular function. [1,11] Prolactin is also involved in female breast enlargement during pregnancy, stimulating milk production during lactation. [1,11] Elevation in serum prolactin has been hypothesized to be a result of dopamine-2 (D_2) receptor binding, wherein adverse-effect profiles emerge when psychotropic agents sustain a D_2 occupancy. [1] Individual differences exist for the fluctuation in serum prolactin levels; the consortium position on the upper limit demarking hyperprolactinemia has, however, been suggested to be approximately 10 - 25μg/L for both men and women. [1,22] The consequences of increased serum prolactin levels vary in severity across SGAs. Symptoms that may develop in women as a result of hyperprolactinemia include: galactorrhea, infertility, migraine, amenorrhea, and breast tenderness or engorgement. Likewise, men may experience reduced libido, fatigue, erectile dysfunction, gynecomastia, and galactorrhea. [1,23]

In addition, there is growing concern about the long-term effects that changes in serum prolactin levels may have for children and adolescents receiving antipsychotic treatment as they approach adulthood. [28] In a study that examined the ensuing reproductive and sexual adverse events experienced by children and adolescents receiving antipsychotic treatment, results implicated female gender ($\geq$ 13 years) with comorbid obesity, metabolic and/or endocrine disorders with greater risk for developing hyperprolactinemia [28], an event associated with ensuing reproductive and sexual adverse events. [28] Moreover, the use of risperidone and aripiprazole in paediatric populations has increased with the broad-spectrum application of SGAs in reducing irritability in children and adolescents with autism and other pervasive developmental disorders. [29] It has been reported that hyperprolactinemia manifests in up to 71% of the schizophrenic and autistic paediatric population treated with SGAs (i.e. risperidone) within 5-10 weeks following treatment initiation. [29]

Risperidone appears to be associated with a sustained elevation in serum prolactin levels resulting in symptomatic hyperprolactinemia unlike quetiapine, olanzapine, and clozapine which have minimal effect on prolactin levels. [23] A recent study investigating the relationship between sexual dysfunction and serum prolactin levels with quetiapine versus risperidone found that risperidone significantly increased prolactin levels, which correlated to increases in sexual disturbance. [25] Similarly, the most frequently reported adverse effect associated with treatment-emergent hyperprolactinemia for both men and women was diminished sexual desire (≈40%). [26] In a study comparing haloperidol with quetiapine in schizophrenic subjects (n=35), prolactin concentrations were persistently lower in those treated with quetiapine as compared to those treated with haloperidol. [29] Evidence in children has also demonstrated significantly fewer hyperprolactinaemic events in those treated with quetiapine versus risperidone. [30]

Clozapine interacts with the D_1, D_2, histamine, and 5-HT_2 receptors affecting pre- and post-synaptic dopamine response and function. [31] *In vitro* studies have indicated that high concentrations of clozapine may directly inhibit prolactin release. [31] Moreover, clozapine therapy demonstrated a reduction in hyperprolactinemia by 16-80% over a 6-week trial. [32] At treatment initiation, olanzapine displays a dose-dependent association with prolactin elevation. [33] In a double-blind trial comparing olanzapine to placebo over a six week period, olanzapine-treated groups differed significantly from the placebo group at 2-weeks when doses exceeded 10mg/day. [33] However, the same olanzapine-treated groups exhibited prolactin elevations comparable to those in the placebo group by week 6. [33]

A comparison study evaluating prolactin elevation in aripiprazole-treated groups demonstrated that the oral administration of aripiprazole versus haloperidol results in the decreased release of prolactin *in vivo*. [34] This result may be attributable to aripiprazole's partial agonistic effect at the D_2 and 5-HT_{1A} receptors in addition to its antagonistic effect at the 5-HT_{2A} receptors. [35, 36]

Transient elevations in prolactin levels are observed with ziprasidone during treatment initiation. [36] Ziprasidone appears to exert agonistic properties at $5HT_{1A}$ receptors. [36] Similarly, the only significant difference found in short-term trials evaluating prolactin levels and lurasidone treatment was the mean change from baseline. [37] Results of these studies showed a dose-dependent increase in prolactin concentrations at treatment initiation, particularly in women. [37]

Few reports of hyperprolactenaemic events in association with asenapine are available, with hyperprolactinemia occurring in only approximately 4-9% of asenapine recipients when compared to approximately 2% of placebo recipients. [38]

Treatment-emergent hyperprolactinemia can be established by treatment cessation, allowing for exclusion of alternative hyperprolactinemia diagnoses (e.g. pituitary microadenoma, oral contraceptive use). [1] The management of SGA-induced hyperprolactinemia may involve dose reduction and/or switching, use of a dopamine agonist (i.e. bromocriptine), or concomitant oral contraceptive use (for females) to eliminate symptoms related to estrogen deficiency (e.g. migraine, fatigue, hot flashes). [1,23]

Blood Dyscrasias

Leukopenia/Neutropenia

Most SGAs have insufficient controlled data to support definitive conclusions about the specific incidence and severity of adverse haematological events. Notwithstanding this paucity of data, studies scrutinizing the haematological toxicity of clozapine provide evidence for differential risk in persons exhibiting genetic variations involving metabolites that target peripheral blood neutrophils. [39] Additional reports suggest that clozapine-induced adverse haematological events [e.g. agranulocytosis, neutropenia, leukopenia) normally occur within an 18-week period from treatment initiation. [40] Several case reports have also suggested risks associated with olanzapine and quetiapine therapy. [41, 42] Variations in characteristic human leukocyte antigen (HLA) groups (e.g. DQB1*0502, DQA1*0102) have been implicated in olanzapine-induced leukopenia/neutropenia, which may also be associated with clozapine-induced haematotoxicity. [43] The concomitant use of quetiapine and valproate has been associated with increased occurrence of leukopenia/neutropenia compared to either treatment alone. [44] Polypharmacotherapy is a frequent and increasing practice in treating mood disorder populations; it may exacerbate existing inherent tendencies towards poor disease outcomes and/or additional adverse events. The therapeutic usefulness of agents promoting leukocytosis (i.e. lithium), and/or rapid granulocyte production (i.e. filgrastim) in the management of blood dyscrasias has, however, not yet been sufficiently studied. [45]

Agranulocytosis

Declines in white blood cell (WBC) and absolute neutrophil granulocyte (ANC) counts from the normal range (4.0–11.0 $\times 10^9$/L WBC and 2.5–7.5 $\times$ 10^9/L ANC) may result in agranulocytosis. [46] Clozapine-induced agranulocytosis has been comprehensively reviewed elsewhere [46], with an estimate of approximately 1% -2% of persons receiving clozapine therapy developing agranulocytosis. [41,46] Agranulocytosis consists of signs and symptoms including high fever, fatigue, and mucosal necroses in the throat, perianal, and genital regions. [41] Given that most available data describing atypical antipsychotic-associated agranulocytosis were obtained from case reports and short-term studies focusing on clozapine, few reports have investigated the emergence of agranulocytosis with other SGAs. The possible occurrence of neutropenia/agranulocytosis has been described with quetiapine and olanzapine. [41] Some reports suggest that clozapine therapy continuation despite neutropenia is possible with adjunct granulocyte colony-stimulating factor (i.e. filgrastim) injections. [41] However, it is recommended that SGA therapy is promptly discontinued once neutropenia/agranulocytosis is determined. Persons discontinuing clozapine therapy following neutropenia/agranulocytosis have been evinced to show a favourable response to aripiprazole [41]. All product monographs for SGAs in the US include safety information warning about risk of blood dyscrasias with all SGAs.

Reproductive Health and Safety

Pregnancy

The data available describing the effective management of psychotic disorders during pregnancy with SGAs, and their potential teratogenicity, is insufficient for definitive conclusions to be drawn about their reproductive toxicity. [1] Nevertheless, no definitive evidence has shown increased risk for birth defects or other potential adverse events during pregnancy as a result of SGA treatment. [47,48] Second generation antipsychotic agents are largely classified by the US Food and Drug Administration (FDA) as category C, with the exception of clozapine and, more recently, lurasidone classified as category B (Table 1). Other risks associated with SGA treatment, including weight gain and associated metabolic disturbances, must be considered in the selection of psychotropic medication in pregnancy to improve maternal psychiatric illness while also reducing potential teratogenic effects. [1,47,49]

Clozapine is associated with increased risk for iatrogenic weight gain as well as metabolic disturbances, which may result in gestational metabolic complications during pregnancy. [1,50] Case reports have described neonatal seizures/convulsions, floppy infant syndrome, birth defects, and hypotonia with clozapine. [1,47,50] Overdose on clozapine is evidenced to produce fatal poisoning in the newborn during pregnancy. [47]

Few studies have demonstrated adverse outcomes with the use of risperidone during pregnancy, with no reports of congenital abnormalities or teratogenic risk. [47,51] However, it is known that risperidone is able to cross the placental barrier, estimated at 49.2% ± 33.9% (SD). [50,51] Recent evidence suggests that risperidone may modify fetal-placental blood flow by affecting the contractility of the human umbilical artery which is involved in fetal-placental circulation. [51] Risperidone appears to antagonize histamine and serotonin responses producing a dose-dependent vasorelaxant effect in human vascular smooth muscle. [51] The specific effects of the increased blood flow through the fetal-placental barrier as a result of risperidone treatment during pregnancy remains unclear. [51]

Lurasidone, first approved by the FDA in 2010 for schizophrenia, demonstrated its effectiveness in four placebo-controlled trials over a six-week period. [52] Three of the four trials were assessed to be superior to placebo with a 40 mg/day dosage regimen. [52] The FDA has assigned lurasidone Pregnancy Class B, despite no well-controlled clinical trials for this SGA in women during pregnancy. Adverse events that may affect fetal development resulting from lurasidone therapy in pregnancy include extrapyramidal reactions or withdrawal symptoms, particularly during the third trimester.

The human toxicity data for other SGAs (e.g. quetiapine, ziprasidone, aripiprazole) in pregnancy, resulting in fetal toxicity, is insufficient to provide definitive recommendations for the management of psychotic disorders during pregnancy. [1]

Lactation

No evidence is available for the risk-to-benefit profile of SGA treatment during breastfeeding. [1,53] However, contraindications have been set for clozapine and olanzapine due to their liability to produce adverse events (e.g. extrapyramidal reactions, transient neurodevelopmental delay, hematologic complications) in nursing infants. [53] An accumulation of measurable amounts of clozapine in the plasma and tissue of the brain in nursing infants has been reported with continued clozapine therapy during breastfeeding. [1] The successful use of risperidone, quetiapine, and olanzapine has been reported during breast feeding, however, conclusive evidence has yet to be provided for the safety of these SGAs in nursing infants. [54] For a comprehensive and systematic review of the risk of using SGA therapy in breastfeeding, with recommendations for the maintenance of an appropriate pharmacologic regimen, see *Gentile.* [53]

Summary

The adverse event profile of SGAs overlaps with first-generation agents (e.g. NMS, QTc prolongation, hyperprolactinemia). In addition, SGAs as a class are often associated with other adverse events (e.g. weight gain and metabolic abnormalities). The initial exuberance for SGAs has been somewhat tempered with available evidence supporting the assertion that SGAs as a class of agents may offer a greater therapeutic index when compared to first-generation agents in most patients. Notwithstanding their appreciable efficacy, the hazards associated with SGAs in some cases may entirely offset their therapeutic advantage. There is an insufficient data base regarding adverse events of SGAs when prescribed in combination with each other and/or with other psychotropic agents (e.g. anticonvulsants). Moreover, commonly encountered drug interactions associated with the increasing trend towards polypharmacotherapy often results in abstruse clinical situations wherein inappropriate co-prescriptions for comorbid psychiatric and medical disorders lead to adverse events, non-adherence, and/or treatment discontinuation.

Drug Interactions

Individuals using SGAs are often co-prescribed other medications for comorbid psychiatric and medical disorders. Moreover, the use of over-the-counter as well as complimentary/alternative medicines is common practice amongst individuals with psychiatric disorders. For a detailed summary of drug interactions associated with SGAs, we would recommend referencing the product monograph information for each respective SGA. Herein, we review the basic principles of drug biotransformation with SGAs which provides the basis for predicting potential drug interactions (Table 4). [55]

Many SGAs will become generic in formulation over the next few years. This may become an issue of relevance for many patients where medication acquisition costs represent a barrier to treatment access. It has not been determined whether or not, despite bioequivalence, if generic antipsychotics are identical in efficacy, tolerability, and safety to trade-name SGAs.

Table 4. Drug and Food Interactions: Drug Interactions with Second-Generation Antipsychotics

Drugs (X) Interacts with:	Second-Generation Antipsychotics (A)[a]	Comments
Antiarrhythmic (e.g. quinidine)	X↑ A↑	Increases quinidine-like effects with dysrhythmias; increases clozapine and risperidone levels.
Anticholinergic	X↑	Added anticholinergic effect. Consider amantadine; variable effects seen on metabolism, plasma level, and efficacy of antipsychotic.
Anticoagulant (warfarin)	X↑ A↑	Increased PT ratio or INR response with quetiapine.
Anticonvulsant	A↓	Increased clearance and decreased antipsychotic plasma level with carbamazepine.
Antidepressants:		
MAO inhibitor	X↓	Hypotension may result; MAO inhibitors may trigger movement disorders.
SSRI	A↑	May increase movement disorders and plasma level. Fluvoxamine least likely to increase antipsychotic level.
TCA	X↑ A↑	Possible toxicity or hypotension; TCAs may diminish movement disorders.
Antihypertensives	X↑	Increased hypotension.
Caffeine	A↓	Increased psychosis in high doses, 600-1000 mg; increased plasma levels of clozapine.

Drugs (X) Interacts with:	Second-Generation Antipsychotics (A)a	Comments
CNS Depressant (e.g. alcohol, antihistamines, hypnotics)	X↑ A↑	CNS depression.
Estrogen	A↑	Potentiates hyperprolactinemic effect.
Grapefruit Juice	A↑	Increased plasma level of quetiapine due to inhibited metabolism via CYP34A. AVOID.
Lithium	X↑ A↑	Possibly increased risk of agranulocytosis and seizures with clozapine.
Nicotine	A↓	Decreased blood levels.
Sympathomimetic (e.g. epinephrine, norepinephrine)	X↓	Hypotension.

[a] ↑ = increase; ↓ = decrease.

Table adapted from: [55]

Drug Selection

There are several factors that a clinician needs to consider in the selection and sequencing of SGAs. All of the antipsychotics are FDA approved for use in schizophrenia; however, differential licensing exists across mood disorders (e.g. bipolar disorder, major depressive disorder) as well as pediatric conditions. Clinicians are encouraged to familiarize themselves with product monograph licensing information for SGA selection.

The profile of tolerability and safety is often the leading factor in choosing antipsychotic treatment. In some cases, the adverse event profile of an SGA may be utilized for its therapeutic advantage. For example, in patients with prominent sleep complaints as well as anxiety and psychomotor agitation, the sedating profile of some agents (i.e. quetiapine) may be of advantage, perhaps for short-term use. In most cases, however, adverse events are perceived as a barrier to acceptance, increasing the likelihood of noncompliance. The propensity to weight gain and metabolic disturbance is a significant issue in the selection of treatment. This observation has provided the basis for increased utilization of agents with lower weight gain and metabolic hazard (e.g. asenapine, lurasidone, ziprasidone, aripiprazole).

Patients with treatment resistant schizophrenia and/or suicidality should be considered for clozapine therapy. Patients who are non-adherent and/or prefer parental agents (i.e. first-generation antipsychotics) may be considered for depot SGAs. Patient preferences, history of response, as well as family attitude towards treatment are other major factors influencing treatment selection. Individuals receiving SGAs are often co-prescribed other medications and/or are utilisers of over-the-counter agents as well as complementary and alternative medicines. The selection and dosing of antipsychotics would therefore be influenced by other concomitantly administered treatments. Clinicians are also encouraged to familiarize themselves with "black box" warnings with antipsychotic agents wherein their use is not recommended (i.e. SGAs in patients with dementia-related psychosis).

Conclusion

The SGAs are a highly prescribed and utilized class of medications. They are garnering many FDA approvals in a myriad of psychiatric conditions in addition to being utilized in an off label manner. This chapter was designed to discuss side effects not elsewhere discussed in this book and offer clinicians suggestions regarding SGA selection in clinical practice.

References

[1] McIntyre RS, Konarski JZ. Tolerability profiles of atypical antipsychotics in the treatment of bipolar disorder. *J Clin Psychiatry* 2005;66 Suppl 3:28-36.

[2] Correll CU, Leucht S, Kane JM. Lower risk for tardive dyskinesia associated with second-generation antipsychotics: a systematic review of 1-year studies. *Am J Psychiatry* 2004 March;161(3):414-25.

[3] Pae CU. A review of the safety and tolerability of aripiprazole. *Expert Opin Drug Saf* 2009 May;8(3):373-86.
[4] Tandon R. Safety and tolerability: how do newer generation "atypical" antipsychotics compare? *Psychiatr Q* 2002;73(4):297-311.
[5] Nelson JC, Pikalov A, Berman RM. Augmentation treatment in major depressive disorder: focus on aripiprazole. *Neuropsychiatr Dis Treat* 2008 October;4(5):937-48.
[6] Ballard C, Creese B, Corbett A, Aarsland D. Atypical antipsychotics for the treatment of behavioral and psychological symptoms in dementia, with a particular focus on longer term outcomes and mortality. *Expert Opin Drug Saf* 2011 January;10(1):35-43.
[7] Liauw SS, McIntyre RS. Atypical antipsychotic tolerability and switching strategies in bipolar disorder. *Expert Opin Pharmacother* 2010 December;11(17):2827-37.
[8] Farmer CA, Aman MG. Aripiprazole for the treatment of irritability associated with autism. *Expert Opin Pharmacother* 2011 March;12(4):635-40.
[9] Schneider LS, Dagerman KS, Insel P. Risk of death with atypical antipsychotic drug treatment for dementia: meta-analysis of randomized placebo-controlled trials. *JAMA* 2005 October 19;294(15):1934-43.
[10] Centorrino F, Price BH, Tuttle M, Bahk WM, Hennen J, Albert MJ, Baldessarini RJ. EEG abnormalities during treatment with typical and atypical antipsychotics. *Am J Psychiatry* 2002 January;159(1):109-15.
[11] Haddad PM, Dursun SM. Neurological complications of psychiatric drugs: clinical features and management. *Hum Psychopharmacol* 2008 January;23 Suppl 1:15-26.
[12] Amann BL, Pogarell O, Mergl R, Juckel G, Grunze H, Mulert C, Hegerl U. EEG abnormalities associated with antipsychotics: a comparison of quetiapine, olanzapine, haloperidol and healthy subjects. *Hum Psychopharmacol* 2003 December;18(8):641-6.
[13] Gortney JS, Fagan A, Kissack JC. Neuroleptic malignant syndrome secondary to quetiapine. *Ann Pharmacother* 2009 April;43(4):785-91.
[14] Trollor JN, Chen Z, Sachdev PS. Neuroleptic malignant syndrome associated with atypical antipsychotic drugs. CNS *Drugs* 2009; 23(6):477-492.
[15] Feldman AM, McNamara D. Myocarditis. *N Engl J Med* 2000 November 9;343(19):1388-98.
[16] Ucok A, Gaebel W. Side effects of atypical antipsychotics: a brief overview. *World Psychiatry* 2008 February;7(1):58-62.
[17] Yang FD, Wang XQ, Liu XP, Zhao KX, Fu WH, Hao XR, Zhang XL, Huang GS, Qu SC, Bai JS, Huang XF, Kosten TR, Zhang XY. Sex difference in QTc prolongation in chronic institutionalized patients with schizophrenia on long-term treatment with typical and atypical antipsychotics. *Psychopharmacology* (Berl] 2011 July;216(1):9-16.
[18] Nielsen J. The safety of atypical antipsychotics: does QTc provide all the answers? *Expert Opin Drug Saf* 2011 May;10(3):341-4.
[19] Alvarez PA, Pahissa J. QT alterations in psychopharmacology: proven candidates and suspects. *Curr Drug* Saf 2010 January;5(1):97-104.
[20] Sala M, Vicentini A, Brambilla P, Montomoli C, Jogia JR, Caverzasi E, Bonzano A, Piccinelli M, Barale F, De Ferrari GM. QT interval prolongation related to psychoactive drug treatment: a comparison of monotherapy versus polytherapy. *Ann Gen Psychiatry* 2005 January 25;4(1):1.

[21] Ray WA, Chung CP, Murray KT, Hall K, Stein CM. Atypical antipsychotic drugs and the risk of sudden cardiac death. *N Engl J Med* 2009 January 15;360(3):225-35.

[22] Henderson DC, Doraiswamy PM. Prolactin-related and metabolic adverse effects of atypical antipsychotic agents. *J Clin Psychiatry* 2008;69 Suppl 1:32-44.

[23] Haddad PM, Wieck A. Antipsychotic-induced hyperprolactinaemia: mechanisms, clinical features and management. *Drugs* 2004;64(20):2291-314.

[24] David SR, Taylor CC, Kinon BJ, Breier A. The effects of olanzapine, risperidone, and haloperidol on plasma prolactin levels in patients with schizophrenia. *Clin Ther* 2000 September;22(9):1085-96.

[25] Knegtering H, van den Bosch R, Castelein S, Bruggeman R, Sytema S, van OJ. Are sexual side effects of prolactin-raising antipsychotics reducible to serum prolactin? *Psychoneuroendocrinology* 2008 July;33(6):711-7.

[26] Rettenbacher MA, Hofer A, Ebenbichler C, Baumgartner S, Edlinger M, Engl J, Kaser S, Kemmler G, Malik P, Tschoner A, Fleischhacker WW. Prolactin levels and sexual adverse effects in patients with schizophrenia during antipsychotic treatment. *J Clin Psychopharmacol* 2010 December;30(6):711-5.

[27] Jerrell JM, Bacon J, Burgis JT, Menon S. Hyperprolactinemia-related adverse events associated with antipsychotic treatment in children and adolescents. *J Adolesc Health* 2009 July;45(1):70-6.

[28] Caccia S, Clavenna A, Bonati M. Antipsychotic drug toxicology in children. *Expert Opin Drug Metab Toxicol* 2011 May;7(5):591-608.

[29] Atmaca M, Kuloglu M, Tezcan E, et al. Quetiapine is not associated with increase in prolactin secretion in contrast to haloperidol. *Arch Med Res* 2002. 33(6):562-565.

[30] Stevens JR, Kymissis PI, Baker AJ. Elevated prolactin levels in male youths treated with risperidone and quetiapine. *J Child Adolesc Psychopharmacol* 2005. 15(6):893-900.

[31] Lamberts SW, van Koetsveld PM, Hofland LJ. The effect of clozapine on prolactin secretion at the level of the lactotroph. *Life Sci* 1990. 46(14):1013-1019.

[32] Goodnick PJ, Rodriguez L, Santana O. Antipsychotics: impact on prolactin levels. *Expert Opin Pharmacother* 2002. 3(10):1381-1391.

[33] Crawford AM, Beasley CM Jr, Tollefson GD. The acute and long-term effect of olanzapine compared with placebo and haloperidol on serum prolactin concentrations. *Schizophr Res* 1997. 26(1):41-54.

[34] Cosi C, Carilla-Durand E, Assie MB, et al. Partial agonist properties of the antipsychotics SSR181507, aripiprazole and bifeprunox at dopamine D2 receptors: G protein activation and prolactin release. *Eur J Pharmacol* 2006. 535(1-3):135-144.

[35] Lawler CP, Prioleau C, Lewis MM, et al. Interactions of the novel antipsychotic aripiprazole (OPC-14597] with dopamine and serotonin receptor subtypes. *Neuropsychopharmacology* 1999. 20(6):612-627.

[36] Madhusoodanan S, Parida S, Jimenez C. Hyperprolacinemia associated with psychotropics - a review. *Hum Psychopharmacol Clin Exp* 2010. 25:281-297.

[37] Samalin L, Garnier M, Llorca PM. Clinical potential of lurasidone in the management of schizophrenia. *Therapeutics and Clinical Risk Management* 2011. 7:239-250.

[38] Weber J, McCormack PL. Asenapine. *CNS Drugs* 2009. 23(9):781-792.

[39] Flanagan RJ. Fatal toxicity of drugs used in psychiatry. *Hum Psychopharmacol* 2008 January;23 Suppl 1:43-51.

[40] Nongpiur A, Praharaj SK, Sarkar S, Das B. Delayed Onset of Clozapine-Induced Leucopenia. *Am J Ther* 2010 August 19.

[41] Stergiou V, Bozikas VP, Garyfallos G, Nikolaidis N, Lavrentiadis G, Fokas K. Olanzapine-induced leucopenia and neutropenia. *Prog Neuropsychopharmacol Biol Psychiatry* 2005 July;29(6):992-4.

[42] Shankar BR. Quetiapine-induced leucopenia and thrombocytopenia. *Psychosomatics* 2007 November;48(6):530-1.

[43] Buchman N, Strous RD, Ulman AM, Lerner M, Kotler M. Olanzapine-induced leukopenia with human leukocyte antigen profiling. *Int Clin Psychopharmacol* 2001 January;16(1):55-7.

[44] Rahman A, Mican LM, Fischer C, Campbell AH. Evaluating the incidence of leukopenia and neutropenia with valproate, quetiapine, or the combination in children and adolescents. *Ann Pharmacother* 2009 May;43(5):822-30.

[45] Nooijen PM, Carvalho F, Flanagan RJ. Haematological toxicity of clozapine and some other drugs used in psychiatry. *Hum Psychopharmacol* 2011 March;26(2):112-9.

[46] Chandrasekaran PK. Agranulocytosis monitoring with Clozapine patients: to follow guidelines or to attempt therapeutic controversies? *Singapore Med J* 2008 February;49(2):96-9.

[47] McCauley-Elsom K, Kulkarni J. Managing psychosis in pregnancy. Aust N Z J *Psychiatry* 2007 March;41(3):289-92.

[48] Einarson A, Boskovic R. Use and safety of antipsychotic drugs during pregnancy. *J Psychiatr Pract* 2009 May;15(3):183-92.

[49] Gentile S. Clinical utilization of atypical antipsychotics in pregnancy and lactation. *Ann Pharmacother* 2004 July;38(7-8):1265-71.

[50] Gentile S. Antipsychotic therapy during early and late pregnancy. A systematic review. *Schizophr Bull* 2010 May;36(3):518-44.

[51] Iveli MF, Rebolledo A, Martin P, Enrique N, Roldan Palomo AR, Rimorini L, Salemme S, Milesi V. Risperidone inhibits contractions induced by serotonin and histamine and reduces K+ currents in smooth muscle of human umbilical artery. *Reprod Sci* 2010 September;17(9):854-60.

[52] Hussar DA, Shah A. New drugs. Azilsartan medoxomil, belimumab, and lurasidone hydrochloride. *J Am Pharm Assoc* (2003] 2011 May;51(3):444-7.

[53] Gentile S. Infant safety with antipsychotic therapy in breast-feeding: a systematic review. *J Clin Psychiatry* 2008 April;69(4):666-73.

[54] McCauley-Elsom K, Gurvich C, Elsom SJ, Kulkarni J. Antipsychotics in pregnancy. *Journal of Psychiatric and Mental Health Nursing* 2010. 17:97-104.

[55] McIntyre RS. Psychotropic drugs fast facts: antipsychotics. In: Roger S. McIntyre, Sidney H. Kennedy, editors. *Psychotropic drugs fast facts: antipsychotics*. New York: W.W. Norton & Company; 2008; 1-48.

In: Antipsychotic Drugs
Editors: T.L. Schwartz, J. Megna and M.E. Topel
ISBN: 978-1-62100-071-6

Chapter 15

CLOZAPINE: ADVERSE EFFECTS AND THEIR MANAGEMENT

Mohammad M. Iqbal [1]***, Mariela Herrera Rojas*** [2] ***and James L. Megna*** [3]*

[1] Clinical Assistant Professor, SUNY Upstate Medical University, Syracuse, NY, US
Clinical Director, Auburn Mental Health Unit, Central NY Psychiatric Center, NY, US
[2] Clinical Assistant Instructor, Cleveland Clinic Foundation, Cleveland, OH, US
[3] Director, Inpatient Psychiatry; Associate Professor, Department of Psychiatry;
Associate Professor, Department of Medicine,
SUNY Upstate University Hospital, Syracuse, NY, US

ABSTRACT

Introduction: Clozapine is often noted to be one of the most effective antipsychotics with the ability to help those suffering from schizophrenia when other agents have failed. It is also known to promote a myriad of side effects ranging from mild to those with significant morbidity and mortality.

Conclusion: This chapter reviews the usual side effects and their management when clozapine is deployed and used to treat resistant schizophrenia symptoms.

INTRODUCTION

Clozapine is the oldest of the second-generation antipsychotics, first introduced in the 1970s to the European Market but withdrawn years later due to the development of severe neutropenia and death in 18 and 8 patients, respectively. It was reintroduced in the mid-1980s. [1] It is FDA-approved for use in treatment-resistant schizophrenia in adults and for reduction of risk of recurrent suicidal behavior in schizophrenia or schizoaffective disorder in adults. [2, 3, 4]. However, it is used in several clinical scenarios, including treatment-resistant

---

* 750 East Adams Street, Syracuse, NY 13210, USA; megnaj@upstate.edu

psychosis and schizoaffective disorder, non-treatment-resistant schizophrenia or schizoaffective disorder, prevention and treatment of tardive dyskinesia, bipolar disorder resistant to conventional treatment, aggressiveness and violence in psychiatric patients, as well as psychosis, aggressiveness and violence in patients with mental retardation, Parkinson's Disease or Dementia with Lewy bodies. It also has been reported to be clinically beneficial for adolescents with intermittent explosive disorder, bipolar disorder, and posttraumatic stress disorder. [2, 5-9].

The receptor profile of clozapine is characterized by a relatively low dopamine D2 and D1 blockade, high dopamine D4 blockade, high 5HT2c antagonism, antimuscarinic effect, antihistaminergic effect and antiadrenergic effect (anti-α1>anti-α2). [2, 10, 11]. The action of clozapine at these receptors is related to some of its side effects. In general terms, clozapine has a markedly low incidence of extrapyramidal symptoms (EPS) comparable to that seen with placebo, has the lowest incidence of tardive dyskinesia among all available antipsychotics as of 2009 (excluding aripiprazole, which didn't have enough evidence), and has the second lowest likelihood to elevate prolactin and cause sexual side effects after aripiprazole. [2, 4, 11, 12]. In fact, a double-blind, randomized study reported a decrease in prolactin levels associated with clozapine. [13] Side effects of sedation, antimuscarinic symptoms, postural hypotension, agranulocytosis, and seizures have been reported as more common with clozapine than with other atypical antipsychotics. [14] A recent review confirmed that clozapine is associated with increased risk of seizures and agranulocytosis, but differences among the atypical antipsychotics in other serious harms were not clearly shown. [3] The reported discontinuation rate due to adverse effects has been estimated as 17%, and it has been found to be higher than the odds of discontinuing drug due to adverse events with olanzapine. [3, 15]. However, in a recent review, clozapine and olanzapine were found to result in lower rates of discontinuation of drug for any reason over periods of up to 2 years in patients with schizophrenia, and limited evidence indicated that clozapine may have longer time to discontinuation than olanzapine. [3]

This chapter reviews the adverse effects of clozapine, as well as the strategies for minimizing and managing them.

Serious Reactions

Agranulocytosis

Agranulocytosis (absolute neutrophil count [ANC] <500/mm^3) and neutropenia (ANC <1500/mm^3) are the most feared adverse effects of clozapine. [2] The cumulative incidence of both agranulocytosis and neutropenia has been estimated to be 0.8% over 15 months. [5] The reported incidence ranges from 0% to 5.9% in different studies with 1 to 5 years follow up, with larger database studies reporting rates of 0.4 to 0.8%. [3] The mortality rate of agranulocytosis is estimated as 3-4% of cases, since patients are susceptible to neutropenic sepsis. [4, 16]. Benign neutropenia occurs more frequently than agranulocytosis. Transient neutropenia occurs frequently as well [22% of patients in one report), and is characterized by a drop in the neutrophil count with return to normal values with continued clozapine treatment. Morning pseudo-neutropenia can also occur, which normalizes in the afternoon and is due to a diurnal variation in the number of circulating neutrophils. [17]

The risk of agranulocytosis increases with age and is also somewhat higher amongst patients younger than 21 years old compared to those between 21-40 years old. [2, 18, 19]. It is an idiosyncratic and not dose-dependent effect. [2, 5]. Predisposing risk factors include older age, female gender, and African-American and Asian ethnic groups. The risk also has been reported as higher in patients of Ashkenazi Jewish descent with the haplotype HLA-B38, DR4, DQw3. [4, 5]. A genetic basis for clozapine-induces agranulocytosis is also suggested by reports of this side effect in monozygotic twins diagnosed with schizophrenia. [20] The risk can also increase by co-administration of medications such as carbamazepine, captopril, propylthiuracil, sulfonamides, procainamide, ticlopidine, tocainide, or other medications that carry a risk for blood dyscrasia. [2, 4, 5, 21].

The exact mechanism of action is unknown, but proposed mechanisms leading to bone marrow damage include immune-mediated and/or a toxic process caused by clozapine metabolites. [5] The cytotoxicity would be mediated by formation of an electrophilic nitrenium metabolite that binds to neutrophil proteins and results in a decrease in cell function and ultimately, cell death. Genetic risk factors as mentioned above could also account for some cases. [4, 5, 20].

The most frequent period of occurrence is during the first 6-18 weeks of treatment and 95% of the cases occur within the first 6 months of treatment, with highest incidence in the first 3 months. [2,5,19,22] However, the risk persists for much longer periods, with only five case reports of occurrence at 6 years or more of treatment with clozapine, and in three of them there was concomitant use of additional psychotropics with risk for blood dyscrasia. [5] Blood monitoring schedule is mandatory on a weekly basis during the first 6 months in the US, but this varies across countries with the minimal time period of weekly monitoring being 18 weeks. When acceptable values of white blood count ($\geq$3500/mm^3) and ANC ($\geq$2000/mm^3) are maintained during the weekly monitoring period, the guidelines vary across countries, with most recommending white blood count (WBC) and ANC every other week or at least monthly for 6 months. Then, it can be reduced to monthly monitoring if there has not been any interruption of treatment due to leucopenia. [2, 5].

Clozapine is contraindicated if WBC<3500/mm^3, ANC<1500/mm^3, and if there is a history of myeloproliferative disorder or clozapine-associated agranulocytosis. [2] If during treatment WBC<3500/mm^3, or WBC is between 3000-3500/mm^3 with ANC>1500/mm^3, CBC should be repeated twice weekly. If WBC <3000/mm^3 or ANC <1500/mm^3, clozapine should be stopped and close monitoring should be started including daily hematologic check. Treatment could be resumed if WBC returns to a level >3000/ mm^3 and/or ANC returns to a level >1500 mm^3. If WBC <2000/mm^3 or ANC <1000/mm^3 clozapine should be stopped and the recommendation is not to rechallenge. If WBC drops 30% from a previous level or there is substantial drop in WBC (>3000/ mm^3] the WBC should be repeated. If WBC continues to fall clozapine should be stopped and the patient should be monitored for fever, sore throat, weakness, or other signs of infection, and appropriate referrals should be made [2,5] Weekly monitoring should be continued for at least 1 month after discontinuation of clozapine for any reason. Mild to moderate neutropenia (ANC < 1500/mm^3 and >500/mm^3) recovers usually in 2-8 days and occurs in 1.8% of treated patients. Agranulocytosis has an incidence of 0.78% and usually lasts for 14-21 days. Due to the phenomenom of benign ethnic neutropenia, approximately 20% of African American patients are deemed ineligible for clozapine, since their normal WBC levels generally range from 2800-9500/mm³, significantly lower than the range for Caucasians (3600-9500/mm³). Therefore, it has been suggested that the appropriateness of the clozapine guidelines should be re-evaluated in this population. [5]

Agranulocytosis is considered a medical emergency, and management includes reverse isolation and prophylactic antibiotics. Granulocyte colony stimulation factor (G-CSF) and granulocyte-macrophage colony stimulation factor are options for treatment. It is reversible in most cases after prompt discontinuation of clozapine. [2, 5, 15].

There have been reports of attempts to rechallenge patients with poor response to other antipsychotics with a second clozapine trial after the occurrence of clozapine-associated neutropenia or agranulocytosis. [5,23] In a retrospective study of 53 cases rechallenged, amongst the cases that developed blood dyscrasia (38%) on rechallenge, 85% occurred more quickly and more severely than it did with the first clozapine trial, and in 65% of cases it lasted longer after discontinuation of clozapine than when it was discontinued for the first time. [24] G-CSF or filgrastim, a G-CSF analog, can be added during re-challenge but its efficacy is questionable with inconsistent findings in case reports. The optimal dosage, frequency, and duration of administration during clozapine rechallenge have not been formally evaluated. [4, 5, 23, 25, 26]. Lithium can also be used during rechallenge since it causes a reversible leukocytosis which can potentially antagonize any neutropenia. However this should be done with extra vigilance to detect masked blood dyscrasias that might lead to catastrophic agranulocytosis. Lithium treatment is titrated up to a plasma level around 0.4 mmol/L and continued for 1 to 2 weeks. If the WBC is back to normal, clozapine is restarted with the routine recommended monitoring. A retrospective chart review of 25 patients who were rechallenged with lithium showed only one case developing a second episode of neutropenia. Transient neurotoxic side effects have been reported with the combination of clozapine and lithium. [5, 17, 27].

A recent review analyzed 14 reports of cases rechallenged with clozapine after developing neutropenia during a prior clozapine treatment. It identified a total of 112 patients, 69.6% were successfully rechallenged without development of a blood dyscrasia after 20-96 weeks follow up. In the patients who had an unsuccessful rechallenge, neutropenia reoccurred within a mean of 4.3 weeks (range 0.9 to 156 weeks), and 44.1% developed a more severe dyscrasia in the agranulocytic range during the second exposure. 35 patients were treated with lithium and 94.3% tolerated the rechallenge. 11 patients were given G-CSF and 63.6% were successfully rechallenged. [23]

The same review found 15 cases of patients rechallenged with clozapine after developing agranulocytosis with a first clozapine trial. Only 3 were able to continue treatment with clozapine after rechallenge, 3 patients had a reoccurrence of agranulocytosis (two at 4 weeks and one at 104 weeks), 2 patients developed a less severe neutropenia upon rechallenge, and in 9 cases the rechallenge led to the recurrence of agranulocytosis or leukocytosis without a timeframe of appearance or a severity of the abnormality reported. [23].

Seizure Disorder

Patients with schizophrenia have an increased incidence of seizure or epilepsy, and the occurrence of seizures is more common with use of clozapine (3%) than with the use of typical antipsychotics [28]. Two studies, with at least 2 years of follow-up reported rates of seizures associated with clozapine as 2.9% (n=1418, treatment period 3.8 years) and 4.2% (n=96, treatment period 13 years). [3, 29].

Clozapine lowers the seizure threshold and produces significant changes in the electroencephalogram (EEG). EEG changes were reported in 61.5% and 53% of patients treated with clozapine in a retrospective study (n=283) and a prospective study (n=50), respectively. Almost all patients develop background slowing in the theta and delta ranges. Rare rhythms include spikes (or spike and wave complexes) and frontal intermittent delta activity. Other reported changes described in a retrospective study included slight (22.5%) to moderate (10.1%) diffuse slowing and non-paroxysmal waves (39.8%) or sharp waves (16.2%), while potential signs of increased bioelectrical cerebral activity were rarely noted including paroxysmal activity (4.3%) or severe diffuse slowing (0.2%). [5, 30, 31].

Most of clozapine-associated seizures are generalized tonic-clonic seizures, but myoclonic and atonic seizures constitute about one quarter of the reported cases. Subtle types of seizures, including myoclonic, atonic, or partial seizures, might be difficult to recognize and may be underreported, and may be a precursor of tonic-clonic seizures. There have been reports of prolonged postictal encephalopathy following a clozapine-induced seizure. [4, 5, 32].

The rate of seizure disorder associated with clozapine increases over time, with a cumulative risk reaching 9% at 3 years in one study (n=1418) and reported as 10% after 3.8 years of treatment in different reviews. [2, 3, 5, 29, 33].

The risk for seizures and EEG abnormality associated with clozapine increases with higher doses (4.4% risk of seizures with doses ≥ to 600 mg/day, 2.7% with doses between 300mg/day and 599 mg/day, and 1% with low doses <300 mg/day). The incidence is associated with plasma levels, with higher risk correlated with concentrations >1300 ng/ml. However, seizures can occur with doses as low as 37.5 mg daily and the plasma level can be used as a guide but not as a definite predictor of seizures. Rapid titration, concurrent use of other epileptogenic drugs, preexisting seizures, slow drug metabolism, metabolic factors, drug-drug interactions (and other substances such as nicotine and caffeine) probably mediated by CYP1A2 inhibition, and neurological abnormalities also increase the risk for seizures. The risk may be decreased with EEG monitoring, low starting doses/slower dose titration, maintenance of minimal effective dose, avoidance of complex drug combinations, divided daily doses to avoid high peak plasma levels, and doses <600 mg/day. [2, 3, 4, 5, 32-35].

The higher epileptogenicity of clozapine in comparison to other antipsychotics might be explained by its selectivity for mesolimbic dopamine receptors. An anticholinergic etiology has also been noted as a hypothetic mechanism. [2, 5, 15].

An isolated seizure is not considered a reason to discontinue treatment, but the dosage can be reduced by about 40-50%, or the treatment can be interrupted with more gradual dose titration. Any other seizure-provoking factors (such as sleep deprivation, alcohol withdrawal, or pro-convulsant over-the-counter drugs, such as antihistamines) should be eliminated. Therapeutic drug monitoring is recommended with onset of seizures, or an alternative antipsychotic agent might be employed. If seizures persist, the standard of practice is prophylactic treatment with occurrence of a second seizure, with sodium valproate as the drug of choice. Other choices include lamotrigine, gabapentin, and topiramate, when side effects or changes in the metabolism of clozapine occur with combination of clozapine and valproate. Valproate generally reduces the plasma level of clozapine and can interfere with its therapeutic efficacy. Conversely, with discontinuation of valproate the plasma level of clozapine can increase while the seizure threshold of the patient may be lowered. In cases of myoclonic seizures, clonazepam may be used. Carbamazepine is contraindicated because of concerns for development of agranulocytosis. [2, 5, 32, 36, 37].

Neuroleptic Malignant Syndrome (NMS)

The rate of NMS is 1% with typical antipsychotics and few cases have been reported with clozapine, mostly in males, with very few fatalities. In a critical analysis of 19 reported cases, the relation to clozapine was not clear, or the full criteria for NMS were not met. The mortality rate in patients who develop NMS can reach 20-30%. [2, 38-42] In a review 21 cases of NMS were reported with clozapine treatment, 15 of those having a diagnosis of schizophrenia. This side effect has not been found to be dose-dependent. [43] Most cases in the study occurred within the first 14 days of clozapine treatment. The risk increases with concomitant use of other drugs, especially lithium or other antipsychotics (eg, droperidol, mesoridazine, thioridazine). [2, 4, 40, 44, 45].

NMS associated with clozapine is usually atypical, characterized by fewer EPS, slower elevation of creatine kinase, less frequent occurrence of fever and rigidity, and very common diaphoresis and tachycardia compared to NMS induced by other causes. [2, 4, 46].

The mechanism is not fully clear, it is considered to be due to a sudden blockade of D2 receptors, which might explain why it is not common with clozapine treatment since clozapine only binds to D2 receptors loosely. [4, 10].

Management of mild cases can be done on psychiatric units with medical support. Cases with extremely high temperature, autonomic instability, renal failure, elevated creatine kinase, rhabdomyolisis or respiratory difficulties require intensive care. Early recognition and prompt discontinuation of antipsychotics are key. Benzodiazepines like lorazepam could be tried initially in most cases since they are useful in reversing catatonia and are easy to administer. Trials of bromocriptine, amantadine, or other dopaminergic drugs can be used as a next step in moderate cases. (2] Dantrolene is particularly useful when there is significant rigidity and hyperthermia, and it rapidly reduces extreme temperature elevations in many cases. Medications are effective during the first few days of treatment while ECT remains effective late in the course when other interventions have failed. ECT may be preferred for cases where idiopathic lethal catatonia cannot be ruled out, for refractory NMS, and in patients with residual catatonic state or cases with persistent psychosis after NMS has resolved. [2, 47-49]. Development of NMS should not prevent treatment rechallenge after resolution of symptoms. [4] A recent review reported five cases of rechallenge with clozapine after the occurrence of NMS and all five cases were successful in a follow up range of 16-52 weeks. [23].

Mortality

In April 2005 the U.S. Food and Drug Administration (FDA) issued a black box warning that the use of atypical antipsychotics to treat behavioral disturbances in patients with dementia was associated with greater mortality. This was based on analyses of trials performed with olanzapine, aripiprazole, risperidone, or immediate-release quetiapine reporting a rate of death of about 1.6 to 1.7 times that of placebo, mainly due to heart-related events or infections. The U.S. FDA concluded that the relationship was due to pharmacological effects common to all atypical antipsychotics, which led to include those that had not been systematically studied in this population, including clozapine. [3]

Other studies didn't show an increase in mortality in patients taking clozapine. One cohort study, including 55 nursing homes in 5 US states, found an increase in mortality with conventional antipsychotics (n=3205, adjusted hazard ratio 1.26, 95% CI 1.13 to 1.42] compared to risperidone (used as reference), while clozapine, olanzapine, and immediate-release quetiapine didn't show an increased mortality compared to risperidone (adjusted hazard ratios 0.94, 0.95, and 1.05, respectively; 95% CI's 0.49 to 1.79, 0.8 to 1.12, and 0.8 to 1.39, respectively). [50] Another retrospective review found clozapine (n=561) associated with a lower, but not statistically significant, all-cause mortality rate [1.78%) compared to a group of patients (n=4918) taking other psychiatric drugs (2.13%). However, in the group of patients taking clozapine mortality due to sudden death was 3.8 times higher than that found in non-clozapine treated patients. [51].

COMMON REACTIONS

Hypersalivation

Hypersalivation has been reported to occur in 30-80% of patients on CLZ. [5,52].

Evidence from 4 studies shows that clozapine results in higher rates of hypersalivation than olanzapine (pooled risk difference 0.16, 95% CI 0.09 to 0.42, NNH=6). In another study showing an even higher risk of hypersalivation with clozapine, the risk difference was 0.42, with 95% CI 0.10 to 0.20 and NNH 2 [3]

Possible mechanisms include activation of M4-muscarinic receptors [2, 53, 54], blockade of α2-adrenoreceptors [2,55], decreased laryngeal peristalsis [5], and/or interference with the swallowing reflex causing pooling of saliva [2,52,56]. A prospective study showed a significant increase in salivary flow rate between the first 2 and 3 weeks of treatment, followed by a plateau. The salivary flow rate change was not dose-dependent. [5]

Sialorrhea is considered to be bothersome and socially stigmatizing, [5] Patients complain of excessive drooling, wet pillow, choking sensation at night, and aspiration of excessive saliva. [52] Salivary gland swelling [57, 58] and aspiration pneumonia [59] have been reported.

Management includes recommendations to use a towel on the pillowcase and to chew gum during the day. [2, 60] Pharmacologic agents, used based on case reports or open-label studies, include benztropine [2, 60], pirenzepine [2, 61], glycopyrrolate, biperiden, trihexyphenidyl, diphenhydramine, propantheline, doxepin, local anticholinergics (sublingual or intranasal ipatropium spray), transdermal scopolamine [5], α2-adrenergic agonists (clonidine patch, lofexidine) [2,4,5] amisulpride, and amitriptyline at doses of 75-100 mg/day. [62] Most of the medications mentioned to treat sialorrhea have limited efficacy or unwanted side effects. [5] Botulinum injections into the parotid gland have been successful in refractory cases. [63] In stabilized patients a reduction in the dose of clozapine may reduce hypersalivation. [2].

Metabolic

Clozapine has been associated with different risks factors for cardiovascular diseases including weight gain, hypertriglyceridemia, increased total cholesterol levels, hypertension, obesity, higher insulin levels, insulin resistance, hyperglycemia, and type 2 diabetes mellitus. [5, 12].

Clozapine is reported as the antipsychotic associated with the highest risk of metabolic syndrome. [5] A head-to-head meta-analysis of the metabolic side effects of second-generation antipsychotics in randomized controlled trials found that olanzapine showed more weight gain, cholesterol and glucose elevation than all other atypical antipsychotics, except for clozapine where no difference with olanzapine was demonstrated. [64].

In a retrospective cohort study (n=108, mean duration of treatment 2.8 years), comparing different atypical antipsychotics, an increase in the prevalence of metabolic syndrome based on ATP III criteria was seen with clozapine (+50%), olanzapine (+41%), risperidone (+12%), and immediate-release quetiapine (+10%), but not with aripiprazole (no change in prevalence from baseline). [65] A different study found similar results with a prevalence of metabolic syndrome of 48% in the clozapine-treated sample. [66] The development of metabolic syndrome is dose dependent, with a relationship between clozapine serum concentrations and metabolic outcomes, suggestive of a causal effect. [5]

In the treatment of patients with schizophrenia, the American Psychiatric Association and the American Diabetes Association recommend baseline assessment of body weight, waist circumference, blood pressure, blood glucose, lipid panel, and documentation of family history of obesity, diabetes, dyslipidemia, hypertension, and cardiovascular disease. Also, weight gain should be monitored monthly during the first trimester of treatment, followed by biochemical analysis after the first three months, and then on a yearly basis. [5,67,68] Metformin has shown some effectiveness in treating atypical antipsychotic-induced metabolic syndrome. A randomized controlled trial of patients on stable clozapine treatment assessed the effect of adding metformin or placebo for 14 weeks on metabolic syndrome in patients with schizophrenia, schizophreniphorm disorder, or bipolar disorder (n=61). Metabolic syndrome was reduced from 25% to 14 % in the metformin group while there was no change in the placebo group. [69].

Weight Gain

An increase in weight greater than 10% from baseline was seen in 20% of patients taking clozapine during 12 weeks to 12 months of follow up [2, 70-72], most frequently in the first 4 to 12 weeks [2, 71, 73] but it can occur during more prolonged treatment. [2, 71-73]. Indeed, patients gain most of their weight during the early months of treatment, followed by a lower rate of weight gain for several years. The average weight gain in patients taking clozapine is reported as 8 kg. [5]

In a meta-analysis, clozapine was associated with significantly more weight gain than was haloperidol (mean weight gain difference 3.4 kg, 95% CI 2.0 to 4.9, $p<0.0001$), but didn't show a significant difference compared to low-potency first-generation drugs [mean weight gain difference 0.3 kg, 95% CI -1.6 to 2.2, $p=0.753$). [74] Clozapine, along with olanzapine, is more likely to cause weight gain when directly compared to the other SGAs.

[3,12] In comparison with olanzapine, most studies have not shown a significant difference. [3] Reports differ with comparison studies finding that clozapine is the antipsychotic associated with the highest risk of weight gain. [5] However, a longer-term [2 year) multicenter, randomized, international trial [n=980) reported a significant difference in favor of clozapine compared with olanzapine in the proportion of patients with weight gain (31.3% of patients in clozapine group, 55.6% of patients in the olanzapine group, p<.001). [75] In different trials comparing mean weight gain in patients taking clozapine or risperidone, the increase in weight was reported in ranges between 2.4 kg and 6.52 kg in patients taking clozapine, and 0.2 kg to 2.3 kg in patients taking risperidone. [76-79] A head-to-head meta-analysis reported that clozapine produced about three kilograms more weight gain than risperidone (MD 2.9 kg) [64]

In children and adolescents clozapine has also being associated with a more substantial risk of weight gain, along with olanzapine. In this population, clozapine increased weight in 50-60% of children and adolescents in the first few months of treatment and it reaches a plateau at 1 year.

Likely mechanisms include antagonism of D2 receptor, antihistaminergic activity, antimuscarinic effect, antagonism on 5HT2C receptors, increased leptin secretion, decreased ghrelin and adiponectin serum levels, and smoking cessation. [2,5,68,81-83] These mechanisms lead to increased appetite, energy intake and storage, metabolic and endocrine alterations, reduced energy expenditure and increased utilization, and lower physical activity. Factors associated with more weight gain include younger age at clozapine initiation, lower baseline body mass index (BMI), adiponectin level, and dose used. Clinical response, as well, has been associated with clozapine-induced weight gain, although this is an inconsistent finding amongst studies, with higher significance in most long-term studies. Findings also suggest that early changes in leptin secretion may predict long-term weight gain in patients taking clozapine. [5]

Genetic factors also have been estimated to account for 60-80% of antipsychotic-induced weight gain, including, but not limited to, polymorphisms in the serotoninergic receptor-2c (HTR2c) coding gene [5,68,84], serotoninergic receptor-2a (HTR2a) coding gene and leptin coding gene. The strongest evidence has been identified for an association between the polymorphism -759C/T of the HTR2c coding gene and antipsychotic-induced weight gain [5,68]. This polymorphism was identified as an important genetic factor associated with clozapine-induced weight gain. [68,84] However, this finding is inconsistent among different studies [68]. Many other genes have been studied as factors that might account for antipsychotic-induced weight gain. These genes code for substances involved in the regulation of food intake, which include promelanin concentrating hormone, Adrenergic alpha-1A, alpha-2A, beta-2 and beta-3 receptors, Cannabinoid receptor 1, Neuropeptide Y, Neuropeptide Y receptor Y5, Ghrelin precursor, Galanin, Histamine receptor, Apolipoproteins A1, A2, A4, B, and E, Paraoxonase 1, Scavenger receptors class B1 and B2, Steroid regulatory element binding proteins F1 and F2,, Propiomelanocortin, and Adiponectin. [68]

Prevention of weight gain can be achieved with diet and exercise, with recommendations to weigh patients at baseline and monthly for the first three months of treatment, and a strict dietary regimen should be started immediately if weight gain occurs at high rate (>2 kg within 2 weeks). [2,83]

Baseline screening and regular follow-up monitoring are advised. [68] The first treatment approach for significant weight gain should be switching to another medication with a lower weight gain liability. Referral to an endocrinologist may also be warranted, and patients should be advised on healthy life style adjustments [5], including dietary suggestions and behavioral strategies. [68] Adjunctive drug treatments have been assessed to counteract weight gain and addition of a medication when an antipsychotic agent is initiated, or during ongoing therapy to prevent weight gain, is another option. [5,68] Along this line, medications studied in the treatment of antipsychotic-induced weight gain include serotoninergic agents (fenfluramine) [2, 68, 85], orlistat [2, 68, 86], amantadine [2, 68, 87, 88], sibutramine [68], reboxetine [68], histamine H2 antagonists (nizatidine, cimetidine by lowering of appetite or suppression of gastric acid secretion) [2,68,89-91], rosiglitazone [68], aripiprazole [68], and topiramate. [92-95] In general, the effectiveness of these drugs has been shown to be poor and only a few randomized, placebo-controlled clinical trials have been conducted. For example, a randomized controlled trial of patients on stable clozapine treatment assessed the effect of adding metformin or placebo on body weight of patients with schizophrenia, schizophreniphorm disorder, or bipolar disorder (n=61). Body weight decreased by an average of 4 pounds in the metformin group and was unchanged with placebo. [68, 69]. However, non pharmacological strategies should be preferred given the variable results of pharmacologic intervention. [5].

Glucose Dysregulation and Dyslipidemia

A high propensity to induce glucose dysregulation, diabetes mellitus, and dyslipidemia has been reported with clozapine. [2,96-102] Clozapine treatment has been linked in case reports to the development of abnormal glucose tolerance, hyperglycemia, type 2 diabetes mellitus, and diabetic ketoacidosis. [5]

Type 2 diabetes mellitus can occur during treatment with clozapine, especially in patients with risk factors for diabetes. [103] Different studies show a significantly increased risk of developing diabetes mellitus with clozapine (odds ratio 1.18) and olanzapine (range odd ratios 1.03 to 5.8), but not with risperidone (range odds ratios 0.97 to 2.2) or immediate-release quetiapine (odds ratio 0.99), while no data were available on other, newer, atypical antipsychotics. [5] Compared with typical antipsychotics, there was an increased risk of diabetes with clozapine (RR 1.39), olanzapine (RR 1.28), and immediate-release quetiapine (RR 1.28), while risperidone didn't show a statistically significant increase in risk. [104] Head-to-head studies have found non-statistically significant differences between clozapine and olanzapine and between clozapine and risperidone. [105, 106].

In patients with schizophrenia, a naturalistic study found a rate of new-onset type 2 diabetes mellitus, defined as a fasting blood glucose $\geq$126 mg/dl, of 67% in patients treated with clozapine. Amongst the atypical antipsychotics, it has the highest association with hyperglycemia. [5]

Diabetic ketoacidosis in a retrospective database analysis was reported in 12.25/10,000 cases for clozapine, 10.72/10,000 cases for olanzapine, 5.64/10,000 cases for immediate-release quetiapine, and 6.04/10,000 cases for risperidone. [107]

Factors related to new-onset type 2 diabetes mellitus, or diabetic ketoacidosis, in patients taking atypical antipsychotics include younger age, lower rate of overweight at baseline, longer duration of treatment [5], and African American ethnicity. [2,103] It is not dose dependent. [2,103]

In a case-control study, compared with conventional antipsychotics, the risk of developing or exacerbating diabetes mellitus in patients with bipolar disorder was significantly higher for clozapine (hazard ratio 7.0, 95% CI 1.7 to 28.9), risperidone (hazard ratio 3.44, 95% CI 2.8 to 4.2), olanzapine (hazard ratio 3.2, 95% CI 2.7 to 3.8), and immediate-release quetiapine (hazard ratio 1.8, 95% CI 1.4 to 2.4), but not for ziprasidone (hazard ration 1.68, 95% CI 0.84 to 3.36). [108]

In a recent review update showing results from a small short term [6 weeks) trial, olanzapine and clozapine were associated with significantly greater increases in triglycerides (+31.23 mg/dL and +36.28 mg/dL, respectively) than immediate-release quetiapine and risperidone (+11.64 mg/dL and +3.87 mg/dL, respectively). The review update also analyzed a case-control study that found no differences in the risk of elevated serum cholesterol among immediate-release quetiapine and clozapine, olanzapine, or risperidone at 12-, 24-, or 52-week exposures. [3]

Mechanisms for glucose dysregulation include weight gain, insulin resistance, increased appetite, increased adipose tissue, and endocrine changes. [2 ,5, 109]. The appearance of metabolic syndrome itself may cause insulin resistance and type 2 diabetes mellitus. A subgroup of patients presents with diabetic ketoacidosis independent of weight gain and independent of insulin sensitivity, which suggests a direct diabetogenic effect of clozapine. Clozapine antagonism at peripheral M3 muscarinic receptors impairs cholinergic-stimulated insulin secretion, while clozapine antagonism at serotonin and histaminic receptors may alter secretion or utilization of insulin and growth hormone. Dopamine D2 receptor antagonism might also affect lipid and glucose metabolism by disinhibition of prolactin secretion. [5] Insulin resistance can result from 5HT1a antagonism which decreases pancreatic β-cell responsiveness and this in turn can lead to inhibition of glucose-stimulated insulin release and hyperglycemia. [2, 5, 110, 111]. An increase in basal insulin secretion might result from an induction of concentration dependent insulin resistance with clozapine. [5]

The mechanisms accounting for antipsychotic-induced dyslipidemia have been less studied. As with diabetes, weight gain can cause new onset dyslipidemia with atypical antipsychotics, but in other cases, dyslipidemia has occurred without any weight gain and the effect size of various atypical antipsychotics on weight doesn't always correlate with the extent of disturbance in lipid metabolism. [112] The development of glucose intolerance could be involved in the effects of antipsychotics on lipid levels because insulin resistance is associated with an abnormal physiology of serum lipids. [113] Interferences with leptin have also been mentioned as a direct mechanism. [114]

Prevention can be achieved with adequate information provided to patients about these adverse effects in order to prevent excessive weight gain, recommendations to monitor blood glucose and lipids before treatment and at regular intervals, nutritional advice, and regular physical exercise. Appropriate selection of medications should be based on the relative adverse effect profiles balanced with drug efficacy, considering patient risk factors such as propensity to gain weight, family or personal history of diabetes or hyperlipidemia, and elevated fasting serum glucose, lipid, or insulin levels. [2, 115, 116].

Sedation, Drowsiness and Fatigue

Sedation is the most frequently reported adverse effect of clozapine, with frequency between 10% and 58% in different studies. [2, 4, 37, 117, 118]

In a meta-analysis clozapine was significantly more sedating than haloperidol (RR 1.5 with 95% CI 1.01-2.23 and p=0.043) and more sedating than low-potency first-generation antipsychotic drugs as a group (RR 1.32 with 95% CI 1.10-1.59 and p=0.003). The NNH for clozapine was 5. [74] In a recent analysis of different antipsychotics, clozapine resulted in higher rates of somnolence than risperidone (pooled risk difference 0.11, 95% CI 0.03 to 0.20, NNH=9) and higher rates of somnolence than olanzapine (pooled risk difference 0.12, 95% CI 0.05 to 0.19, NNH=8), and even higher in one longer-term trial (risk difference 0.21, 95% CI 0.15 to 0.27, NNH=5). [5]

Sedation gradually diminishes over 4-6 weeks. [2]

It is related to clozapine's potent antihistaminergic effect. [4]

Management can be effected by using higher doses at night, doing a slower titration, or decreasing the dose. Some medications with dopaminergic activating effect such as modafinil [2], dextroamphetamine, methylphenidate, L-dopa [4] and bupropion [2] can improve the wakefulness state. However, their use is not recommended routinely since they can worsen psychosis and/or movement disorders. They are reserved only for severe and persistent cases. [4].

Orthostatic Hypotension

Orthostatic hypotension occurs in 9% of clozapine patients, usually early in the treatment course and gradually diminishes, with tolerance usually developed by 4-6 weeks. However, it may also appear with a dosage increase. [2,4, 119, 120].

The mechanism is thought to be alpha1-adrenergic antagonism. [4]

Orthostatic blood pressures should be checked when a patient is started on clozapine and whenever the dose in increased. [2, 15]

A slow titration is recommended to avoid this side effect. Prevention can be effected by advising patients to rise slowly from a sitting (or lying) to a standing position, increasing fluid and salt intake, using support stockings, tilting upward the head of the bed at night, and taking divided doses of clozapine rather than a single dose. [2, 121]. If that fails, medications such as fludrocortisone [2, 122] or ephedrine [2, 123. can be used, but caution is recommended due to their side effects. [4]. Discontinuation of clozapine should be considered if hypotension is severe or refractory. [2].

Other Adverse Effects

Extrapyramidal Symptoms (EPS)

In a meta-analysis, clozapine was associated with much fewer EPS side effects than haloperidol based on the need for antiparkinsonian medication (RR 0.17 with 95% CI 0.03-

0.88, p=0.035, NNT 2 for clozapine) and fewer side effects than low-potency first generation antipsychotics at doses equivalent to >600 mg of chlorpromazine daily based on at least one extrapyramidal side effect (RR 0.66 with 95% CI 0.48-0.91 and p=0.010). This difference was reduced but still maintained its significance when only studies using prophylactic antiparkinsonian drugs were included. [74] It is known that clozapine's reduced EPS liability does not explain its greater efficacy. [124]

The low incidence of EPS associated with clozapine might be explained by its greater activity at mesolimbic (opposed to striatal) dopamine receptors and its lower affinity for D2 receptors. [3].

Eosinophilia

Rates of eosinophilia range from 0.2% up to 23% for females and 7% for males. [4] As of 2004, there had been 4 deaths reported worldwide from 25 cases of eosinophilic cardiomyopathy. [125] All developed within 4 weeks of initiation. There has also been suggestion of a clozapine-induced eosinophilic colitis syndrome. [126]

Discontinuation of clozapine is recommended for an eosinophil count >3000/mm^3 and re-challenge can be done when the count falls to <1000/mm^3. [125]

The symptoms are significantly reduced by prompt identification and treatment. Corticosteroids, local and systemic, are used to manage several allergic conditions and to reduce the number of eosinophils. [2].

Other Blood Dyscrasias

Leukocytosis has been reported to appear in 0.6% of patients treated with clozapine. Other blood disorders include thrombocytopenia, thrombocytosis, acute leukemia, and SLE-like syndrome. The manufacturer recommends discontinuing clozapine when the platelet count falls below 100,000/mm^3 and resuming therapy when the count returns to the normal range. If thrombocytopenia recurs, clozapine should be discontinued permanently. Some authors recommend routine monitoring of platelets along with the monitoring of WBC. [17].

Delirium

Delirium in patients taking clozapine is due to anticholinergic activity and usually occurs in susceptible populations, such as eldery or those with organic cognitive deficits [2,4,15], in patients with concomitant medications with potential to precipitate delirium [2,128], or in patients on higher clozapine doses. [4]

Management includes a reduction in the dose, a decreased rate of dose titration and limited absolute dose, if necessary. [129] If it occurs during withdrawal, it resolves with reinstitution of clozapine. [130,131].

Obssessive-Compulsive Symptoms

No definitive relation has been found between obsessive-compulsive symptoms and clozapine use. [2,132] It has been reported to occur in 10% of schizophrenic patients taking clozapine. [2,133].

The proposed mechanism is the serotoninergic antagonistic property of clozapine [2,134]. It is a dose-related effect. [4]

Management is done by decreasing dosage [135] or by adding a selective serotonin reuptake inhibitor [136] other than fluoxetine and fluvoxamine, since these two medications cause interactions in the metabolism of clozapine and increase clozapine plasma levels. [4,5].

Myocarditis and Cardiomyopathy

There have been several case reports of myocarditis associated with clozapine. Estimated rates range from 0.01 and 0.2% [2,137], but in recent studies up to 66% of patients on clozapine treatment developed non-specific findings consistent with possible myocarditis. It is the most common cardiac side effect of clozapine. [5] A large adverse event study used the World Health Organization database and found that only clozapine, but not olanzapine, immediate-release quetiapine, and risperidone, was significantly associated with myocarditis or cardiomyopathy [231 clozapine reports compared with 89 reports for all other antipsychotics). [138] The heterogeneous and non-specific presenting features, and the absence of a pathognomonic finding, make it difficult to diagnose this condition which is worrisome since it can be fatal in a minority of cases, especially if it is not recognized and treated in a timely manner. [4,5] It can develop at any time during treatment but is more common in the first one (80% of cases) to two (90% of cases) months, and it doesn't seem to be dose-dependent. [5]

The mechanism is unknown. Hypotheses proposed include a type 1 IgE-mediated acute hypersensitivity reaction, clozapine-mediated cytokine release, and hyper-catecholaminemia. [4,5]

The risk of developing dilated cardiomyopathy in patients taking clozapine may be at least 5 times higher than that in the general population. [2,137,139] Eight patients developed cardiomyopathy in an Australian study that reported 15 cases of myocarditis. Five patients with myocarditis and one patient with cardiomyopathy died. Clozapine doses ranged from 100-725 mg daily. Myocarditis developed early in treatment [15 days median, range between 3-21 days) while cardiomyopathy symptoms took months to develop (12 months median, range between 2-36 months). [12, 140]. Dilated cardiomyopathy carries a high morbidity and mortality (50% survival rate at 5 years). [5]

Clozapine is contraindicated in patients with severe cardiac disease. A cardiac evaluation is recommended before starting treatment for patients with a personal or family history of heart disease. Early recognition is prompted by active monitoring for myocarditis during the first 4 weeks of treatment to prevent dangerous sequelae, mainly fulminant myocarditis and dilated cardiomyopathy. The appearance of tachycardia, chest pain, dyspnea, fever, flu-like symptoms, or eosinophilia is considered an indication for ECG and serum troponin, creatin-kinase-MB, and C-Reactive Protein measurement. [5] Management includes admission for observation, discontinuation of clozapine, and treatment with corticosteroids [2, 138, 141], beta-blockers, angiotensin-converting enzyme inhibitors, and diuretics. [5]. Rechallenge with clozapine is not recommended since in most patients it results in recurrent myocarditis. [5] A recent review reported four patients who developed myocarditis during treatment with clozapine were rechallenged, and three didn't develop any major adverse drug effects after follow up for a mean of 27 weeks. The remaining patient did have a reoccurrence of myocarditis after 1.2 weeks. [23].

Deep Venous Thrombosis (DVT)

12 cases of DVT and thromboembolism were reported in association with clozapine [2,142], and this potentially fatal complication is more likely to occur in the first 3 months of treatment. [4] Between Feb 1999 and Dec 1999 there were 99 case reports, with objective evidence in 39% of the cases. 51% were females, median age was 38 years (range 17-70 years), median daily dose 400 mg (range 12.5-900 mg/day), and the median duration of exposure 3 months (range 2 days to 6 years). [2,143] A survey conducted in Germany and Switzerland didn't find any significant difference in the reported cases of thromboembolism occurring in clozapine-treated patients compared with patients treated with other antipsychotics, or with no antipsychotics, and the authors concluded that treatment with clozapine was not a risk factor for thromboembolism. [2,144]

Clozapine therapy should be discontinued if a reaction is evident. [2].

Tachycardia

Twenty five percent of patients on clozapine therapy develop tachycardia, but it is rarely of clinical significance [2,14], with an average increase in the heart rate of 10-15 beats per minute. [4]

It might be secondary to anticholinergic effects that cause vagal inhibition, and/or a reflex tachycardia secondary to hypotension. [2,146] It is dose-dependent, and doses >300 mg/day increase heart rate by 20-25 beats per minute. [2,147] Tachyphylaxis typically develops within 4-6 weeks of treatment initiation. [4]

Management is recommended if it persists or distresses the patient, after non pharmacological approaches such as a lower dose or slower titration fail. [2,15] The drug of choice is a cardio-selective beta-blocker, which may also minimize orthostatic hypotension due to alpha blockade. [2, 4, 121].

EKG Changes

New-onset electrocardiographic changes were reported in 24.5% of patients starting clozapine, generally in the titration phase. These included left atrial enlargement, right and left ventricular hypertrophy, ST-T wave abnormality, nonspecific T wave change, and a single case of QT interval prolongation. No changes in the course of treatment were required. [148] Clozapine may increase the QTc interval, but the effect is dose dependent and is equivalent to that of olanzapine or haloperidol. [12] One study failed to replicate this since it found that clozapine did not prolong the QTc interval. [2, 12, 149].

Constipation

Clozapine-associated constipation occurs frequently, in 14-60% of patients, according to different reports. [2,5,15] This side effect is more likely to occur in sedentary patients or in patients taking other constipating drugs. The mechanism is probably related to the peripheral anticholinergic effect and serotoninergic 5HT3 antagonism. [5]

It may have serious consequences, reported to be as high as 33%, such as paralytic ileus, necrotizing colitis, gastric outlet obstruction, colonic perforation with peritonitis, fatal aspiration of feculent vomitus as a result of bowel obstruction, bowel infarction, and death. Clozapine has also been associated with eosinophilic colitis. A literature review reported 102 cases of suspected life-threatening clozapine associated gastrointestinal hypomotility, with a mortality rate of 27.5%, and considerable morbidity generally related to bowel resection. Risk factors identified included recent start of clozapine, high clozapine dose or high serum level, concomitant use of anticholinergic agents, or intercurrent illness. [5]

Prevention is recommended with high-fiber diet, adequate fluid intake [2], avoidance of excessive calcium [5], and exercise [2]. Other proposed recommendations included radiographic and physical exam before the start of treatment, daily monitoring for bowel movements, vomiting, and abdominal pain, and a dietitian consult. Slower rates of titration might prevent this side effect. [5] Management depends upon severity and is achieved with stool softeners, laxatives (bulk-forming preferred), cathartics, or enemas. [2,15,150] It should be treated especially when it is prolonged, or associated with other symptoms such as abdominal pain or distention, and fever. [5].

Nausea

Nausea is experimented by approximately 11% of patients treated with clozapine. It occurs usually late in the course of therapy. [2,120]

Suggested mechanisms include delayed gastric emptying due to anticholinergic effect, an increase in salivation and food intake, and/or due to direct effects on the hypothalamus. [4]

Recommended management includes using metoclopramide, antacids, or H2-blocker therapy. [2,22] Cimetidine should be avoided due to interaction with clozapine metabolism leading to an increase in clozapine plasma concentrations. [151].

Hepatic Effects

Hepatitis associated with clozapine is usually not significant clinically. [5] Aminotransferase increase with clozapine was reported in 37.8% of patients compared with 16.6% of patients treated with haldol in one study. [2,4,152] In another study, there was an increase of 31% from baseline value [2, 153]. This elevation is usually mild and transient and without clinical sequelae [2], and usually resolves within the initial 3 months of treatment. [4]

Icteric hepatits is estimated to occur in 0.06% of patients. [5] There have been only few case reports of acute severe hepatitis. [154-156] The mechanism of clozapine associated hepatits is unknown. [5]

Monitoring of liver function tests has been recommended in early phases of treatment. [2,15] If persistent elevation of transaminases occurs, it is reversible with gradual dose titration or withholding the medication. [157] Once liver function tests return to normal, therapy can be resumed at a lower dose. [4].

Pancreatitis

An association between treatment with clozapine and pancreatitis is not definitely proven. [5] It is considered very rare, only a few cases of clozapine-associated pancreatitis have been reported and more than half were asymptomatic. [2,158-160] However, it can have a severe outcome. 95) This adverse effect is reported more commonly in children than in adults. [2,161] The mechanism for clozapine-induced pancreatitis is unknown. It might be related to apoptosis induced by a clozapine metabolite, with consequent activation of cytokines and immunoglobulins. [5] Some authors suggest monitoring pancreatic enzymes routinely, at least in the first months of clozapine therapy. [5].

Acute Interstitial Nephritis (AIN)

Although very rare, the risk of AIN seems higher during clozapine treatment compared to treatment with other antipsychotics. Early involvement of a nephrologist is recommended if this reaction is suspected. [5].

Urinary Incontinence/Enuresis

Clozapine-associated nocturnal enuresis is reported in 0.23% to 41% of patients. [2, 5, 162, 163] It is often embarrassing, therefore, it may be under-reported.

Potential mechanisms include anticholinergic effects and alpha-adrenergic antagonism [2,163,164]. Also, the side effect of sedation might impair patients from waking up during sleep to empty their bladder. [5]

Management includes avoiding fluid intake in the evening, voiding before bedtime and in the middle of the night, and using enuresis alarms. [2,15] If these fail, medications such as ephedrine, alpha-adrenergic agonists [2, 163, 164], intranasal desmopressin [2, 165, 166], amitriptyline, trihexiphenidyl(5), and oxybutinin [2] have been used.

Clozapine Withdrawal

Symptoms of withdrawal can occur after abrupt discontinuation of clozapine. When clozapine is discontinued the dose should be tapered, ideally over 2 weeks. [2] If withdrawal occurs it is managed with anticholinergic agents and benzodiazepines, usually in high intramuscular doses, especially when the patient presents with catatonia. [2].

Fever

Patients treated with clozapine can develop a mild to high-grade fever [5], rarely higher than 38°C [4], usually in the first 10-15 days after start of treatment [5]. It occurs in approximately 5% of patients. [4] The mechanism is not clear but it seems to be mediated by pyrogenic cytokines [5], specifically increasing plasma levels of soluble IL-2 receptor, TNF-alpha and soluble TNF receptors p55 and p75. [4].

It is usually benign, but it is important to rule out agranulocytosis with infection, NMS, or myocarditis. [5] Clinical guidelines establish that if a patient develops a fever of 38°C without specific symptoms a routine workup with physical exam, WBC with differential and a urinalysis should be obtained. Depending on clinical presentation, a chest X-ray, creatine phosphokinase, and blood cultures can be indicated. [4]

Rare Effects

Less frequent and/or less serious side effects include tremor, headache, sweating, cataplexy, hypertension, hypothermia, stiffness, confusion, dry mouth, nasal congestion, and periodic paralysis. [2, 60, 96, 149].

Conclusion

Clozapine is the only antipsychotic that has shown to be effective in reducing psychotic symptoms in patients with treatment-resistant schizophrenia and the only antipsychotic proven to have an anti-suicide effect in patients with schizophrenia spectrum disorders. It constitutes, therefore, an important choice in the repertoire of antipsychotics for the treatment of schizophrenia, even though it carries risks for potentially life-threatening complications and other adverse effects. It has an unique tolerability profile among the second-generation antipsychotics and adherence to the medication tends to be high, despite the need of close monitoring of WBC and the adverse effects. Since at least approximately 30% of patients with schizophrenia will not respond appropriately to any other antipsychotic medication, discussion on rechallenging treatment after a serious adverse effect occurs is currently ongoing. It is important to be aware of possible severe complications associated with this medication in order to ensure prompt recognition and management.

REFERENCES

[1] Crilly J. The history of clozapine and its emergence in the US market: a review and analysis. *Hist Psychiatry*. 2007;18(1):39-60.

[2] Iqbal MM, Aneja A, Rahman A, Megna JL, Yasmin L, Schwartz TL, Osmany S, Alam MA. Therapeutic options in the treatment of clozapine-induces adverse effects. *J PharmTechnol*. 2004(20) 155-164.

[3] McDonagh M, Peterson K, Carson S, Fu R, Thakurta S. Drug Class Review: Atypical Antipsychotic Drugs: Final Update 3 Report [Internet]. Portland (OR): Oregon Health & Science University. 2010.

[4] Fitzsimons J, Berk M, Lambert T, Bourin M, Dodd S. A review of clozapine safety. *Expert Opin Drug Saf.* 2005;4(4):731-744.

[5] Raja M. Clozapine Safety, 35 Years Later. *Curr Drug Saf.* 2011;6(3) 164-184.

[6] Hummel B, Dittmann S, Forsthoff A, Matzner N, Amann B, Grunze H. Clozapine as add-on medication in the maintenance treatment of bipolar and schizoaffective disorder. A case series. *Neuropsychobiology*. 2002;45 Suppl 1:37-42.

[7] Hammock R, Levine WR, Schroeder SR. Brief report: effects of clozapine on self-injurious behavior of two risperidone nonresponders with mental retardation. *J Autism Dev Disord*. 2001;31:109-113.

[8] Meltzer HY. Treatment of suicidality in schizophrenia. *Ann N Y Acad Sci*. 2001;932:44-60.

[9] Buckley P, Bartell J, Donenwirth K, Lee S, Torigoe F, Schulz SC. Violence and schizophrenia: clozapine as a specific antiaggressive agent. *Bull Am Acad Psychiatry Law*. 1995;23(4):607-611.

[10] Kapur S, Seeman P. Does fast dissociation from the dopamine D2 receptor explain the action of atypical antipsychotics?: A new hypothesis. *Am J Psychiatry*. 2001;158(3):360-9.

[11] Richelson E. Neuroleptic affinities for human brain receptors and their use in predicting adverse effects. *J Clin Psychiatry*. 1984;45(8):331-6.

[12] Buchanan RW, Kreyenbuhl J, Kelly DL, Noel JM, Boggs DL, Fischer BA, Himelhoch S, Fang B, Peterson E, Aquino Pr, Keller W; Schizophrenia Patient Outcome Research Team (PORT). The 2009 schizophrenia PORT psychopharmanological treatment recommendations and summary statements. *Schizophr Bulletin*. 2010;36 (1) 71-93.

[13] Volavka J, Czobor P, Cooper TB, Sheitman B, Lindenmayer JP, Citrome L, McEvoy JP, Lieberman JA. Prolactin levels in schizophrenia and schizoaffective disorder patients treated with clozapine, olanzapine, risperidone, or haloperidol. *J Clin Psychiatry*. 2004;65(1):57-61.

[14] Haddad PM, Sharma SG. Adverse effects of atypical antipsychotics: differential risk and clinical implications. *CNS Drugs*. 2007;21(11):911-36

[15] Young CR, Bowers MB Jr, Mazure CM. Management of the adverse effects of clozapine. Schizophr Bull. 1998;24(3):381-90.

[16] Gerson SL. G-CSF and the management of clozapine-induced agranulocytosis. *J Clin Psychiatry*. 1994;55 Suppl B:139-42.

[17] Herceg M, Muzinic L, Jukic V. Can we prevent blood dyscrasia (leucopenia, thrombocytopenia) and epileptic seizures induced by clozapine. *Psychiatr Danub.* 2010;22(1):85-9.
[18] Alvir JM, Lieberman JA. Agranulocytosis: incidence and risk factors. J Clin Psychiatry. 1994;55 Suppl B:137-8.
[19] Alvir JM, Lieberman JA, Safferman AZ, Schwimmer JL, Schaaf JA. Clozapine-induced agranulocytosis. Incidence and risk factors in the United States. *N Engl J Med.* 1993;329(3):162-7.
[20] Yagcoglu AE, Ilhan BC, Goktas MT, Babaoglu MO, Uz E, Yazc MK. Agranulocytosis related to clozapine in monozygotic twins and association with allelic variants of multidrug resistant gene MDR1. *J Clin Psychopharmacol.* 2011;31(2):247-9.
[21] Lieberman JA, Kane JM, Johns CA. Clozapine: guidelines for clinical management. *J Clin Psychiatry.* 1989;50(9):329-38.
[22] Lieberman JA, Safferman AZ. Clinical profile of clozapine: adverse reactions and agranulocytosis. *Psychiat Q.* 1992;63(1):51-70.
[23] Manu P, Sarpal D, Muir O, Kane JM, Correll CU. When can patients with potentially life-threatening adverse effects be rechallenged with clozapine? A systematic review of the published literature. *Schizophr Res.* 2011, in press.
[24] Dunk LR, Annan LJ, Andrews CD. Rechallenge with clozapine following leucopenia or neutropenia during previous therapy. *Br J Psychiatry.* 2006;188:255-63.
[25] Harris SC, Mattox B. Clozapine-rechallenge resulting in agranulocytosis: Treatment with granulocyte colony-stimulating factor (G-CSF). *J Pharm Practice.* 2010;23(2):183.
[26] Majczenko TG, Stewart JT. Failure of filgrastrim to prevent severe clozapine-induced agranulocytosis. *South Med J.* 2008;101(6):639-40.
[27] Kanaan RA, Kerwin R. Lithium and clozapine rechallenge: a retrospective case analysis. *J Clin Psychiatry.* 2006;67(5):756-60.
[28] Devinsky O, Pacia SV. Seizures during clozapine therapy. *J Clin Psychiatry.* 1994;55 Suppl B:153-6
[29] Lindstrom LH. A retrospective study on the long-term efficacy of clozapine in 96 schizophrenic and schizoaffective patients during a 13-year period. *Psychopharmacology.* 1989;99 Suppl:S84-6.
[30] Gunter W, Baghai T, Naber D, Spatz R, Hippius H. EEG alterations and seizures during treatment with clozapine. A retrospective study of 283 patients. *Pharmacopsychiatry.* 1993;26(3):69-74.
[31] Freudenreich O, Weiner RD, McEvoy JP. Clozapine-induced electroencephalogram changes as a function of clozapine serum levels. *Biol Psychiatry.* 1997;42(2):132-7.
[32] Wong J, Delva N. Clozapine-induced seizures: recognition and treatment. *Can J Psychiatry.* 2007;52(7):457-63.
[33] Devinsky O, Honigfeld G, Patin J. Clozapine-related seizures. *Neurology.* 1991;41(3):369-71.
[34] Haller E, Binder RL. Clozapine and seizures. *Am J Psychiatry.* 1990;147(8):1069-71.
[35] Karper LP, Salloway SP, Seibyl JP, Krystal JH. Prolonged postictal encephalopathy in two patients with clozapine-induced seizures. *J Neuropsychiatry Clin Neurosci.* 1992;4(4):454-7.

[36] Hill D. The relationship between schizophrenia and epilepsy. *Folia Psychiatr Neurol Neurochir* 1948;51:95-111.
[37] Baldessarini RJ, Frankenburg FR. Clozapine. A novel antipsychotic agent. N Engl J Med. 1991;324(11):746-54.
[38] Dalkilic A, Grosch WN. Neuroleptic malignant syndrome following initiation of clozapine therapy. *Am J Psychiatry*. 1997;154(6):81-2.
[39] Tsai G, Crisostomo G, Rosenblatt ML, Stern TA. Neuroleptic malignant syndrome associated with clozapine treatment. *Ann Clin Psychiatry*. 1995;7(2):91-5.
[40] Karagianis JL, Phillips LC, Hogan KP, LeDrew KK. Clozapine-associated neuroleptic malignant syndrome: two new cases and a review of the literature. *Ann Pharmacother*. 1999;33(5):623-30
[41] Campellone JV, McCluskey LF, Greenspan D. Fatal outcome from neuroleptic malignant syndrome associated with clozapine. *Neuropsychiatry Neuropsychol Behav Neurol*. 1995;8:70-3.
[42] Hasan S, Buckley P. Novel antipsychotics and the neuroleptic malignant syndrome: a review and critique. *Am J Psychiatry*. 1998;155(8):1113-6.
[43] Ananth J, Parameswaran S, Gunatilake S, Burgoyne K, Sidhom T. Neuroleptic malignant syndrome and atypical antipsychiotic drugs. *J Clin Psychiatry*. 2004;65(4):464-70.
[44] Rosebush P, Stewart T. A prospective analysis of 24 episodes of neuroleptic malignant syndrome. *Am J Psychiatry*. 1989;146(6):717-25.
[45] Caroff SN, Mann SC. Neuroleptic malignant syndrome. *Med Clin North Am*. 1993;77(1):185-202.
[46.Sachdev P, Kruk J, Kneebone M, Kissane D. Clozapine-induced neuroleptic malignant syndrome: review and report of new cases. *J Clin Psychopharmacol*. 1995;15(5):365-71.
[47] Davis JM, Caroff SN, Mann SC. Treatment of neuroleptic malignant syndrome. *Psychiatry Ann*. 2000;30:325-31.
[48] Caroff SN, Mann SC, Keck PE Jr. Specific treatment of the neuroleptic malignant syndrome. *Biol Psychiatry*. 1998;44(6):378-81.
[49] Caroff SN, Mann SC, Keck PE Jr, Francis A. Residual catatonic state following neuroleptic malignant syndrome. *J Clin Psychopharmacol*. 2000;20(2):257-9
[50] Liperoti R, Onder G, Landi F, Lapane KL, Mor V, Bernabei R, Gambassi G. All-cause mortality associated with atypical and conventional antipsychotics among nursing home residents with dementia: a retrospective cohort study. *J Clin Psychiatry*. 2009;70(10):1340-7.
[51] Modai I, Hirschmann S, Rava A, Kurs B, Barak P, Lichtenberg P. Sudden death in patients receiving clozapine treatment: a preliminary investigation. *J Clin Psychopharmacol*. 2000;20(3):325-7.
[52] Davydov L, Botts SR. Clozapine-induced hypersalivation. *Ann Pharmacother*. 2000;34(5):662-5.
[53] Zorn SH, Jones SB, Ward KM, Liston DR. Clozapine is a potent and selective muscarinic M4 receptor agonist. *Eur J Pharmacol*. 1994;269(3):R1-2
[54] Szabadi E. Clozapine-induced hypersalivation. *Br J Psychiatry*. 1997;171-89.
[55] Berlan M, Montastruc J-M, Lafontan M. Pharmacological prospects for alpha 2-adrenoreceptor antagonist therapy. *Trends Pharmacol Sci*. 1992;13(7):227-82.

[56] Pearlmen C. Clozapine, nocturnal sialorrhea, and choking. *J Clin Psychopharmacol.* 1994;14(4):283.

[57] Robinson D, Fenn H, Yesavage J. Possible association of parotitis with clozapine. *Am J Psychiatry.* 1995;152(2):297-8.

[58] Brodkin ES. Pelton GH, Price LH. Treatment of clozapine-induced parotid gland swelling. *Am J Psychiatry.* 1996;153(3):445.

[59] Hinkes R, Quesada TV, Currier MB, Gonzalez-Blanco M. Aspiration pneumonia possibly secondary to clozapine-induced sialorrhea. *J Clin Psychopharmacol.* 1996;16(6):462-3.

[60] Bourgeois JA, Drexler KG, Hall MJ. Hypersalivation and clozapine. Hosp Community Psychiatry. 1991;42(11):1174.

[61] Rogers DP, Shramko JK. Therapeutic options in the treatment of clozapine-induced sialorrhea. *Pharmacotherapy.* 2000;20(9):1092-5.

[62] Copp PJ, Lament R, Tennent TG. Amitriptyline in clozapine-induced sialorrhea. *Br J Psychiatry.* 1991;159:166.

[63] Steinlechner S, Klein C, Moser A, Lencer R, Hagenah J. Botulinum toxin B as an effective and safe treatment for neuroleptic-induced sialorrhea. *Psychopharmacology* (Berl). 2010;207(4):593-7.

[64] Rummel-Kluge C, Komossa K, Schwarz S, Hunger H, Schmid F, Asenjo Lobos C, Kissling W, Davis JM, Leucht S. Head-to-head comparisons of metabolic side effects of second generation antipsychotics in the treatment of schizophrenia: A systematic review and meta-analysis. *Schizophrenia Res.* 2010;123:225-33.

[65 .De Hert M, Schreurs V, Sweers K, Van Eyck D, Hanssens L, Sinko S, Wampers M, Scheen A, Peuskens J, van Winkel R.. Typical and atypical antipsychotics differentially affect long-term incidence rates of the metabolic syndrome in first-episode patients with schizophrenia: a retrospective chart review. *Schizophr Res.* 2008;101(1-3):295-303.

[66] Hägg S, Lindblom Y, Myörndal T, Adolfsson R. High prevalence of the metabolic syndrome among a Swedish cohort of patients with schizophrenia. *Int Clin Psychopharmacol.* 2006;21(2):93-8.

[67] American Diabetes Association/American Psychiatric Association. Consensus development conference on antipsychotic drugs and obesity and diabetes. *Diabetes Care.* 2004;27: 596-601.

[68] Megna JL, Schwartz TL, Siddiqui UA, Herrera Rojas M. Obesity in adults with serious and persistent mental illness: A Review of postulated mechanisms and current interventions. *Ann Clin Psychiatry.* 2011;23(2):131-40.

[69] Carrizo E, Fernandez V, Connell L, Sandia I, Prieto D, Mogollon J, Valuena D, Fernandez I, de Baptista EA, Baptista T. Extended release metformin for metabolic control assistance during prolonged clozapine administration: a 14 week, double-blind, parallel group, placebo-controlled study. *Schizophr Res.* 2009; 113(1): 19-26.

[70] Wirshing DA, Wirshing WC, Kysar L, Berisford MA, Goldstein D, Pashdag J, Mintz J, Marder SR. Novel antipsychotics: comparison of weight gain liabilities. *J Clin Psychiatry.* 1999;60(6):358-63.

[71] Bustillo JR, Buchanan RW, Irish D, Breier A. Differential effect of clozapine on weight: a controlled study. *Am J Psychiatry.* 1996;153(6):817-9.

[72] Leadbetter R, Shutty M, Pavalonis D, Vieweg V, Higgins P, Downs M. Clozapine-induced weight gain: prevalence and clinical relevance. Am J Psychiatry. 1992;149(1):68-72.
[73] Hummer M, Kemmler G, Kurz M, Kurzthaler I, Oberhauer H, Fleischhacker WW. Weight gain induced by clozapine. *Eur Neuropsychopharmacol*. 1995;5(4):437-40.
[74] Leucht S, Corves C, Arbter D, Engel RR, Li C, Davis JM. Second-generation versus first-generation antipsychotic drugs for schizophrenia: a meta-analysis. *Lancet*. 2009;373(9657): 31-41.
[75] Meltzer HY, Alphs L, Green AI, Altamura AC. Anand R, Bertoldi A, Bourgeois M, Chouinard G, Islam MZ, Kane J, Krishnan R, Lindenmayer JP, Potkin S. Clozapine treatment for suicidality in schizophrenia: International Suicide Prevention Trial (InterSePT). *Arch Gen Psychiatry*. 2003;60(1):82-91.
[76] Atmaca M, Kuloglu M, Tezcan E, Ustundag B. Serum leptin and triglyceride levels in patients on treatment with atypical antipsychotics. *J Clin Psychiatry*. 2003;64(5):598-604.
[77] Azorin JM, Spiegel R, Remington G, Vanelle JM, Pere JJ, Giguere M, Bourdeix I. A double-blind comparative study of clozapine and risperidone in the management of severe chronic schizophrenia. *Am J Psychiatry*. 2001;158(8):1305-1313.
[78] Bondolfi G, Dufour H, Patris M, May JP, Billeter U, Eap CB, Baumann P. Risperidone versus clozapine in treatment-resistant chronic schizophrenia: a randomized double-blind study. The Risperidone Study Group. *Am J Psychiatry*. 1998;155(4):499-504.
[79] Czobor P, Volavka J, Sheitman B, Lindenmayer JP, CItrome L, McEvoy J, Cooper TB, Chakos M, Lieberman JA. Antipsychotic-induced weight gain and therapeutic response: a differential association. *J Clin Psychopharmacol*. 2002;22(3):244-251.
[80] Wetterling T, Mussigbrodt HE. Weight gain: side effect of atypical neuroleptics? *J Clin Psychopharmacol*. 1999;19(4):316-21.
[81] George TP, Sernyak MJ, Ziedonis DM, Woods SW. Effects of clozapine on smoking in chronic schizophrenic outpatients. *J Clin Psychiatry*. 1995;56(8):344-6.
[82] Hughes JR, Hatsukami DK, Mitchell JE, Dahlgren LA. Prevalence of smoking among psychiatric outpatients. *Am J Psychiatry*. 1986;143(8):993-7.
[83] Wetterling T. Ziprasidone: a new atypical antipsychotic. *J Clin Psychiatry*. 1996;57:40-5.
[84] Reynolds GP, Zhang Z, Zhang X. Polymorphism of the promoter region of the serotonin 5-HT(2C) receptor gene and clozapine-induced weight gain. *Am J Psychiatry*. 2003;160(4):677-9.
[85] Goodall E, Oxtoby C, Richards R, Watkinson G, Brown D, Silverstone T. A clinical trial of the efficacy and acceptability of D-flenfuramine in the treatment of neuroleptic-induced obesity. *Br J Psychiatry*. 1988;153:208-13.
[86] Schwartz TL, Jindal S, Simionescu M, Nihalani N, Azhar N, Tirmazi S, Hussein J. Effectiveness of orlistat versus diet and exercise for weight gain associated with antidepressant use: a pilot study. *J Clin Psychopharmacol*. 2004;24(5):555-6.
[87] Floris M, Lejeune J, Deberdt W. Effect of amantadine on weight gain during olanzapine treatment. *Eur Neuropsychopharmacol*. 2001;11(2):181-2.
[88] Baruch R, Poulin M, Thakur A, Karagianis J, Raskin J. Amantadine induces weight loss in patients treated with olanzapine. *Schizophr Res*. 2002;53:159.

[89] Stoa-Birketvedt G. Effect of cimetidine suspension on appetite and weight in overweight subjects. *BMJ*. 1993;306(6885):1091-3.

[90] Stoa-Birketvedt G, Paus PN, Ganss R, Ingebretsen OC, Florholmen J. Cimetidine reduces weight and improves metabolic control in overweight patients with type 2 diabetes. *Int J Obes Relat Metab Disord*. 1998;22(11):1041-5.

[91] Sacchetti E, Guarneri L, Bravi D. H(2) antagonist nizatidine may control olanzapine-associated weight gain in schizophrenic patients. *Biol Psychiatry*. 2000;48(2):167-8.

[92] Gordon A, Price LH. Mood stabilization and weight loss with topiramate. *Am J Psychiatry*. 1999;156(6):968-9.

[93] Norton J, Potter D, Edwards K. Sustained weight loss associated with topiramate. *Epilepsia* 1997;38:58.

[94] Dursun SM, Devarajan S. Clozapine weight gain, plus topiramate weight loss. *Can J Psychiatry*. 2000;45(2):198.

[95] Chengappa KN, Levine J, Rathore D, Parapally H, Atzert R. Long-term effects of topiramate on bipolar mood instability, weight change and glycemic control: a case series. *Eur Psychiatry*. 2001;16:186-90.

[96] Wu G, Dias P, Chun W, Li G, Kumar S, Singh S. Hyperglycemia, hyperlipidemia, and periodic paralysis: a case report of new side effects of clozapine. *Prog Neuropsychopharmacol Biol Psychiatry*. 2000;24(8):1395-400.

[97] Koponen H, Saari K, Savolainen M, Isohanni M. Weight gain and glucose and lipid metabolism disturbances during antipsychotic medication: a review. *Eur Arch Psychiatry Clin Neurosci*. 2002;252(6):294-8.

[98] Lindermayer JP, Czobor P, Volavka J, Citrom L, Sheitman B, McEvoy JP, Cooper TB, Chakos M, Lieberman JA. Changes in glucose and cholesterol levels in patients with schizophrenia treated with typical or atypical antipsychotics. *Am J Psychiatry*. 2003;160(2):290-6.

[99] Wirshing DA, Boyd JA, Meng LR, Ballon JS, Marder SR, Wirshing WC. The effects of novel antipsychotics on glucose and lipid levels. *J Clin Psychiatry*. 2002;63(10):856-65.

[100] Leonard P, Halley A, Browne S. Prevalence of obesity, lipid and glucose abnormalities in outpatients prescribed clozapine. *Ir Med J*. 2002;95(4):119-20.

[101] Meltzer HY. Putting metabolic side effects into perspective: risks versus benefits of atypical antipsychotics. *J Clin Psychiatry*. 2001;62:35-41.

[102] Nasrallah HA. Pharmacoeconomic implications of adverse effects during antipsychotic drug therapy. *Am J Health Syst Pharm*. 2002;59(22 Suppl 8):S16-21.

[103] Wirshing DA, Spellberg BJ, Erhart SM, Marder SR, Wirshing WC. Novel antipsychotics and new onset diabetes. *Biol Psychiatry*. 1998;44(8):778-83.

[104] Smith M, Hopkins D, Peveler RC, Holt RI, Woodward M, Ismail K. First-v. second-generation antipsychotics and risk for diabetes in schizophrenia: systematic review and meta-analysis. *Br J Psychiatry*. 2008;192(6):406-11.

[105] Daumit GL, Goff DC, Meyer JM, Davis VG, Nasrallah HA, McEvoy JP, Rosenheck R, Davis SM, Hsiao JK, Stroup TS, Lieberman JA. Antipsychotic effects on estimated 10-year coronary heart disease risk in the CATIE schizophrenia study. *Schizophr Res*. 2008;105(1-3):175-87.

[106] Ollendorf DA, Joyce AT, Rucker M. Rate of new-onset diabetes among patients treated with atypical or conventional antipsychotic medications for schizophrenia. *MedGenMed*. 2004;6(1):5
[107] Ramaswamy K, Kozma CM, Nasrallah H. Risk of diabetic ketoacidosis after exposure to risperidone or olanzapine. *Drug Saf*. 2007;30(7):589-99.
[108] Guo JJ, Keck PE Jr., Corey-Lisle PK, Li H, Jiang D, Jang R, L'Italien GJ. Risk of diabetes mellitus associated with atypical antipsychotic use among patients with bipolar disorder: A retrospective, population-based, case-control study. *J Clin Psychiatry*. 2006;67(7):1055-61.
[109] Griffiths J, Springuel P. Atypical antipsychotics: impaired glucose metabolism. *CMAJ*. 2001;165(7):947-9.
[110] Uvnas-Moberg K, Ahlenius S, Alster P, Hillegaart V. Effects of selective serotonin and dopamine agonists on plasma levels of glucose, insulin, and glucagon in the rat. *Neuroendocrinology* 1996;63(3):269-74.
[111] Wozniak KM, Linnoila M. Hyperglycemic properties of serotonin receptor antagonists. *Life Sci*. 1991;49(2):101-9.
[112] Pramyothin P, Khaodhiar L. Metabolic syndrome with the atypical antipsychotics. *Curr Opin Endocrinol, Diabetes* Obes. 2010, 17(5):460-466.
[113] Monteleone P, Martiadis V, Maj M. Management of schizophrenia with obesity, metabolic, and endocrinological disorders. *Psychiatr Clin North Am*. 2009;32(4): 775-94.
[114] de Leon J, Diaz FJ. Planning for the optimal design of studies to personalize antipsychotic prescriptions in the post-CATIE era: The clinical and pharmacoepidemiological data suggest that pursuing the pharmacogenetics of metabolic syndrome complications (hypertension, diabetes mellitus and hyperlipidemia) may be a reasonable strategy. *Schizophr Res*. 2007, 96(1-3): 185-97.
[115] Baptista T, Kin NM, Beaulieu S, de Baptista EA. Obesity and related metabolic abnormalities during antipsychotic drug administration: mechanisms, management and research perspectives. Pharmacopsychiatry. 2002;35(6):205-19.
[116] Wirshing DA, Pierre JM, Erhart SM, Boyd JA. Understanding the new and evolving profile of adverse drug effects in schizophrenia. *Psychiatr Clin North Am*. 2003;26(1):165-90.
[117] Kane J, Honigfeld G, Singer J, Meltzer H. Clozapine for the treatment-resistant schizophrenic. A double-blind comparison with chlorpromazine. *Arch Gen Psychiatry*. 1988;45(9):789-96.
[118] Claghorn J, Honigfeld G, Abuzzahab FS Sr, Wang R, Steinbook R, Tuason V, Kleman G. The risks and benefits of clozapine versus chlorpromazine. J Clin Psychopharmacol. 1987;7(6):377-84.
[119] Safferman A, Lieberman JA, Kane JM, Syzmanski S, Kinon B. Update on the clinical efficacy and side effects of clozapine. *Schizophr Bull*. 1991;17(2):247-61.
[120] Marinkovic D, Timtijevic I, Babinski T, Totic S, Paunovic VR. The side effects of clozapine: a four year follow-up study. *Progr Neuropsychopharmacol Biol Psychiatry*. 1994;18(3):537-44.
[121] Cleophas TJM, Kauw FHW. Pressor responses from noncardioselective beta-blockers. *Angiology* 1988;39(7 Pt 1):587-96.

[122] Testani M. Clozapine-induced orthostatic hypotension treated with fludrocortisone. *J Clin Psychiatry*. 1994;55(11):497-8.

[123] Patterson TS. In: Yesavage J, ed. Clozapine: a compendium of selected readings. Standford, CA: Sandoz *Pharmaceuticals*, 1992:136-8.

[124.Tandon R, Belmaker RH, Gattaz WF, Lopez-Ibor JJ Jr, Okasha A, Singh B, Stein DJ, Olie JP, Fleischhacker WW, Moeller HJ. World Psychiatric Association Pharmacopsychiatry Section statement on comparative effectiveness of antipsychotics in the treatment of schizophrenia. *Schizophr Res*. 2008;100(1-3) 20-38.

[125] Chatterton R. Eosinophilia after commencement of clozapine treatment. Aust N Z J Psychiatry. 1997;31(6):874-6.

[126] Friedberg JW, Frankenburg FR, Burk J, Johnson W. Clozapine-caused eosinophilic colitis. *Ann Clin Psychiatry*. 1995;7(2):97-8.

[127] Barbui C, Campomori A, Bonati M. Clozapine and blood dyscrasias different from agranulocytosis. *Can J Psychiatry*. 1997;42(9):981-2.

[128] Gaertner HJ, Fischer E, Hoss J. Side effects of clozapine. *Psychopharmacology*. 1989;99(Suppl):S97-100.

[129.Szymanski S, Jody D, Leipsig R, Masiar S, Lieberman N. Anticholinergic delirium caused by retreatment with clozapine. *Am J Psychiatry*. 1992;148:1752.

[130] Stanilla JK, de Leon J, Simpson GM. Clozapine withdrawal resulting in delirium with psychosis: a report of three cases. *J Clin Psychiatry*. 1997;58(6):252-5.

[131] Simpson GM, Varga E. Clozapine-a new antipsychotic agent. *Curr Ther Res Clin Exp*. 1974;16(7):679-86.

[132] Ghaemi SN, Zarate CA Jr, Popli AP, Pillay SS, Cole JO. Is there a relationship between clozapine and obsessive-compulsive disorder?: a retrospective chart review. *Compr Psychiatry* 1995;36(4):267-70.

[133] Baker RW, Chengappa KN, Baird JW, Steingard S, Christ MA, Schooler NR. Emergence of obsessive compulsive symptoms during treatment with clozapine. *J Clin Psychiatry*. 1992;53(12):439-42.

[134] Patil VJ. Development of transient obsessive-compulsive symptoms during treatment with clozapine. *Am J Psychiatry*. 1992;149(2):272.

[135] Levkovitch Y, Kronnenberg Y, Gaoni B. Can clozapine trigger OCD?. J Am Acad Child Adolesc *Psychiatry*. 1995;34(3):263.

[136] Cassidy SL, Thaker GK. Addition of fluoxetine to clozapine. *Am J Psychiatry* 1993;149:1900-1.

[137] Warner B, Alphs L, Schaedelin J, Koestler T. Clozapine and sudden death. *Lancet* . 2000;355(9206):842.

[138] Coulter DM, Bate A, Meyboom RHB, Lindquist M, Edwards IR. Antipsychotic drugs and heart muscle disorder in international pharmacovigilance: data mining study. *BMJ*. 2001;322(7296):1207-9.

[139] Walker AM, Lanza LL, Arellano F, Rothman KJ. Mortality in current and former users of clozapine. *Epidemiology* 1997;8(6):671-7.

[140] Kilian JG, Kerr K, Lawrence C, Celermajer DS. Myocarditis and cardiomyopathy associated with clozapine. *Lancet*. 1999;354(9193):1841-5.

[141] Wynne J, Braunwald E. The cardiomyopathies and myocarditides. In: Braunwald E, Fauci AS, Kasper DL, Hauser SL, Longo DL, Jameson JL, eds. Harrison's principles of internal medicine. 15th ed. New York: McGraw-Hill, 2001:1359-65.

[142] Hagg S, Spigset O, Soderstrom TG. Association of venous thromboembolism and clozapine. *Lancet* 2000;355(9210):1155-6.

[143.Knudson JF, Kortepeter C, Dubitsky GM, Ahmad SR, Chen M. Antipsychotic drugs and venous thromboembolism. *Lancet*. 2000;355(9210):1155-6.

[144] Wolstein J, Grohmann R, Ruther E, Hippius H. Antipsychotic drugs and venous thromboembolism. *Lancet*. 2000;356(9225):252.

[145] Kraus T, Haack M, Schuld A, Hinze-Selch D, Kuhn M, Uhr M, Pollmacher T. Body weight and leptin plasma levels during treatment with antipsychotic drugs. *Am J Psychiatry*. 1999;156(2):312-4.

[146] Rechlin T, Claus D, Weis M. Heart rate variability in schizophrenic patients and changes of autonomic heart rate parameters during treatment with clozapine. *Biol Psychiatry*. 1994;35(11):888-92.

[147] Ereshefsky L, Watanabe MD, Tran-Johnson TK. Clozapine: an atypical antipsychotic agent. *Clin Pharm*. 1989;8(10):691-709.

[148] Kang UG, Kwon JS, Ahn YM, Chung SJ, Ha JH, Koo YJ, Kim YS. Electrocardiographic abnormalities in patients treated with clozapine. *J Clin Psychiatry*. 2000;61(6):441-6.

[149] Casey D. Side effect profiles of new antipsychotic agents. J Clin Psychiatry. 1996;57:40-5.

[150] Lennard-Jones JE. Clinical management of constipation. *Pharmacology*. 1993;47(Suppl 1):216-23.

[151] Jann MW, Grimsley SR, Gray EC, Chang WH. Pharmacokinetics and pharmacodynamics of clozapine. *Clin Pharmacokinet*. 1993;24(2):161-76.

[152] Hummer M, Kurz M, Kurzthaler I, Oberbauer H, Miller C, Fleischhacker WW. Hepatotoxicity of clozapine. *J Clin Psychopharmacol*. 1997;17(4):314-7.

[153] Gaertner HJ, Fischer E, Hoss J. Side effects of clozapine. *Psychopharmacology* 1989;99 Suppl:S97-100.

[154] Kellner M, Wiedemann K, Krieg JC, Berg PA. Toxic hepatitis by clozapine treatment. *Am J Psychiatry* 1993;150(6):985-6.

[155] Larsen JT, Clemensen SV, Klitgaard NA, Nielsen B, Brosen K. Clozapine-induced toxic hepatits. *Ugeskr Laeger* 2001;163(14):2013-4.

[156] Thompson J, Chengappa KN, Good CB, Baker RW, Kiewe RP, Bezner J, Schooler NR. Hepatitis, hyperglycemia, pleural effusion, eosinophilia, hematuria and proteinuria occurring early in clozapine treatment. *Int Clin Psychopharmacol* 1998;13(2):95-8.

[157] Lieberman JA. Maximizing clozapine therapy: managing side effects. J Clin Psychiatry. 1998;59 Suppl 3:38-43.

[158] Bergemann N, Ehrig C, Diebold K, Mundt C, von Einsiedel R. Asymptomatic pancreatitis associated with clozapine. *Pharmacopsychiatry*. 1999;32(2):78-80.

[159] Jubert P, Fernandez R, Ruiz A. Clozapine-related pancreatitis. *Ann Intern Med*. 1994;121(9):722-3.

[160] Martin A. Acute pancreatitis associated with clozapine use. *Am J Psychiatry*. 1992;149:714.

[161] Sepulveda VAC, Lopez AE, Yanez LP, Ramirez CR, Escobar PB, Madrazo DGA. Sodium diphenylhydantoin as a probable cause of pancreatitis. *Rev Gastroenterol Mex* 1999;64(4):186-9.

[162] Aranowitz JS, Safferman AZ, Lieberman JA. Management of clozapine-induced enuresis. *Am J Psychiatry*. 1995;152(3):472.

[163] Fuller MA, Borovicka MC, Jaskiw GE, Simon MR, Kwon K, Konicki PE. Clozapine-induced urinary incontinence: incidence and treatment with ephedrine. *J Clin Psychiatry*. 1996;57(11):514-8.

[164] Steingard S. Use of desmopressin to treat clozapine-induced enuresis. *J Clin Psychiatry*. 1994;55(7):325-6.

[165] Richardson DW, Robinson AG. Desmopressin. *Ann Intern Med*. 1985;103(2):228-9.

[166] Frankenburg FR, Kando JC, Centorrino F, Gilbert JM. Bladder dysfunction associated with clozapine therapy. *J Clin Psychiatry* 1996;57(1):39-40.

INDEX

A

B

C

D

E

F

G

H

N

O

P

Q

R

S

T

U

V

W

Y

Z